Spirituality, Values and Mental Health

616·89

Spirituality, Values and Mental Health

Jewels for the Journey

Edited by Mary Ellen Coyte, Peter Gilbert and Vicky Nicholls

Foreword by John Swinton, Professor in Practical Theology and Pastoral Care, University of Aberdeen

Jessica Kingsley Publishers
London and Philadelphia

The editors and publishers are grateful to the proprietors listed below for
permission to quote the following material:
'The Well of Grief' by David Whyte from *Where Many Rivers Meet* (1990) by David Whyte. Printed with
permission from Many Rivers Press, Langley, Washington. www.davidwhyte.com 'Wild Wind' by Rose
Snow, from *From the Ashes of Experience: Reflections of Madness, Survival and Growth* by Phil Barker, Peter
Campbell and Ben Davidson. Copyright © John Wiley and Sons Limited. Reproduced with permission.
'Just Be' by Sue Holt, from *Poems of Survival* (2003) by Sue Holt.
Printed with permission from Chipmunkapublishing.

First published in 2007
by Jessica Kingsley Publishers
116 Pentonville Road
London N1 9JB, UK
and
400 Market Street, Suite 400
Philadelphia, PA 19106, USA

www.jkp.com

Library of Congress Cataloging in Publication Data
Spirituality, values, and mental health : jewels for the journey / edited by Mary Ellen Coyte, Peter Gilbert, and
Vicky Nicholls ; foreword by John Swinton.
  p. ; cm.
Includes bibliographical references and index.
ISBN-13: 978-1-84310-456-8 (alk. paper) 1. Mental health services. 2. Spirituality--Health aspects. 3.
Values--Health aspects. 4. Spiritual care (Medical care)
  [DNLM: 1. Mental Health Services. 2. Spirituality. 3. Caregivers. 4. Social Values. WM 61 S7599 2008] I.
Coyte, Mary Ellen, 1958- II. Gilbert, Peter, 1950- III. Nicholls, Vicky.
  RA790.S73 2008
  362.2--dc22
                                                                                    2007014415

British Library Cataloguing in Publication Data
A CIP catalogue record for this book is available from the British Library

ISBN 978 1 84310 456 8

Printed and bound in Great Britain by
Athenaeum Press, Gateshead, Tyne and Wear

ACKNOWLEDGEMENTS

Mary Ellen, Peter and Vicky are grateful to people too many to mention, but would like to thank, most especially, those who inspired us, spoke to our souls, walked with us on the journey. Many of those who have done so, are featured in this book, either as contributors of chapters, reflections or poems.

We are especially grateful to Stephen Jones, editor at Jessica Kingsley, for his good humour and patience with us and this mammoth and complex project of 24 chapters and as many reflections. We owe a debt to Professor John Swinton for his seminal *Spirituality and Mental Health Care: The Forgotten Dimension*, to which we hope this is, in some ways, an offspring and development. Our thanks are also due to Professor Anthony Sheehan, in his capacity as the generator of the National Institute for Mental Health in England (NIMHE), for initiating the Spirituality and Mental Health Project and being a constant source of inspiration. Paddy Cooney has continued his support as the Lead Director for CSIP. It has been a great pleasure working with Martin Aaron, the Chair of the National Spirituality and Mental Health Forum, Dr Christine King, the Vice Chancellor of Staffordshire University, and Dr Sarah Eagger, the Chair of the Special Interest Group for the Royal College of Psychiatrists and her colleagues.

We are, of course, indebted to our long-suffering partners and families who over the last 18 months have had to put up with cries of: 'which version of Chapter X is the final one?'

Finally, our thanks to you, reader for taking the trouble to pick up this book, read it and engage with the ideas, thoughts and feelings which our valued friends and colleagues have generated.

Mary Ellen Coyte
Peter Gilbert
Vicky Nicholls

The editors would like to thank Sarah-Jane Wren for her sensitive illustrations which have greatly enriched the book.

CONTENTS

FOREWORD

My journey within the field of spirituality and mental health has been an interesting one. It began 30-odd years ago on the day that I wandered into my first psychiatric ward, a student psychiatric nurse with not much of a clue about anything. In this strange land of madness, medication and control, spirituality was not a priority and the idea of spiritual care as a discrete aspect of nursing was not really on the agenda either in terms of education or practice. It's not so much that it was avoided, it simply wasn't an issue.

Certainly patients often spoke about spirituality, but we were taught to interpret this primarily in terms of their particular illness. Religion and spirituality, we were taught, should be treated with great caution and best avoided altogether. So, most of us did. Of course we had chaplains, but we paid little attention to what they did or why they did it. The main chaplaincy issue for us as nurses seemed to revolve around whose turn it was to take patients to the chapel on Sunday and whether or not it was *really* necessary for nurses to stay with them. Surely we had more important things to do than to waste time hanging around a chapel? What has religion or the things of the spirit to do with mental health nursing? No one told us, and we didn't really care…and yet, I and many others always had a sense of dis-ease about the way that mental health care was provided, or perhaps it was the way that certain aspects of care were *not* provided or catered for.

It was clear, however, that those patients who did attend chapel received something deep and sometimes something deeply healing from their spiritual encounter. Spending time in worship with people who were encountering deeply disturbing experiences and who were struggling to make sense of their lives and being with them as they received a measure of peace through the words, rituals and symbols, challenged me deeply and reminded me constantly of the rich and deep nature of the personhood of people experiencing profound forms of mental illness. I carried that dis-ease and worked alongside it for the whole of my nursing career. Whether I always responded constructively to its challenge in my practice I'm not sure, I hope so, but it was difficult and resistance was always on the horizon.

Some 19 years later I returned to that same hospital in a different role, as a community mental healthcare chaplain working with the mental health rehabilitation team in a long stay ward. (By then we had moved away from talking about mental illness and had begun to focus on mental health.) My continuing dis-ease had led me into a whole new career. My role was to work with people with enduring mental health problems who were leaving the hospital for the community. I was charged with the task of helping people to find a spiritual community where they could develop meaningful relationships, find acceptance and have their spiritual needs effectively met. However, it soon became clear that there was (and is) no such 'community' understood as a safe, morally congruent place which accepts and values people with their problems and differences. When governments talk about 'community' and 'community care', they tend to define the term 'community' primarily as life outside the institution. But life outside the institution can be a frightening and isolating place, particularly for those whom society labels as different and 'unlovable'. I very quickly realized that religious communities could be just as exclusive and excluding and stigmatizing as any other aspect of society. There was clearly a huge task to be undertaken both within the institutions and society. I decided then to dedicate the rest of my time to working with people with disabilities and mental health problems to enable the possibility of change, acceptance and the recognition of the importance of spirituality in both its religious and non-religious forms as a vital source for maintaining people's humanness and inclusive citizenship.

Now here I am some 30 years on from my reluctant encounters in the hospital chapel, and things have changed – not least my career path! In 2001 I wrote a book entitled *Spirituality and Mental Health Care: Rediscovering a 'Forgotten' Dimension*. There I argued that mainstream mental healthcare services had, to their detriment, forgotten the importance of spirituality for mental health and urged a return to the spiritual roots that underpin the caring professions. Reflecting on the argument of that book in 2007 it is clear from the wealth of literature and research that surrounds the field today that that which had been forgotten has certainly been remembered. All of the health and social care professions are beginning to recognize the significance of spirituality for the lives of people with mental health problems, as are service users who are finding a powerful voice in the midst of the complexities of debates within this field of enquiry. In Scotland, for example, all of the health care trusts have formal departments of spiritual care and significant government legislation to back them up. Throughout the UK there is a posi-

tive movement towards taking spirituality seriously within healthcare practices. The fact that the Royal College of Psychiatrists special interest group
contains over 400 psychiatrists and is one of their most popular SIGs
indicates some important shifts in what has historically been one of the
professions that have tended to resist the incorporation of spirituality.
Things are certainly changing.

This volume of essays is an important contribution to the ongoing
debate around the relationship between spirituality and mental health care.
It covers some fascinating and important ground, drawing on empirical
research, personal narrative and, most importantly, retaining a continuous
focus on the empowerment of service users. While taking seriously research
and reflection undertaken on people experiencing mental health problems,
the volume retains a fundamental focus on research and reflection done *with*
and *by* people with these life experiences. This genuinely collaborative and
creative approach to spirituality and mental health is the way forward for the
field. We all have different gifts and perspectives. It is only when we draw
them together and learn what it means to live and work peaceably together
that the field of spirituality and mental health can truly become a source for
good. This volume begins to show us a way in which this idea can become a
reality. I look forward to seeing where the thinking and reflection presented
here takes me and all of its readers as we move on to the next phase of our
journey. My dis-ease is beginning to recede.

John Swinton
Centre for Spirituality, Health and Disability
University of Aberdeen
January 2007

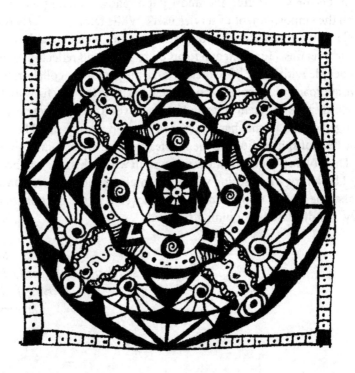

SECTION A
CONTEXT

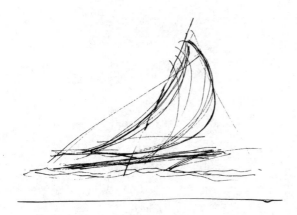

CHAPTER I

THE SPIRITUAL FOUNDATION: AWARENESS AND CONTEXT FOR PEOPLE'S LIVES TODAY

Peter Gilbert

I am sitting down here...

I am sitting on a rock looking out to sea. Not any rock; it is the mottled pink and blue granite of a natural breakwater, jutting out into St Ouen's Bay on the island of Jersey, UK. This is my homeland; part of my identity and, just as the poet Rumi urges us to touch and connect with the waters of our own essence, so I come, when I can, to hear and see and touch and taste the waves of blue-green water as they caress the shore – lapping as they have done for thousands of years.

I am sitting on a rock...where are you, reader? I really want to know, because this book will only have been worth writing if it touches you and the wells of your being, profoundly. All of us who have contributed hope that we can make connections for and with you. You are unique, reader, but we also share a common humanity which stretches back across the generations to the dawn of time.

I am on the beach alone, but, paradoxically, you and all my sisters and brothers are here with me. Our identities are somehow interlinked – we stand both as unique and together, or we drift atomized and alone.

The long search

Ellison states that 'It is the *spirit* of human beings which enables and motivates us to search for meaning and purpose in life...the spiritual dimension does not exist in isolation from the psyche and the soma, but provides an integrative force' (Ellison 1983, pp.331–2). Concentration camp survivor and psychotherapist, Viktor Frankl, from his profound experience of humans in extremis, including in the Nazi concentration camps, propounds that our search for meaning is the primary motivation in our lives (Frankl 1959, p.105).

Philosophers, anthropologists, physical and social scientists, all agree that humankind is a species which engages in a search for meaning, and this often results in a reaching out for a sense of the transcendent or the Other, an essence which many call God, the Gods, or the Spirit of the Universe. This search can become all the more urgent at times of mental ill-health or distress, which many now term a spiritual crisis.

For decades, we have been told that humans are purely rational and material beings, but there has been a huge, popular and academic interest in spirituality (see Anderson 2003; Bianchi 2002; Francis and Robbins 2005; Heelas and Woodhead 2005; Howard and Welbourn 2004; MacKinlay 2006; Nash and Stewart 2002; Swinton 2001; Tacey 2004; Webster 2002; Wilber 2000). We have been informed that religion was dead, but in the post 9/11 world, the concept and practical aspects of religion are moving up the agenda, so that, in the popular medium, in December 2005, BBC2 screened a series with Professor Robert Winston: *The Story of God* (Winston 2005), while in January 2006, Professor Richard Dawkins presented a Channel 4 programme, *The Root of all Evil? The God Delusion* (9 January 2006). In the less accessible medium of research studies for Government, the Mercia Group (Beckford *et al.* 2006) sees faith as one of the prime forms of identity in modern society.

Art and spirituality were, of course, intrinsically linked well before the age of television. Nigel Spivey (Spivey 2005) describes the human desire to depict life, and something beyond life, even at the daybreak of time on earth, as a species of consciousness. In many parts of the world, cave paintings demonstrate a natural preoccupation with the means of survival, i.e. hunting, but they demonstrate more than that. Some drawings appear to show the importance of shamans, who were believed to be a link between the living and the dead. Their role was to mediate between humans in a fragile ecosystem and the almost overwhelming powers of nature – powers that we feel just as sharply today in a technocratic age, through tsunamis and earthquakes. Commentators have also pondered over the inaccessibility of some of these cave paintings, such as the ones at Cabarets in France, and surmised that the artist was not so much demonstrating their prowess to their contemporaries, but engaging in a ritual purpose, the art then being a libation to that Other, which humans both yearn for and fear (Bowker 2002, pp.8–23; Spivey 2005, Chapter 2; Winston 2005, Chapter 1).

So the long search, which for many has taken place at the extremities of existence, under threat of natural disaster, physical or mental ill-health, starvation, the snuffing out of life itself, appears to be a thread woven from our inception to the present day. Perhaps, at the beginning of the 20th century, we had a notion that we would find the answer to everything in time. Now, at the beginning of the 21st century, we seem to be like a child reaching out to the sun or moon and finding the light trickling through our fingers, but no nearer to our grasp. Professor Winston, introducing his television series (BBC Radio 4, *Start the Week*, 28 November 2005) put it like this: 'The more we understand about science, the less we actually understand the universe...so much of particle physics doesn't make complete rational sense' (see also Davies 2006). Many may feel, as does the philosopher A.C. Grayling, that 'the concept of God...is a gerrymandered affair', but if the concept is 'an invention of man', it is 'because humans are spiritual creatures, and spirituality matters' (Grayling 2002, p.119).

The spirit moves

When an individual reaches a point in their life where they are challenged by a major physical or mental illness, or a period of profound psychological distress (see Chapter 4), then the search for meaning, which seems to be inherent in all of us, though possibly dormant all the time, becomes ignited. It is then that human beings do something, which apparently no other animals do; we tell ourselves, or each other stories. As Michael Ondaatje wrote in *The English Patient*:

> We die containing a richness of lovers and tribes, tastes we have swallowed, bodies we have plunged into and swum up as if rivers of wisdom, characters we have climbed into as if trees, fears we have hidden in as if caves. I wish for all this to be marked on my body when I am dead. I believe in such cartography – to be marked by nature, not just to label ourselves on a map like the names of rich men and women on buildings. We are communal histories, communal books... All I desired was to walk upon such an earth that had no maps. (Ondaatje 1992, p.261)

We know from the first histories that before the creation of writing, stories, and especially powerful, iconic myths, were related by wandering players. Perhaps the most incandescent period of human history is when the illumination of the face of the storyteller around the hearth is captured in the writings of the scribe, in Homer, Bede, and other literary creators of peoples. Karen Armstrong (Armstrong 2005) charts the history of myths, from the

Neanderthal graves to the present day, and gives us five important components of myth:

- They are usually rooted in the experience of death and the fear of extinction.
- Ideas are carried out in ritual.
- The most powerful myths are about extremity – they force us to go beyond our experience.
- Myths show us how we should behave.
- Mythology speaks of another plane that exists alongside our own world (Armstrong 2005).

The telling and re-telling of myths tells us a huge amount about the preoccupations of society. Basia Spalek's work on crime victims, for example, not only charts the modern dimensions of victimhood (Spalek 2006), but could also easily look back to Aeschylus, in whose Oresteia, the concept of retribution by blood, is transmuted into the modern city state's rule of law.

Modern myth-makers such as J.R.R. Tolkien, Ursula Le Guin, Philip Pullman, C.S. Lewis, Jeanette Winterson and Terry Pratchett, all introduce, in their various ways, the human search for the Other. Pratchett talks about 'the small gods' (Pratchett 1993). Gods whose size depends on belief: 'Because what gods need is belief, and what humans want is gods' (p.11). Pullman, whose trilogy *His Dark Materials* depicts a world without God, recently wrote:

> We need a story, a myth that does what the traditional religious stories did. It must *explain*. It must satisfy our hunger for a *Why?* …there are two kinds of *Why?* and our story must deal with both. There is the one that asks *What brought us here?* and the other that asks *What are we here for?* (quoted in Watkins 2004, p.250)

Scientists, (e.g. Clarke 2005; see also Cox, Campbell and Fulford 2007; Davies 2006; Winston 2005; Zohar and Marshall 2000) appear to agree that 'human beings are spiritual animals' (Armstrong 1999). Danah Zohar, a physicist, details research in neuroscience which demonstrates that there is an area of the brain – popularly known as 'the God spot', which, when stimulated, opens the door to mystical experiences. Of relevance here, is that, while research shows that between 30 and 70 per cent of the population experiences at least one occasion of 'great euphoria and well-being, accompanying deep insight that brings new perspectives to life' (p.99), people with experience of mental distress seem particularly touched by, and in touch with, this phenomenon. Zohar and Marshall (2000) quote the poet Stephen Spender and his salute to colleague poets whose mental distress interacted with their poetic muse:

> I think continually of those who were truly great. Who, from the womb, remembered the soul's history...whose lovely ambition was that their lips, still touched with fire, should tell of the Spirit clothed from head to foot in song. (p.107)

Biologist Richard Dawkins speaks of a range of experiences and artefacts, such as the Grand Canyon and visiting the Great Fossils in the National Museum of Kenya, as experiences of 'the sacred' (Rogers 2004, pp.135–7). Dawkins ends by saying that 'Poetic imagination is one of the manifestations of human nature' and that one of the duties of scientists is 'to explain that, and I expect that one day we shall'. But, as humans have been wrestling with mystery for millennia, perhaps we need to *know* more than we need to know?

Naming names

People tend to know what religion is, though defining it usually ends in tears, but spirituality can be somewhat intangible. Swinton and Pattison (2001) define spirituality as:

> *Spirituality* can be understood as that aspect of human existence which relates to structures of significance that give meaning and direction to a person's life and helps them deal with the vicissitudes of existence. It is associated with the human quest for meaning, purpose, self-transcending knowledge, meaningful relationships, love and a sense of the holy. It may, or may not, be associated with a specific religious system. (pp.24–25)

In conversation with people I sometimes describe a person's spirituality as at its base what makes them tick, and keeps them going in times of mental distress. Colleagues in Bradford put it more poetically:

> It can refer to the essence of human beings as unique individuals, 'what makes me, me, and you, you'. So it is the power, energy and hopefulness in a person. It is life at its best, growth and creativity, freedom and love. It is what is deepest in us – what gives us direction, motivation. It is what enables a person to survive bad times, to overcome difficulties, to become themselves. (Quoted in NIMHE/MHF 2003, p.14)

Table 1.1 The central features of spirituality

Meaning	The ontological significance of life; making sense of life situations; deriving purpose in existence.
Value	Beliefs and standards that are cherished; having to deal with the truth, beauty, worth, of a thought, object or behaviour; often discussed as 'ultimate values'.
Transcendence	Experience and appreciation of a dimension beyond the self; expanding self-boundaries.
Connecting	Relationships with self, others, God(s)/higher power and the environment.
Becoming	An unfolding of life that demands reflection and experience; includes a sense of who one is and how one knows.

Swinton 2001, p.25.

 ## The Diamond of Self and Others

THE OTHER
- God/Gods
- Philosophy
- Belief systems

SELF
- Identity
- Self-awareness
- Being grounded in
  core values
- Gaining a balance
  between 'being' and
  'becoming'

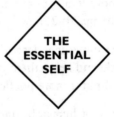
THE
ESSENTIAL
SELF

OTHER PEOPLE
- Family
- Friends
- Colleagues
- Network of support

THE PHYSICAL WORLD
- Landscape
- Seascape
- The animal world
- Minerals, flowers, etc.

Figure 1.1 The Diamond of Self and Others (Gilbert 2005)

It is clear then, that individuals, to gain a sense of wholeness, need to relate to themselves, other people, the physical world around them, and a sense of the Other, which may for many people be God or gods (see Figure 1.1 – The Diamond of Self and Others).

The whole concept of self in both psychology and religion is a tricky one. Buddhists would counsel that Western approaches over emphasize the self, which turns into self-absorption and selfishness, but on the other hand 'self-confidence based on a strong self' is necessary for self-awareness and compassion (Dalai Lama 1997, p.9; see also Haidt 2006).

'*Religion*' encompasses many aspects encompassed in the description of spirituality, usually in the context of belief in a transcendent being or beings, and with a meta-narrative which seeks to explain the origins of the world and those living in it and the questions which face human beings around life, suffering, death and re-awakening in this world or another.

Religion can provide a 'world view', which is acted out in narrative, doctrine, symbols, rites, rituals, sacraments and gatherings; and the promotion of ties of mutual obligation. It creates a framework within which people seek to understand and interpret and make sense of themselves, their lives and daily experiences, and what might happen after death.

Faith communities can be welcoming, integrative and supportive, while some others can be exclusive and stigmatizing of people experiencing mental ill-health.

Where have all the flowers gone?

There is a tendency to talk loosely of a decline in religion in Western society but, in fact, the picture is much more complicated than that. A journey off the motorway into Birmingham, England, may well show a complex picture of some Christian churches converted into bookshops or cafés, but a burgeoning number of mosques, Hindu temples and Sikh gurdwaras. From history and sociology come other complexities. Religious belief and practice has always been an enigmatic and contested area; times of ostensibly strong religious observance, e.g. in Victorian England, may have had as much to do with social conformity as genuine belief (Hunt 2002). One of the manifestations of religion is its ability to create meaning, not just for the individual, but 'through a shared world view of the nature of reality and man's [sic] place in the cosmic realm' (Hunt 2002, p.5).

Surveying the scene

The European Values Study, the 1999 poll undertaken by Opinion Research Business; the *Soul of Britain* polls of 1987 and 2000; and a *News 24* survey in 2005, all seem to point paradoxically to a decline in the sense of a specific, personal, Christian God; an overwhelming percentage still wishing to claim some form of religious affiliation or spiritual dimension; and a growth in allegiance to a number of other religious groupings (see e.g. Brown 2001; Davie 1994; Harries 2002, pp.ix–x; Hunt 2002). Grace Davie, who surveyed religion in Britain since 1945, talks about a separation of *belief* and *belonging.* There is still widespread belief in a spiritual dimension or a spiritual force, but it is often not expressed through institutional allegiance.

The recent national census of inpatients in mental health hospitals and facilities in England and Wales (CHAI/CSIP/Mental Health Act Commission/NIMHE, November 2005) showed that only 20.4 per cent were unaffiliated to a religious grouping, and 1.9 per cent declared themselves atheist or agnostic. Perhaps a number of others merely put down a religious grouping as a matter of habit, but still, it is interesting that this appears to form part of their identity. As Professor Kamlesh Patel, who drove the survey, as Chair of the Mental Health Act Commission, put it:

> If you don't know who I am, how are you going to provide a package of care for me to deliver something? When you do not know how important my religion is to me, what language I speak, where I am coming from, how are you going to help me cope with my mental illness? And that is what I am trying to get over to people; the first step is about *identity*. It is absolutely fundamental to the package of care we offer an individual. (Mulholland 2005, p.5, my emphasis)

Identity – who am I, who are you?

Sociologist Zygmunt Bauman in his book on identity (Bauman 2004), speaks of the tension in terms of national identity he has in being Polish by birth and British by adoption. One of Bauman's contentions is that 'the thought of "having an identity" will not occur to people as long as "belonging" remains their fate, a condition with no alternative' (p.12). As identity becomes more mobile, fluid, liquid; as we move into an era of what I call 'travelling identity', where we engage both in constructing ourselves and being re-formed, identity is the issue of the age.

As we see further on in this chapter, many stages of history have seen that most people lived 'surrounded by others with whom they shared a faith, a tradition, a way of life, a set of rituals and narratives of memory and hope'

(Sacks 2002). Now, however, with the major wars and disruptions of the 20th century, and a mass movement of peoples probably not seen since the fall of the Roman Empire, 'We live', as Chief Rabbi Jonathan Sacks, puts it, 'in the conscious presence of difference' (p.10). For Sacks, the 20th century was dominated by the politics of *ideology* while we are now into the politics of *identity*.

In an age of what some call late Modernity, others Postmodernity, and Bauman 'Liquid Modernity' (Bauman 1997 and 2000), people increasingly have to create their own identity and travel with it, like a snail with its mobile house, poking one's head out of the shell every so often, to test whether one's identity still makes sense! Raphael Mozades, writing in *The Guardian* (2005), questions our tick-box approach to ethnicity. In describing the many branches of his family tree and his life experiences, he concludes:

> I'm Black and I'm brown and I'm a brother and I'm Indian and I'm Jewish and I'm Muslim. White people have told me I'm white, too: after all, I went to Oxford and I talk properly, don't I? Wherever I go, I can't fit in. So I'm everything. But I'm nothing. I fit in, but I'm never at home. I'm not part of a 'community'. (p.26)

This complexity is increasingly expressed in autobiographies such as that by reporter Rageh Omaar (2006), and in novels like Zadie Smith's *White Teeth* (Smith 2001).

Professor John Swinton gave a seminar in 2005 at the Royal College of Psychiatry's Annual Conference in which he pointed to the dissonance which people experience when they see a black speaker with a broad Scottish accent. My own presentation followed on from that: I am white, middle-aged, middle class and I look pretty self-confident. Perhaps you would not immediately guess by looking at me, that while my father's family can trace their way back to a village outside Stafford in the 13th century, some of my mother's family were French Huguenots, French Protestants exiled from their homeland during religious wars, and therefore asylum seekers; others were Scottish Presbyterians, and Portuguese Catholics. You wouldn't immediately know by looking at me, that I experienced an episode of clinical depression a few years ago and was fortunate to recover (see Chapter 10), but the experience of falling into the chasm of depression, and having to claw my way out with the help of friends pulling on ropes, is very much part of my travelling identity – I am who I was, but yet again, I'm not quite the same!

Every world order, philosophy and culture, has its pros and cons, because they are human and being human is a messy business. Journalist

Polly Toynbee once asked why people in Britain are all miserable, pessimistic and cynical. 'Nostalgia, usually a disability of the old, is infecting relatively young people too, as thirty-somethings bewail the mass culture of the moment as something more mass and more crass than it was. Where is "authenticity" the cry goes up' (Toynbee 2005, p.26).

LSE economist and Government adviser, Professor Richard Layard, asks the crucial question: why is it that, on average, people's incomes have doubled in the United States, Britain and Japan, and yet we are no happier than we were 50 years ago? (Layard 2005 a and b). (See also Hutchinson *et al.* 2002; Schwartz 2004.)

Economists and commentators such as Layard (2005) and Hutton (1995) believe that as the grand narratives of stateism so prevalent in the 20th century have given way to a greater privatization of the social realm, governments may have forgotten that humans do not live by bread alone. Layard points to the effect of 'the status race', in that our happiness in our material circumstances is more often than not predicated on our perception of how well-off our neighbour is – a 'status anxiety' (see also De Botton 2004; Marmot 2004) and so that, as Bauman (2000) puts it, there is no finishing line to our satisfaction.

People also wish for security, in the workplace, in the family, and in neighbourhoods and communities; and they wish to be able to trust people. In many places within the old Soviet Union, there is both an appreciation of greater freedom, and some nostalgia for the order, security, consistency and social cohesion of the past. This nostalgia is beautifully portrayed in the film *Goodbye Lenin* (Wolfgang Becker 2004). As Bauman expresses it:

> A cynical observer would say that freedom comes when it no longer matters. There is a nasty fly of impotence in the tasty ointment of freedom, cooked in the cauldron of individualization; that impotence is felt to be all the more odious, discomforting and upsetting, in view of the empowerment that freedom was expected to deliver. (Bauman 2000, p.35)

From Plato to Postmodernism

One of our great problems is that we seem to have great difficulty in holding *difference* in our hands and living with it. We yearn for choice and colour, but only insofar as we have control of them and do not have to mutually engage. We cling to rocks of 'certainty', but can we learn to swim in the sea without either attacking other swimmers, losing ourselves, or clinging to rocks with our eyes tight shut?

Each era gains insights and loses others. In the ancient world, Plato spoke of the necessity of seeing the essential congruence of mind, body, heart and spirit:

> As you ought not to attempt to cure the eyes without the head, or the head without the body, so neither ought you to attempt to cure the body without the soul ... for the part can never be well unless the whole is well. (Quoted in Ross 1997, p.i)

The Enlightenment brought in the reign of reason, but this also had its disadvantages, as mental illness was seen as a threat to reason and a utilitarian approach to society. The Classical Age is an era during which the bounds of nature are thrown back. The gates of the great classical palaces, such as Versailles and Blenheim, are in the form of twisted thorny barbs, guarding the building and courtyard from the great park, which itself keeps untamed nature at bay. The Classical Age is, in all senses, the time when the gates are closed and reason shielded from folly. The great American hospitals for the insane, such as that in Pennsylvania, are modelled on the same pattern as the European palaces, and here again we have the same enclosed symmetry and beauty. The Classical Age is essentially agoraphobic! (see Foucault 2001 and Porter 1987).

The 20th century saw what Bauman calls 'the dream of purity' (Bauman 1997) where nations, harnessing modern technology, produced order of a most fearsome kind: Hitler's Germany, Stalin's Russia, Mao's China, Pol Pot's Cambodia. Hitler's Germany is perhaps the apotheosis of this form, because of its totality; while the Jews were the complete 'strangers' to be excised, everybody seen unfit or unworthy, namely people with mental health needs, people with learning disabilities, etc., were also to be exterminated, and a pathological, secular, religion created (Burleigh 2001).

In the Postmodern world, the threat is perhaps more diffuse. Solid structures have given way to liquid. The State is less oppressive in many places, but also less protective. Individuals have moved from being 'citizens' to 'consumers' and their value is judged very much on their ability to consume. Whereas the Nazi State saw people with disabilities as unproductive, modern society sees them as deficient consumers, unable to respond to the blandishments of the market place and the incentive of status consumption, and so moved to the margins, while the mammoth shopping malls are the temples of the new gods to whom devotees need to go with a propensity to consume.

In a sea without navigation lights, both those with and those without resources, have a tendency to drift in an open boat of identity anxiety. 'Strangers' appear to multiply and the 'haves' tend to protect themselves by withdrawing into a 'drawbridge society' (Hutton 1995, p.332) or behind the 'ramparts of permanently besieged fortresses' (Bauman 1997, p.14).

In a Postmodern world we have greater freedom to tell our own story. The question is, does our story make sense to anyone else? The storytellers around the hearths of the times before the written word, were proponents of what Le Guin (2001) calls 'The Telling', and what Armstrong (2005) calls myths. Their stories would have made sense, giving a structure, a signifi-cance of meaning, to their listeners. Do our stories make sense to those we tell them to? Or are they voices in the air? The grand narratives of the past hold less sway. Although many people have a religious faith, they are less likely to adhere to the whole creed. Faith in science to cure all ills, without creating new ones, has been shaken in its turn: the debates over the appropri-ate energy production for the future, the scare over an avian 'flu pandemic and the uncertainties over the MMR vaccination, being only a few examples. It is perhaps not surprising, that some have turned to a new form of 'cer-tainty' through fundamentalism (see Figure 1.2). As Bauman puts it: 'with the market-induced agony of solitude and abandonment as its only alterna-tive, fundamentalism, religious or otherwise, can count on an ever-growing constituency' (Bauman 1997, p.185). For people in a state of mental distress, or needing to recall and restore, telling their story (see Allan 2006) is an

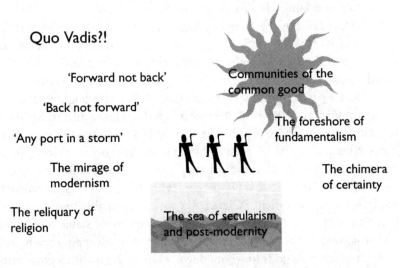

Figure 1.2 Quo Vadis (Gilbert 2006a)

essential part of their creation and recreation of identity, in their journey of recovery and discovery.

Speaking with individuals and groups across the country, a number of questions stand out:

- Can an individual and individualized spirituality reach out in a wider circle of communities, or would such an extension to others contaminate or dilute the very essence of meaning which starts with the existential person?

- Can organizations, in an era of rampant performance measures, move from the transactional to the transformational and so make human services actually human? (see Gilbert 2005 and Chapter 17 in this book).

- Can faith communities retain their unique contribution while creating a congruency and partnership with other constituencies around the positive essentials of a faith-based approach to life and death?

As Bernard Moss points out, 'the issues of religion and spirituality take us to the very heart of what it means to be human and to be living together in society' (Moss 2005, pp.1–2). Individual religion and a faith community will not be right for everyone. Can spiritual or other groups (see Chapter 10) provide the cohesion to build a new form of society? Can we create communities of meaning and the common good which are strong enough to stand the test of tide and time?

We need to be, as Eva Hoffman puts it, 'Keepers of each others' stories' (Hoffman 1998). Hoffman, who moved with her family from Poland to North America, following anti-Jewish pogroms, writes: 'Human beings don't only search for meanings, they are themselves units of meaning; but we can mean something only within the fabric of larger significations.' Through her relationships she speaks of the ability to 'keep creating new maps and tapestries of a shared reality' (p.279).

Gateways and pathways

'Just get the humanity right!' (Dr Joanna Bennett at the inquiry into her brother's death in care). 'There is no health without mental health' (European Commission 2005, p.4).

Mental health services are not created out of thin air. They are constructed out of our values and vision for society, our history, and how we view human nature and the world we live in. As Kathleen Jones, the doyenne of social historians in mental health, puts it: 'The way in which' [people with mental health needs] 'are defined and cared for, is primarily a social response to a very basic set of human problems' and how we answer the questions around liberty, safety, care and inclusion, depends on, 'the values they (societies) hold' (Jones 1972, p.xiii). (See also Chapter 2 and Moss 2006.)

Within the UK, there could be said to be five common strands which run through a range of social issues and services (see Midwinter 1994; Gilbert 2003, Chapter 2), and these form the responses to the challenges which human groups face. These are: (i) the balance between public and private provision; (ii) whether services are organized centrally or locally; (iii) institutional care versus care at home; (iv) services to be provided by cash or in kind; and (v) the tensions between the liberty of the individual and their safety, and the safety of the wider public.

One of humankind's most powerful propensities is to find some rock of 'certainty' and cling to it for dear life! This can be as true of those coming from a rationalist viewpoint, as of those coming from a faith perspective. Rather than opening ourselves to the testing of paradigms, we hug them fearfully to ourselves. When personal experiences (see e.g. Chapters 5, 7 and 15), or research (see Chapter 23), open our eyes to different approaches, we tend to want to turn that new way of working into a 'model' which gives us all the answers and prevents us from having to bear the anxiety of, often unanswerable, questions. While we are happy to refer to the old Victorian asylums as an horrendous failure, we tend to forget that they were, in part, an attempted public response to failures in community capacity and represented a major investment from the society of the time (Gilbert and Scragg 1992). We also forget that we are natural institutional builders. Scandals still rock the system. The death of David 'Rocky' Bennett, a 38-year-old African-Caribbean patient, in a medium secure psychiatric unit, having been restrained by staff, was one of the *causes célèbres* which marked the move towards an action plan on Race Equality in Mental Health Care in Britain (Department of Health 2005). The BBC *Panorama* programme 'Undercover Nurse' in the summer of 2005, showed elderly, frail patients in a Brighton general hospital receiving a lack of care which would have shamed an animal shelter. The response from the Royal College of Nursing to the latter episode was to urge a need to return to some of the fundamental root values of the caring professions, so that technology, necessary in itself, does not supersede humanity.

It is this emphasis on our common humanity, namely, what creates an empathic bond with each other, whatever our personal or cultural differences, as we journey through life and our essential uniqueness as an individual, however great our similarities, which needs to be paid the greatest attention. Both are at the heart of the NIMHE Spirituality and Mental Health Project (see NIMHE/MMF 2003 and Cox *et al.* 2007).

Why is spirituality so important in mental health, and why should it be attended to among the plethora of performance measures?

First, because users and carers are increasingly stating that their spiritual and/or religious needs are an imperative element in their survival and recovery – sometimes the main imperative. In the DVD *Hard to Believe* (Mind in Croydon 2005), a number of people using mental health services talk of a variety of spiritual dimensions which are essential to their well-being. As one puts it: 'My spirituality is the anchor for my soul'. Unfortunately, many people who use mental health services have the same experience as the poet Sue Holt, who writes of having to mask her deepest and most life-affirming beliefs:

I was excited; today was the Lord's birthday,
And I was going home for dinner.
I masked my emotions,
Otherwise they would keep me.
I had to behave myself today,
No talking of God.

(Sue Holt, 'Year 2000 on a Section 3',
my emphasis)

Dr Andrew Powell, founder of the Spirituality and Psychiatry Special Interest Group for the Royal College of Psychiatrists (see Chapter 12) points out in *Hard to Believe*, that while the vast percentage of people with mental health needs place great importance on their spirituality, only about 33 per cent of psychiatrists and psychologists see this as important (see also El-Nimr, Green and Salib 2004). Although social work views itself as a profession with an holistic approach, social work educators such as Gilligan (2003) and Moss (2005) have acknowledged that social work as a profession has often found this element of the user's inner and outer experience difficult to relate to.

Whatever our opinion on approaches to multi-culturalism there is no doubting the fact that an increasing number of Western countries will be multi-cultural in composition. It is not just that many people will have a cultural identity of origin, and then be relating to a different culture in the country which they live, but also there will be an increasing incidence of inter-cultural and inter-faith marriages/partnerships. In the concept of travelling identity, we have the tension of retaining our essential integrity, while also developing as individuals in relation to others and the outside world.

Norman Jones, who settled in Britain from the Caribbean, found that the use of narrative awakened expressions within him which had remained dormant:

> Telling my story to the others reminded me that one of the most important aspects of my faith, is that of my background and culture. I am a Black person and a Black person who originally came from the Caribbean. I am aware of my background and the history of my people... *we need to remember that we have been given the gift to be ourselves.* (Quoted in Reddie 2001, p.116, my emphasis, and see Chapters 3, 6 and 16)

Subsequent to the tragic events of 9/11 in the US and 7/7 in the UK, many people of Asian origin now wish to identify themselves by their religious affiliation than their ethnicity. It is important that services recognize this self-identification without pigeon-holing people. As Nobel economist, Amartya Sen (Sen 2006a) opines, people's construction is complex and multi-faceted.

There is a, perhaps inevitable, reaction against secularism and consumerism, and even against the more liberal approaches of different religious groups in accommodating with secular society.

Young people affiliated to religious groups, are often much more drawn to a firmer framework than their parents were.

For many, secular society is profoundly unsatisfying, and yet the traditional religions are unpalatable. As the Australian David Tacey puts it: 'The ideals of secularism, however well-intended, are inadequate for life, since our lives are not rational and we are hugely implicated in the reality of the sacred, whether or not this is acknowledged' (Tacey 2004, p.12) and again 'the old cultural wineskins cannot contain the new wine of the spirit' (p.18). Therefore, the challenge is to build something that is personal, but which reaches out and is not privatized; and for both services and faith communities, to build a house where all are named, their visions shared and songs heard. With concern being voiced about the mental health of the population at an international (e.g. European Commission 2005) and national (Layard 2005 a and b) levels, the impetus for guidance and policy is broadly seeing a move towards and accent on self-assessment, respect, choice, person-centred planning, well-being and recovery, and user control of care pathways (see NIMHE 2007; SCMH *et al.* 2005) and we need to aim to create a network of narrative, rather than allow policy initiatives which are good in themselves, to further fragment vulnerable people.

The NIMHE Spirituality and Mental Health Project (NIMHE/MHF 2003) (see figure 1.3) aims to bring a raft of grassroots initiatives together in a way which is enabling and facilitative, rather than centrally directed and imposed. It is about both the individual experience of spirituality, and work with communities of belief.

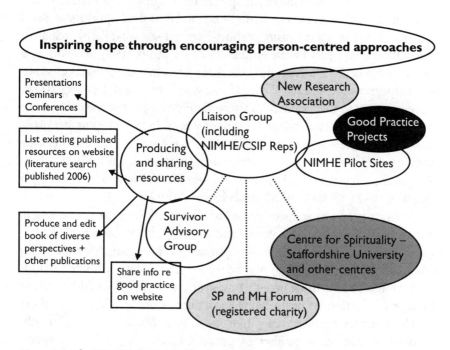

Figure 1.3 The NIMHE Spirituality Project (Gilbert 2006a)

Making meanings

Increasing interest in family roots and heritage has come to the fore in recent years, and if we are indeed in an environment of Bauman's *Liquid Life,* where 'looseness of attachment and revocability of engagement' (Bauman 2005, p.4) are the guiding precepts, then it is not surprising that tracing one's ancestors is such a growth industry. Historians point out that the use of surnames only really became popular from the 13th century; and up until the British Industrial Revolution, people remained remarkably static in both occupational status and geographical location (see Hey 2001). For those

African-Caribbeans who were forced to take the names of their slave-owners (Blackman 2006), and whose stolen and transmuted identity is passed down today, the naming of names has a very specific meaning.

Humans seek progress, but progress comes at a price, and that may be fundamentally the severing of previous relationships. The first Industrial Revolution, and the enclosure of common land for modern agricultural practice, had an effect which is being mirrored today in a second industrial revolution. Arthur Miller's iconic consumerist Willy Loman (Miller 2000), and his plaintive: 'I'm tired to the death' (p.8) as he struggles to meet the requirements of the American Dream, is intensified today as the acquisition of skills and experience has an increasingly short-lived value – what Richard Sennett terms 'the specter [sic] of uselessness' (Sennett 2006, p.99). As work and consumption become increasingly the main, or even only, bringers of value, other aspects of life, or even life itself, can go by the board (Bunting 2005). Governments are always likely to stress 'family values', but the structure of the tax and welfare systems can belie their words. In fact, keeping people in work, getting them into work, and making them mobile so as to meet the needs of work, are a huge imperative. Demographic trends indicate a doubling of the number of single-person households in Britain from 6 to 12 per cent from 1971 to 2005 (ONS 20 February 2006).

We have pressures at the other end of life as well, with the pressure to, in the words of the song: 'Stay young and beautiful, if you want to be loved'. There is also talk of technological improvements increasing life expectancy exponentially (Bunting 2006), and a deep longing for personal immortality.

It would be easy to set up a dichotomy between religious faiths and the concept of the time of death being in the hands of the Divine, and those people who determine to end their own lives. Much more profoundly, however, is that for a number of people experiencing marked physical decline, or acute mental and/or physical suffering, snuffing out the candle of life may be the last element of control one feels one has. If the focus is merely a mechanistic prolongation of physical existence, then that makes little sense to those in pain. As Margaret Lloyd points out: 'Holistic care, however, cannot be achieved without a determined pursuit of an underpinning philosophy which sees human existence in terms other than the currency of the marketplace' (Lloyd 1997, p.103). In these ontological debates, religious and spiritual communities have a legitimate part to play, and it is noticeable that novelists, perhaps especially those who write ostensibly for children, deal with the way that a denial of death denies life as well (see e.g. Le Guin 1973 and Pullman 2001).

While interest in vertical kinship ties increases, actual horizontal ties in the present have tended to atrophy. This is due, not only to globalization and shifting economic structures, but also demography, and even some unintended consequences of welfare initiatives. The influential study of family and kinship in east London by Michael Young and Peter Willmott in 1957, has now been re-visited (Dench, Gavron and Young 2006). The original 1950s study showed considerable community cohesion and support, though this was tempered by the fact that there were the inevitable internecine family squabbles. The more recent picture, however, shows considerable fragmentation of the original working-class community and a feeling of promises betrayed.

If kin is now less important in this fluid, liquid world, then perhaps the answer is in friendship (Pahl 2000; Vernon 2005). Increasingly, we rely on friends, but does friendship in the modern world have the strength to provide a buffer against the winds of fortune, and the corrupting influence of what Pahl calls 'the superficial glad-handedness of much corporate culture' (p.90).

Underpinning all of this is a tension between becoming as quintessentially oneself as possible, grounded and centred and, at the same time, being able to develop, in a more Western mode, to 'become' (see Figure 1.4).

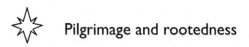 Pilgrimage and rootedness

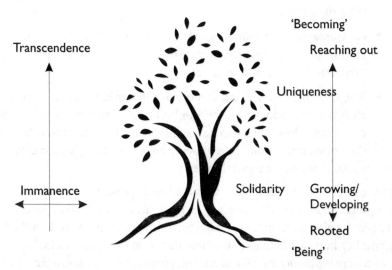

Figure 1.4 Pilgrimage and Rootedness (Gilbert, 2004)

At present, we may well be spending so much time becoming someone or something, that we lose touch with who we actually are. As one of the lay participants in a BBC2 series entitled *The Monastery* put it: 'To follow a spiritual path is not to take the easy way out and withdraw from the world, but rather to choose a different and far more challenging mode of being in the world' (Buxton 2005, pp.8–9).

Government often sees faith communities as a means of promoting social cohesion and social capital (Scottish Executive 2002; Home Office 2004), but faith communities become inconvenient when it comes to globalization, and on a number of moral issues. It is common for Government to push in the direction of on the one hand, family values, social cohesion, keeping welfare and public order costs low through social capital and social inclusion; and on the other hand, promoting increased globalization and profits, labour mobility, consumerism and investing hugely in public order initiatives and incarceration (Spalek 2006).

There are clearly huge increases in material prosperity within most of the Western world, though this is marked by exploitation of people and natural resources, and growing income divides within apparently affluent societies and communities. At the same time, states of perceived well-being have not kept pace with material success. The major changes may well be around the following:

- The lack of a meta-narrative cohesion. Both religion and science have been perceived to fail. 'Multi-culturalism' is often really what Sen (2006a) calls 'plural monoculturalisms' which leaves people in their own silos.

- Consumerism and global capitalism which, in fact, feed on the atomization of humanity, competition in pursuit of a never-ending goal, and built-in obsolescence.

- The lack of a binding ethic: most of the world religions have a clear accent on social justice and building communities, which of course as a downside, can be exclusive. Without an ethical base in the community itself, governments have increasingly to impose social morality and social order.

Jonathan Sacks is perhaps the most erudite exponent of social cohesion through faith communities, because he integrates this within an interaction between secular government, civil law, faith institutions and individual dignity. For him, 'a community is where they *know your name* and where they *miss you when you are not there*. Community is society with a human face' (Sacks 2005, p.54).

At the end of the day, and in the travails of life, we are essentially alone. We connect with ourselves, with other people, and perhaps with a sense of a personal or impersonal God or world spirit. Life is a continuum of aloneness and loneliness, because the sea of life on which we are sailing is one of constant movement and change, of ebb and flow. And, when we reach the Promised Land, is it the land which we sought in the first place; is the Promised Land full of promise, or all too familiar as the land we left behind? The novelist Jeanette Winterson, in her description of love, compares it with the early Celtic pilgrims who drove themselves across alien seas:

> The earliest pilgrims shared a cathedral for a heart…love it was that drove them forth. Love that brought them home again. Love hardened their hands against the oar and heated their sinews against the rain. The journeys they made were beyond common sense; who leaves the hearth for the open sea? Especially without a compass, especially in winter, especially alone. What you risk reveals what you value. In the presence of love, hearth and quest become one. (Winterson 2001, p.81)

It is often love which drives us mad, but the absence of love leaves one sterile. For many people experiencing mental distress, it is the intensity of the experience which gives them hope. It is also at that time, that a sense of God, even a touch of God, comes upon them. Like the lover who has loved and lost, they don't necessarily wish for the *Eternal Sunshine of the Spotless Mind* (film by Gondry 2004) where memories of a spiritual connection can be erased. The intensity of spiritual experience can be as uncomfortable to the religious professional as to the secular professional and, ultimately making space for an exploration of mutual meanings is where we need to have the courage to stay.

On the beach…

Well reader, are we still in touch? I have left the safety of my rock, my granite rock, and am traversing the beach. I need to move, but I feel the loss of safety and security that my marbled perch offered.

The shadow of the valley of despair is behind me and the sun breaks through the clouds over the lighthouse beyond. But I wonder how long the light will last, as the wind whips the stinging grit about my ankles? Will you walk with us through the pages of this book? Will we meet in some forum to discuss our thoughts and make meanings together? The sea is changing colour, from blue to grey. I am here reader, where and how are you?

Bibliography

Allan, C. (2006) *Poppy Shakespeare.* London: Bloomsbury.

Anderson, R.S. (2003) *Spiritual Caregiving as Secular Sacrament.* London: Jessica Kingsley Publishers.

Appiah, K.A. (2005) *The Ethics of Identity.* Princeton: Princeton University Press.

Armstrong, A. (1999) *A History of God.* London: Vintage.

Armstrong, K. (2005) *A Short History of Myth.* London: Canongate.

Bauman, Z. (1997) *Postmodernity and its Discontents.* Cambridge: Polity Press.

Bauman, Z. (2000) *Liquid Modernity.* Cambridge: Polity Press.

Bauman, Z. (2004) *Identity.* Cambridge: Polity Press.

Bauman, Z. (2005) *Liquid Life.* Cambridge: Polity Press.

Beckford, A., Gayle, R., Owen, D., Peach, C. and Weller, P. (2006) *Review of the Evidence Base on Faith Communities – Report for the OPDM.* University of Warwick, May 2006.

Bianchi, E. (2002) *Words of Spirituality: Towards a Lexicon of the Inner Life.* London: SPCK.

Blackman, P.S. (2006) 'Turning the Tide.' Talk to the NIMHE National Conference 'Delivering Race Equality: Research, Policy and Practice', 22 February 2006.

Bowker, J. (ed.) (2002) *The Cambridge Illustrated History of Religions.* Cambridge: Cambridge University Press.

Brown, C.G. (2001) *The Death of Christian Britain.* Abingdon: Routledge.

Bunting, M. (2005) *Willing Slaves: How the Overwork Culture is Ruining Our Lives.* London: Harper Perennial.

Bunting, M. (2006) 'There is no stop button in the race for human re-engineering.' *The Guardian*, 30 January 2006, p.25.

Burleigh, M. (2001) *The Third Reich: A New History.* London: Pan Macmillan.

Buxton, N. (2005) 'Mixed message of The Monastery?' *The Tablet*, 27 August 2005.

Clarke, C. (ed.) (2005) *Ways of Knowing: Science and Mysticism Today.* Exeter: Imprint Academic.

Clarke, I. (ed.) (2001) *Psychosis and Spirituality: Exploring the New Frontier.* London: Whurr Publishers.

Commission for Audit and Inspection (badged with NIMHE, CSIP, MHAC) (2005) *Count Me In: Results of a National Census of In-patients in Mental Health Hospitals and Facilities in England and Wales.* CHAI, November 2005.

Cornah, D. (2007) *The Impact of Spirituality on Mental Health: A Review of the Literature.* London: Mental Health Foundation.

Cottingham, J. (2005) *The Spiritual Dimension: Religion, Philosophy and Human Value.* Cambridge: Cambridge University Press.

Cox, J., Campbell, A., and Fulford, K.W.M. (2007) *Medicine of the Person: Faith, Science and Values in Health Care Provision.* London: Jessica Kingsley Publishers.

Dalai Lama (1997) *The Heart of the Buddha's Path.* London: Thorsons.

Davie, G. (1994) *Religion in Britain Since 1945: Believing Without Belonging.* Oxford: Blackwell.

Davies, P. (2006) *The Goldilocks Enigma: Why is the Universe Just Right for Life.* London: Allen Lane.

De Botton, A. (2004) *Status Anxiety.* London: Hamish Hamilton.

Dench, G., Gavron, K. and Young, M. (2006) *The New East End: Kinship, Race and Conflict.* London: Profile Books.

Department of Health (2005) *Delivering Race Equality in Mental Health Care: an Action Plan for Reform Inside and Outside Services and the Government's Response to the Independent Inquiry into the Death of David Bennett.* London: DoH, 11 January 2005.

Ellison, C.W. (1983) 'Spiritual well-being: conceptualisation and measurement.' *Journal of Psychology and Theology 11*, 4.

El-Nimr, G., Green, L. and Salib, E. (2004) 'Spiritual care in psychiatry: professionals' views.' *Mental Health, Religion and Culture 7*, 2, 165–70.

European Commission/Health and Consumer Protection Directorate-General (2005) *Green Paper: Improving the Mental Health of the Population: Towards a Strategy on Mental Health for the European Union.* Brussels: European Commission, 14 October 2005 com (2005) 484.

Foucault, M. (1967 this edition 2001) *Madness and Civilisation.* London: Routledge.

Francis, L.J. and Robbins, M. (2005) *Urban Hope and Spiritual Health.* Peterborough: Epworth.

Frankl, V. (1959) *Man's Search for Meaning.* New York: Simon and Schuster.

Gilbert, P. (2003) *The Value of Everything.* Lyme Regis. Russell House Publishing.

Gilbert, P. (2004) *It's Humanity, Stoopid!* Inaugural lecture, Staffordshire University, 29 September 2004.

Gilbert, P. (2005) *Leadership: Being Effective and Remaining Human.* Lyme Regis: Russell House Publishing.

Gilbert, P. (2006a) 'Breathing out, breathing in.' In: Social Perspectives Network Study Paper 9: *Reaching for the Spirit.* London: SPN.

Gilbert, P. (2006b) 'Breathing space.' *Community Care* 19–25 January 2006.

Gilbert, P. (2007) 'Spirituality and mental health: practical proposals for action.' In J. Cox *et al.* (2007) *op. cit.*

Gilbert, P. and Scragg, T. (1992) *Managing to Care.* Sutton: BPI.

Gilligan, P.A. (2003) 'It isn't discussed. Religion, belief and practice teaching: missing components of cultural competence in social work education.' *Journal of Practice Teaching in Health and Social Work 5*, 1, 75–95.

Grayling, A.C. (2002) *The Meaning of Things: Applying Philosophy to Life.* London: Phoenix.

Haidt, J. (2006) *The Happiness Hypothesis: Putting Ancient Wisdom and Philosophy to the Test of Modern Science.* London: William Heinemann.

Hard to Believe. DVD, directed by Ben Hole. London: Mind in Croydon, 2005.

Harries, R. (2002) *God Outside the Box: Why Spiritual People Object to Christianity.* London: SPCK.

Heather, P. (2005) *The Fall of the Roman Empire: A New History.* London: Macmillan.

Heelas, P. and Woodhead, L. (2005) *The Spiritual Revolution: Why Religion is Giving Way to Spirituality.* Oxford: Blackwell.

Hey, D. (2001) 'Family names and family history.' *History Today,* July 2001.

Hoffman, E. (1998) *Lost in Translation.* London: Vintage.

Hollins, S. (2005) 'Blessings in abundance.' *The Tablet,* 17 December 2005, p.5.

Holloway, R. (2004) *Looking in the Distance: The Human Search for Meaning.* Edinburgh: Canongate Books.

Holt, S. (2003) *Poems of Survival.* Brentwood: Chipmunka Publishing.

Home Office (2004) *Working Together.* London: Home Office.

Howard, S. and Welbourn, D. (2004) *The Spirit at Work Phenomenon.* London: Azure.

Hunt, S.J. (2002) *Religion in Western Society.* Basingstoke: Palgrave.

Hutchinson, F., Mellor, M. and Olsen, W. (2002) *The Politics of Money: Towards Sustainability and Economic Democracy.* London: Pluto Press.

Hutton, W. (1995) *The State We're In.* London: Penguin Books.

Jones, K. (1972) *A History of the Mental Health Services.* London: Routledge and Keegan Paul.

Layard, R. (2005a) *Happiness: Lessons from a New Science.* London: Allen Lane.

Layard, R. (2005b) *Mental Health: Britain's Biggest Social Problem.* Paper presented to the No 10 Strategy Group, 20 January, 2005.

Le Guin, U. (1973) *The Farthest Shore.* London: Victor Gollancz.

Le Guin, U. (2001) *The Telling.* London: Victor Gollancz.

Lloyd, M. (1997) 'Dying and bereavement, spirituality and social work in a market economy of welfare.' *British Journal of Social Work* 27, 175–90.

Lowe, S. and McArthur, A. (2005) *Is It Just Me or Is Everything Shit?: The Encyclopaedia of Modern Life.* London: Time Warner.

MacKinlay, E. (2006) *The Spiritual Dimension of Ageing.* London: Jessica Kingsley Publishers.

Marmot, M. (2004) *Status Syndrome: How your Social Standing Directly Affects your Health.* London: Bloomsbury.

Midwinter, E. (1994) *The Development of Social Welfare in Britain.* Buckingham: Open University Press.

Miller, A. (2000, first published 1949) *Death of a Salesman.* London: Penguin.

Moss, B. (2005) *Religion and Spirituality.* Lyme Regis: Russell House Publishing.

Moss, B. (2006) *Values.* Lyme Regis: Russell House Publishing.

Mozades, R. (2005) 'Modern identity is not all Black or White – it's a beige thing.' *The Guardian*, 29 December 2005, p.26.

Mulholland, H. (2005) 'Counting on change.' *The Guardian*, 7 December 2005, p.5.

Nash, M. and Stewart, B. (2002) *Spirituality and Social Care: Contributing to Personal and Community Well-being.* London: Jessica Kingsley Publishers.

NIMHE (forthcoming) *Commissioning Guidance on Spirituality and work with Faith Communities.* Leeds: NIMHE.

NIMHE/Mental Health Foundation (Gilbert, P. and Nicholls, V.) (2003) *Inspiring Hope: Recognizing the Importance of Spirituality in a Whole Person Approach to Mental Health.* Leeds: NIMHE.

Omaar, R. (2006) *Only Half of Me: Being a Muslim in Britain.* London: Penguin/Viking.

Ondaatje, M. (1992) *The English Patient.* London: Picador.

Pahl, R. (2000) *On Friendship.* Cambridge: Polity Press.

Porter, R. (1987) *A Social History of Madness.* London: Weidenfield and Nicholson.

Pratchett, T. (1993) *Small Gods.* London: Corgi.

Pullman, P. (2001) *The Amber Spyglass.* London: Scholastic.

Rankin, P. (2006) *Buried Spirituality.* Salisbury: Sarum College Press.

Reddie, A.G. (2001) *Faith Stories and the Experience of Black Elders: Singing the Lord's Song in a Strange Land.* London: Jessica Kingsley Publishers.

Rogers, B. (ed.) (2004) *Is Nothing Sacred?* Abingdon: Routledge.

Ross, L.A. (1997) *Nurses' Perceptions of Spiritual Care.* Aldershot: Avebury.

Sacks, J. (2002) *The Dignity of Difference: How to Avoid the Clash of Civilisations.* London: Continuum.

Sacks, J. (2005) *To Heal a Fractured World: The Ethics of Responsibility.* London: Continuum.

SCHM, LGA, NHSC and ADSS (2005) *The Future of Mental Health: A Vision for 2015.* London: SCMH.

Schwartz, B. (2004) *The Paradox of Choice.* London: Harper Collins.

Scottish Executive Health Department (2002) *Guidelines on Chaplaincy and Spiritual Care in Scotland.* NHS HDL 76, 28 October 2002.

Sen, A. (2006a) *Identity and Violence.* London: Allen Lane.

Sen, A. (2006b) 'Identity crisis.' *The Guardian*, 18 February 2006, p.27.

Sennett, R. (2006) *The Culture of the New Capitalism.* Boston: Yale University Press.

Sheikh, A. and Gatrad, A.R. (2000) *Caring for Muslim Patients.* Oxford: Radcliffe Medical Press.

Smith, Z. (2001) *White Teeth.* London: Penguin.

Spalek, B. (2006) *Crime Victims: Theory, Policy and Practice.* Basingstoke: Palgrave Macmillan.

Spivey, N. (2005) *How Art Made the World.* London: BBC Books.

Swinton, J. (2001) *Spirituality and Mental Health Care: Rediscovering a 'Forgotten' Dimension.* London: Jessica Kingsley Publishers.

Swinton, J. and Pattison, S. (2001) 'Come all ye faithful.' *Health Service Journal,* 20 December 2001, 24–25.

Tacey, D. (2004) *The Spirituality Revolution: the Emergency of Contemporary Spirituality.* Hove: Brunner-Routledge.

Toynbee, P. (2005) 'Let's celebrate the utter bloody goodness of the world today.' *The Guardian,* 30 December 2005, p.26.

Vardy, P. (2003) *Being Human: Fulfilling Genetic and Spiritual Potential.* London: Darton, Longman and Todd.

Vernon, M. (2005) *The Philosophy of Friendship.* Basingstoke: Palgrave.

Watkins, T. (2004) *Dark Matter.* Southampton: Damaris.

Webster, A. (2002) *Wellbeing.* London: SCM Press.

Wilber, K. (2000) *Sex, Ecology, Spirituality: The Spirit of Evolution.* (2nd revised edn) London: Shambhala.

Winston, R. (2005) *The Story of God: A Personal Journey into the World of Science and Religion.* London: Bantam.

Winterson, J. (2001, first published 1992) *Written on the Body.* London: Vintage.

Winterson, J. (2006) *Tanglewreck.* London: Bloomsbury.

Wolpert, L. (2006) *Malignant Sadness: The Anatomy of Depression.* (3rd edn) London: Faber and Faber.

Zohar, D. and Marshall, I. (2000) *SQ: Spiritual Intelligence the Ultimate Intelligence.* London: Bloomsbury.

The Dark has a Friendly Face

The dark has a friendly face
Where each shadow knows its own place
And it sways to the pace of the night
As it rocks its way back into light
It will cover and shelter and hide
All the things that we covet inside
And it stills all the storms of the deep
As the world and its people all sleep.

The dark has a friendly face
When nobody knows where you are
And the sky is as black as my soul
And the whistling breeze reminds me I'm here
And alive and in control.

The dark has a friendly face
As it dwindles its way into dawn
And it tucks itself neatly away
'Til the dusk and the evening are born.

The dark has a friendly face
And it sits up all night like a friend
And it ticks and it tocks into day
When the lull in the chaos will end.

Ju Blencowe

CHAPTER 2

VALUES-BASED PRACTICE: HELP AND HEALING WITHIN A SHARED THEOLOGY OF DIVERSITY

Bill (K.W.M) Fulford and Kim Woodbridge

Values-based practice is a new approach to working with complex and conflicting values that is the basis of a number of policy, training and service
developments in mental health and social care across the UK and
internationally.

Values-based practice, as we outline in this chapter, starts from the principle of respect for *differences* of values (Fulford 2004). As such, it might be
thought to be incompatible with the strongly held values underpinning not
only the great faith traditions but also some forms of secular humanism.
Bioethics, for example, in the form in which it is currently dominant in much
of health and social care, is underpinned by a commitment to such strongly
held values as autonomy and confidentiality. But there are many, and not
only within the great faith traditions, for whom a dogmatic commitment to
their own 'right values' is paralleled by an equally dogmatic rejection of the
values of others: and as the British philosopher (and now Member of the
House of Lords) Baroness O'Neill, explored in a series of Reith Lectures on
the BBC, fanaticism is nowadays increasingly evident in all spheres of life,
both public and private (O'Neill, 2002).

Renewed fanaticism, religious and secular, is only half the story,
however. For alongside the fanatics, there have always been those, and not
least within each of the great faith traditions, who have been able to combine
deep personal convictions with an equal capacity for openness and for
respectful engagement with the often very different values and beliefs of

others. Values-based practice, as we will describe in this chapter, in starting from respect for differences of values, and then relying on 'good process' rather than 'right values' for effective decision-making, provides a framework for drawing on the resources of these more open faith traditions for spiritual help and healing within a shared theology of diversity.

What is values-based practice?

As a new approach to working with complex and conflicting values in health and social care, values-based practice has been developed in a partnership between Warwick Medical School's programme in the Philosophy and Ethics of Mental Health and the London-based NGO, the Sainsbury Centre for Mental Health. A training manual in values-based practice, *Whose Values?* was launched in 2004 by Rosie Winterton as the Minister for State in the Department of Health with responsibility for mental health (Woodbridge and Fulford, 2004). *Whose Values?* has subsequently become the basis for a number of policy, training and service development initiatives in mental health and social care (Fulford, Thornton and Graham 2006a).

As noted above, faced with complex and conflicting values, values-based practice starts from the meta-value of 'respect for differences of values' and relies on good process rather than pre-assigned right values to guide decision-making. Ten key 'pointers' to good process in values-based practice are summarized in Figure 2.1.

Thus, as Figure 2.1 indicates, at the heart of the 'good process' of values-based practice is training in four key skills areas – raising awareness of values and of differences of values, reasoning about values, knowledge of values, and communication skills. *Whose Values?* provides detailed self-training exercises in each of these four skills areas. However, values-based practice also depends on a particular model of service delivery (one that is user-centred and multi-disciplinary), a strong partnership with evidence-based practice (defined by three key theoretical principles), and a sharp shift in 'who decides', from lawyers and ethicists as outside experts, to those directly involved, as users and as providers of services, in particular decision-making situations.

Why do we need values-based practice?

There is a sense in which health and social care have always been values-based. Social care training, in particular, although focusing on 'right values' rather than on processes of the kind defined by values-based practice, has always emphasized the importance of attitudes and values as well as of

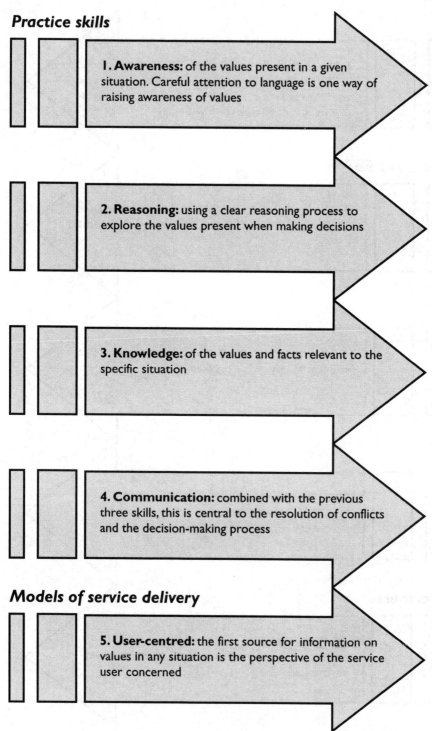

Figure 2.1 Arrow diagram of values-based practice 'process'   (continued on next page)

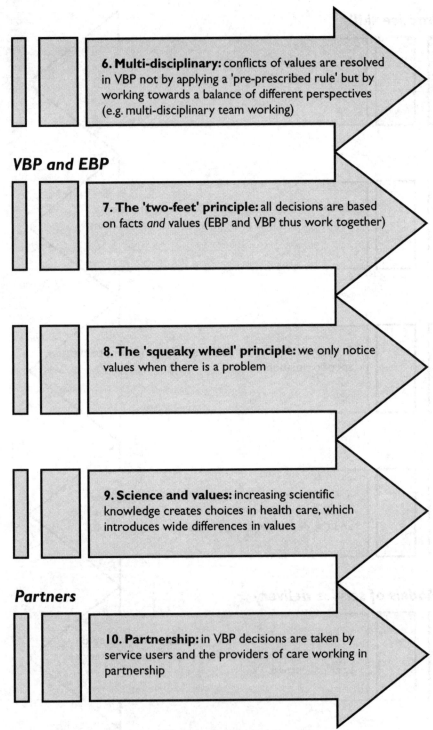

6. Multi-disciplinary: conflicts of values are resolved in VBP not by applying a 'pre-prescribed rule' but by working towards a balance of different perspectives (e.g. multi-disciplinary team working)

VBP and EBP

7. The 'two-feet' principle: all decisions are based on facts *and* values (EBP and VBP thus work together)

8. The 'squeaky wheel' principle: we only notice values when there is a problem

9. Science and values: increasing scientific knowledge creates choices in health care, which introduces wide differences in values

Partners

10. Partnership: in VBP decisions are taken by service users and the providers of care working in partnership

Figure 2.1 cont. Arrow diagram of values-based practice 'process'

knowledge and skills (Banks 1995; Moss 2007); and all professions and many trusts and other organizations have their own lists of values by which they are guided.

The need for values-based practice, then, arises in much the same way as the need for evidence-based practice, i.e. from the growing complexity of modern healthcare. Thus, as those developing evidence-based practice have pointed out (Sackett, Straus, Scott Richardson *et al.* 2000), it is the growing complexity of the evidence base for healthcare that generates the need for more sophisticated tools for drawing on evidence appropriately in decision-making. This is what evidence-based practice, properly understood, is about. Similarly, then, for values-based practice – it is the growing complexity of the values-base of healthcare that generates the need for more sophisticated tools for drawing on values appropriately in decision-making.

The practical importance of values-based practice is illustrated by Figures 2.2 and 2.3. These are derived from a study completed by Kim Woodbridge with East Towers Home Treatment Team based in East London. The team were fully committed to a holistic and user-led approach and worked together in an effective multi-disciplinary way. As part of developing their skills for values-based practice, Woodbridge observed the comments made in routine care review meetings. What this showed was that, although the team *believed* that they were working in a very user-centred way, it was their own values, rather than the values of their clients, that were reflected in their approach to care. Thus, Figure 2.2 shows that an overwhelming majority of the comments in a particular care review meeting reflected the perspectives of the mental health workers, rather than those either of the informal carers or of the users of services concerned.

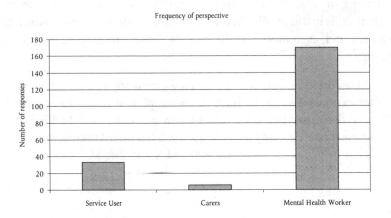

Figure 2.2 Frequency of perspective

Figure 2.3, similarly, shows that, among subjects discussed at the meeting, the most frequent were about medical aspects of care (medication and symptoms), while spirituality, although crucially important to so many people in relation to their well-being, was rarely discussed.

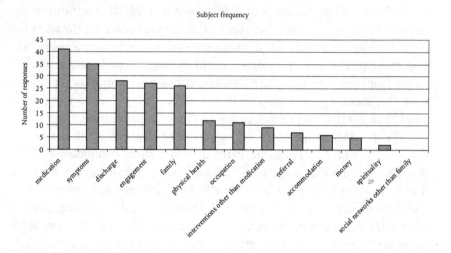

Figure 2.3 Subject frequency

The team were understandably much taken aback by these findings, but it helped to raise awareness of their own values as expressed in practice which is the essential first step in values-based training.

Working with these and other teams, we have had very positive feedback on training in values-based practice. Trainees have described how developing their skills in this area has improved mutual understanding between team members, and, even more significantly, of clients' needs. One trainee put it like this:

> Values-based practice has changed my own work with service users, for example if someone rings up to complain it is easy to become very defensive, but with values-based practice... I'm looking at where they are coming from? Why they felt the need to complain?... It has helped me *to understand more and be more helpful.*

Whose values?

After a training session in values-based practice with a group of doctors, Bill Fulford overheard two senior general practitioners joking 'your values today, my values tomorrow!'

This neatly captures one of the most common misunderstandings about values-based practice, i.e. that, in starting from respect for differences of values, it leads to relativism and 'anything goes'. One reason why this is a *mis*understanding is because human values, although certainly a good deal more diverse than we normally recognize, are very far from 'anything goes'. There are instead many values that people share, both within a given culture and between cultures. One of the outcomes from values-based training can be to help a group establish what their shared values really are.

A second reason why values-based practice does not lead to 'anything goes' is built into the approach itself. In starting from respect for differences of values, values-based practice is somewhat like a political democracy. Democracies differ from totalitarian regimes in starting from 'one person one vote'. But in democracies, this starting point, far from resulting in 'anything goes', leads to clear and strong principles of law and practice.

Box 2.1 illustrates some of the corresponding clear and strong principles of law and practice that can be derived from the values democracy of values-based practice. The Framework of Values shown was adopted in 2004 by the National Institute for Mental Health in England (NIMHE), the section of the Care Services Improvement Partnership (CSIP) in the Department of Health in London responsible for delivering on policy in mental health and social care. Instead of the usual list of values, the Framework starts with three key principles of values-based practice, the '3 Rs' of Recognition, Raising awareness and Respect, and then goes on to spell out the constraints on policy and practice to which the 'democratic' process of values-based practice leads.

The most important of these constraints is that the values of 'each individual service user/client and their communities must be the starting point and key determinant for all actions by professionals'. This key phrase, which was drafted by Simon Allard, as a member of the NIMHE Values Project Group, makes clear the importance of 'walking the talk' on user-centred care. User-centred practice, then, is nothing if it is not user-*values* centred practice (Allott, Loganathan and Fulford 2002). The Framework goes on to spell out a whole series of further positive constraints from values-based practice, that it should be multi-disciplinary, recovery oriented, dynamic, reflexive and so forth.

Notice, furthermore, the crucial point that is spelled out at the heart of the Framework, namely that values-based practice is inconsistent with

Box 2.1 The NIMHE Values Framework

The National Framework of Values for Mental Health

The work of the National Institute for Mental Health in England (NIMHE) on values in mental healthcare is guided by three principles of values-based practice:

1) Recognition – NIMHE recognizes the role of values alongside evidence in all areas of mental health policy and practice.

2) Raising awareness – NIMHE is committed to raising awareness of the values involved in different contexts, the role/s they play and their impact on practice in mental health.

3) Respect – NIMHE respects diversity of values and will support ways of working with such diversity that makes the principle of service-user centrality a unifying focus for practice. This means that the values of each individual service user/client and their communities must be the starting point and key determinant for all actions by professionals.

Respect for diversity of values encompasses a number of specific policies and principles concerned with equality of citizenship. In particular, it is anti-discriminatory because discrimination in all its forms is intolerant of diversity. Thus respect for diversity of values has the consequence that it is unacceptable (and unlawful in some instances) to discriminate on grounds such as gender, sexual orientation, class, age, abilities, religion, race, culture or language. Respect for diversity within mental health is also:

- *user-centred* – it puts respect for the values of individual users at the centre of policy and practice

- *recovery oriented* – it recognizes that building on the personal strengths and resiliencies of individual users, and on their cultural and racial characteristics, there are many diverse routes to recovery

- *multi-disciplinary* – it requires that respect be reciprocal, at a personal level (between service users, their family members, friends, communities and providers), between different provider disciplines (such as nursing, psychology, psychiatry, medicine, social work), and between different organizations (including health, social care, local authority housing, voluntary organizations, community groups, faith communities and other social support services)

- *dynamic* – it is open and responsive to change
- *reflective* – it combines self-monitoring and self-management with positive self-regard
- *balanced* – it emphasizes positive as well as negative values
- *relational* – it puts positive working relationships supported by good communication skills at the heart of practice.

NIMHE will encourage educational and research initiatives aimed at developing the capabilities (the awareness, attitudes, knowledge and skills) needed to deliver mental health services that will give effect to the principles of values-based practice.

---

racism or any other form of discrimination. This follows directly from the central democratic principle of values-based practice of respect for differences. There are of course many other reasons for developing services that are non-discriminatory. But discrimination is inconsistent with any form of values-based practice precisely because discrimination is *intolerant* of diversity.

My values, right or wrong!

Values-based practice, then, is the values equivalent of a political democracy. In starting from respect for differences and relying on good process rather than right values, it is very far from being a recipe for anything goes. But here, surely, someone will say, is the crunch when it comes to the great faiths. Surely it is characteristic of great faiths that they are defined by a commitment to certain *particular* beliefs and values. Is this not precisely what 'having faith' consists in. To *be* a 'believer', you *accept* certain beliefs and values. Is not 'keeping faith' precisely a matter of holding on to the required beliefs and values, come what may – my values 'right or wrong', as it were!

There is of course no arguing with the fanatic. As Bertrand Russell pointed out about the philosophical sceptic (Russell 1940), as long as the sceptic is consistent, there is *literally* no arguing with them! The same is true of the fanatic. And certainly there are many, and not only within dogmatic religion, who are in this way absolutely convinced of their own 'right values'... But, and this is the key BUT, alongside the fanatics in all the great religions, there have developed traditions of openness and inclusiveness among those, no less dedicated to their own chosen faith, but at the same time fully open to and respectful of the beliefs and values of others.

Values, help and healing

A clear example of such an inclusive and open approach is the Christian tradition of spiritual direction. Dating back to the Desert Fathers of the early church, the tradition has been nurtured and carried through to current practice by the Benedictine monks. Spiritual direction depends on combining personal conviction with a total openness to others as the basis of helping them find their own way. Like values-based practice, then, respect for the values and the beliefs of others is the central rule of engagement in spiritual direction.

Spiritual direction, furthermore, again like values-based practice, relies for its effectiveness on a number of well-defined elements of 'good process' rather than pre-assigned right outcomes. A former Benedictine and now parish priest, Robert Atwell, has illustrated how these elements of good process find fresh application in the modern context of pastoral counselling (Atwell and Fulford 2006). They include a deep understanding of such apparently familiar ideas as 'friendship' (a 'meeting of souls') and self-knowledge; but also of the less familiar though no less practically relevant concepts of a 'word of life' (sparking life and hope), 'compunction' (the gift of tears), and discernment (right judgment).

The tradition of spiritual direction also brings a refreshingly positive approach to the realities of human experience: desires, in particular, are not to be suppressed, but, through discernment, become the main springs of action (Sheldrake 1994). As Atwell and Fulford describe, the dominant words in the spiritual vocabulary of the supposedly austere fifth-century Bishop of Hippo, St Augustine, were 'delight', 'desire' and 'love'. 'Healing', too, in this 2,000-year-old and yet wholly contemporary tradition, is a healing equally of bodies as of minds and of memories. And 'direction' itself, the direction of spiritual direction, is not about telling people what to do. It is not even about counselling, as currently understood. It is rather about journeying with, or accompanying, the other; it is about partnership, about self-discovery through relationship.

There are similar resources for help and healing in all the great faith traditions. Thus, the Sikh tradition has a strong commitment to tolerance and inter-faith dialogue derived from the teaching of the 15th-century Guru Nanak, and the custom of feeding the whole community through the communal kitchen called the *langar*, which is a fundamental part of Sikh life today. Judaism speaks of the need for *hessed* – 'loving-kindness', which reaches out to all in the community, and, crucially, outside of one's own community. Chief Rabbi, Dr Jonathan Sacks (Sacks 2005) quotes the prophet Amos as saying: 'let justice well up as waters and righteousness as a mighty stream' (Amos 5:24), and states that Judaism encapsulates the concepts of both *charity* and *justice* in the same word, *tzedakah* (Sacks 2005, p.32), so that Jews are concerned to serve the whole of their society and society at large, as those who have been exiles should empathize with exiles. Muslims speak of the *qalb salim* – *the healthy heart* (see Sheikh and Gatrad 2000, pp.30–32). While the Christian monasteries provided asylum to those with learning disabilities, mental health needs and other conditions such as leprosy, the *maristan* provide care for those with a mental illness in Muslim countries. Zoroastrians have a strong commitment towards social action and improving the local community and society in general (see Gilbert and Kalaga 2007).

At the heart of all these inclusive and respectful approaches within the great faith traditions, therefore, is the idea that true help and healing depends, not on imposing on other people our own beliefs and values, but on helping them to find what is right for them. This is at the heart, similarly, of values-based practice. This is why, therefore, values-based practice, as a secular development within modern health and social care, is entirely consistent with, and indeed often depends critically on, the resources of the great faith traditions to provide help and healing in practice.

Conclusions: values and a shared theology of diversity

In this chapter we have described a new approach to working with complex and conflicting values in health and social care called values-based practice. We have outlined how values-based practice, as a response to the increasingly complex and conflicting values bearing on health and social care, rather than seeking to define 'right values', starts from respect for differences of values and then relies on training in key clinical skills and other elements of good process for effective decision-making.

The most common concern about a values-based approach, as we have indicated, is that it will lead to 'anything goes', of 'my values today, your values tomorrow!' We have shown, however, that the processes of values-based practice, like the corresponding processes of a political democracy, lead to a number of very clear constraints on policy and service development.

This is crucially important. The lesson of history is that it is not relativism but absolutism that is the more at risk of abusive consequences (Glover 1999). And within mental health many of the most serious abuses have arisen, not from those concerned setting out to do harm, but from their absolute conviction that they had 'got it right' (Fulford, Thornton and Graham 2006b). With the renewed rise of fanaticism, therefore, as we continue into the new millennium, it is all the more urgent that we rediscover the resources for openness and inclusiveness within each of the great faith traditions, their shared theology of diversity, that is the basis for true help and healing in mental health and social care.

Acknowledgements

The NIMHE Framework was developed and piloted as one of NIMHE's first initiatives by a small working party, the NIMHE Values Project Group, chaired by Piers Allott, an expert on recovery practice. Figure 2.1 is based on a similar figure in Woodbridge and Fulford, 2004. We are grateful to Peter Gilbert for his many helpful suggestions and information about diverse spiritual traditions.

References

Allott, P., Loganathan, L. and Fulford, K.W.M. (Bill) (2002) 'Discovering hope for recovery.' In 'Innovation in Community Mental Health: International Perspectives'. Special issue of the *Canadian Journal of Community Mental Health 21*, 2, 13–33.

Atwell, R. and Fulford, K.W.M. (2006) 'A Sketch for a Strong Theology of Diversity: Insights from Christian Traditions of Spirituality.' In J.C. Cox, A.C. Campbell and K.W.M. Fulford (eds) *Medicine of the Person: Faith, Science and Values in Health Care Provision*. London: Jessica Kingsley Publishers.

Banks, S. (1995) *Ethics and Values in Social Work*. London: Macmillan.

Fulford, K.W.M. (2004) 'Ten Principles of Values-based Medicine.' In J. Radden (ed.) *The Philosophy of Psychiatry: A Companion*. New York: Oxford University Press.

Fulford, K.W.M., Thornton, T., and Graham, G. (2006a) 'Progress in Five Parts.' In K.W.M. Fulford, T. Thornton and G. Graham (eds) *The Oxford Textbook of Philosophy and Psychiatry*. Oxford: Oxford University Press.

Fulford, K.W.M., Thornton, T., Graham, G. and Hoff, P. (2006b) 'Histories of the Future.' In K.W.M. Fulford, T. Thornton and G. Graham (eds) *The Oxford Textbook of Philosophy and Psychiatry*. Oxford: Oxford University Press.

Gilbert, P. and Kalaga, H. (eds) (forthcoming) *Nurturing Heart and Spirit: Symposium Papers*. Stafford: University of Staffordshire Monograph.

Glover, J. (1999) *Humanity: A Moral History of the Twentieth Century*. London: Jonathan Cape.

Moss, B. (2007) *Values.* Lyme Regis: Russell House Publishing.

O'Neill, O. (2002) *A Question of Trust.* Cambridge: Cambridge University Press.

Russell, B. (1940) *Inquiry into Meaning and Truth.* London: George Allen and Unwin.

Sackett, D.L., Straus, S.E., Scott Richardson, W., Rosenberg, W. and Haynes, R.B. (2000) *Evidence-Based Medicine: How to Practice and Teach, EBM* (2nd edn). Edinburgh and London: Churchill Livingstone.

Sacks, J. (2005) *To Heal a Fractured World: The Ethics of Responsibility.* London: Continuum.

Sheikh, A. and Gatrad, A.R. (eds) (2000) *Caring for Muslim Patients.* Oxford: Radcliffe Medical Press.

Sheldrake, P. (1994) *Befriending our Desires.* London: Darton, Longman and Todd.

Woodbridge, K. and Fulford, K.W.M. (2004) *Whose Values? A Workbook for Values-based Practice in Mental Health Care.* London: Sainsbury Centre for Mental Health.

Softly

Softly I turn the pages of my soul
In the library of forgotten lives;
In my heart a bird of Egypt sings,
Which flies to where my spirit thrives.

In shuttered rooms the poet writes
And conjures images from fountains which
Despite their crystal song of joy
Stream dark waters with their colours rich.

I long to be where fountains pure
Dilute the poison of fevered dreams,
Water the plains of arid hope
Illuminate my life with fluid beams.

Life's dream kingdom, I knew last year,
Was pure as chalcedony rare;
Now, kissing images of stone
I reflect the facets of diamond fear.

Jonathan Ratcliffe

CHAPTER 3

SPIRITUALITY AND MENTAL HEALTH ACROSS CULTURES

Suman Fernando

Introduction

In *Zen Buddhism and Psychoanalysis*, Fromm, Suzuki and de Martino propose that psychoanalysis emerged in the late 19th and early 20th centuries, as an attempt within European cultural history to find a solution to 'Western man's spiritual crisis' – a crisis attributed by them to Europe's 'abandonment of theistic ideas in the 19th century' with 'a big plunge into objectivity' (1960, pp.79–80). Actually, science and religion had started to draw apart in European thinking from the 16th century onwards. By the time Western psychology (the study of the normal 'mind') and psychiatry (study of the 'disordered' or abnormal 'mind') developed, religion had become marginalized in Western academic thinking and so the disciplines that emerged were secular. Ideas about spirituality – a part of the discourse within religion *not science* – were excluded from both psychiatry and Western psychology as these disciplines strove increasingly to become 'scientific'. Clearly though, remnants of spirituality remain in some forms of Western psychotherapy and, of course, spirituality is there in Western traditions of religion.

Cultures in Asia and Africa did not undergo the sort of secularization that occurred in Europe from the 16th century onwards – at least not at that time – and although undoubtedly influenced later by Western secular ideas, appear to have maintained a spiritual dimension to their thinking in many fields, including the medical field, until the present. However, cultures are not static and never just stay in one place. So today, references to cultures as being 'Eastern' or 'non-Western' and 'Western' no longer imply geographical regions but traditions. What can be assumed though is that, unlike the situation in Western modernism, traditionally non-Western ways of thinking accept spirituality as central to human experience.

Whatever the discourse at theoretical levels and within academia, for ordinary people struggling with human problems, both within themselves and in their interactions with others, spirituality and religion have never lost their relevance to what they *feel* mental health is about and even to their ideas of disordered health. In Britain, this feeling is particularly evident among black and minority ethnic (BME) communities, people from cultural backgrounds where religion is much more central to their lives, their mental health and their understanding of human problems. Hence this chapter aims to explore the practical meaning of spirituality in relation to mental health in non-Western traditions, after a brief discussion of what cultural diversity means in a multi-cultural Western society today.

The variation in our society in terms of human behaviour and thinking is self-evident; the issue is about what such diversity means in real life, for ordinary people. What we see easily is a diversity in such things as dress, eating habits, ways of cooking food, music and dance, and so on. However, deeper down – and more important to some people – is a variety in attitudes to, for example, old people, how children should be brought up, correct behaviour, gender and sexuality, choosing partners for marriage, loyalties and family ties and what we do for recreation. Even deeper are the fundamental aspects of human life and living – what we consider to be within our realm of reality: concepts of what is natural and what is supernatural, worldviews about a host of different features of human life, indeed, the very meaning of life. In my view, both mental health and spirituality come into this second level of depth.

A common approach to understanding cultural diversity is to start by defining – or trying to define – the essentials of some aspect of 'culture', by seeing it as essence that can be viewed 'from the outside'. This may be useful for practical purposes, for instance in understanding the diversity of how people dress or the food they eat. In the case of the former, we could define clothing as a means of covering the human body, and then go on to examine how various groups of people, 'cultural groups', have fashioned clothing and the meanings they give to what they wear. However, when it comes to concepts like spirituality or mental health – or indeed to matters like happiness or suffering – we cannot get very far by defining an 'essence'. In these instances if we try to derive an 'essence' we are likely to miss the real meanings of the terms for the people concerned. This is because these matters are inextricably tied up with the historical and social traces that have generated them and continue to do so. In the case of spirituality: 'There is no view from nowhere – no Archimedian point outside of history – from which one could determine a fixed and universal meaning for the term 'spirituality' (Carette and King 2005, p.3).

Mental health

In his classic *Shamans, Mystics and Doctors*, Sudhir Kakar (1984), a Western trained psychotherapist working in India, observed that non-Western cultures have traditions 'concerned with the restoration of what is broadly termed "mental health" in the West' (1984, p.3). He explored these traditions in India by examining and explaining to Western readers the nature of services being provided by some indigenous Indian therapists. Although Indian healers follow a variety of different approaches, they have a common tendency, when compared to Western psychotherapists, to give prominence to the 'sacred'. Kakar writes:

> By 'sacred' I meant not only the Brahman of the mystics, the Krishna of the devotees or the gods of the rituals, but also the spirits of ancestors and forests, the beings that live in enchanted groves, the specters that haunt cremation grounds and the demons who wait at the next crossing. (Kakar 1984, pp.4–5)

Traditional Chinese Medicine (TCM) is generally seen, from a Western standpoint, to be based on physical interventions – the best known being herbal remedies and acupuncture. The problem here is that such a perception is misleading because the mind–body dichotomy is significantly absent in the thinking underlying TCM. In his book *Dragon rises, red bird flies*, Leon Hammer, a Western-trained psychiatrist and practitioner of Chinese Medicine, argues that TCM is more akin to psychology or psychotherapy in the Western idiom than it is to a medical system in Western idiom. He states:

> Chinese medicine, like most psychotherapies, is concerned with an individual's unique physical and emotional state. Chinese medicine and psychology also have systematic classifications of disease; however, the diagnostic and treatment modes of these practices emphasize the distinguishing intrinsic attributes of each individual. (Hammer 1990, p.3)

Thus, both Indian medical traditions and Chinese medicine include ways of intervening that are 'psychological' in the idiom of Western tradition, and I believe that the same conclusion applies to African medical traditions and those from pre-Columbian America. So these 'non-Western' traditions include psychologies or psychotherapies, to use Western terms, if we accept a very broad definition of what they mean. However, I think the situation is somewhat different with respect to psychiatry – basically a Western construction, incorporating aspects of what in other cultures may be seen as a mixture of psychological, medical, ethical, political and spiritual aspects of the human condition. While psychiatry sees the remedy for problems located in the 'mind' as 'therapies', the approximate equivalents to such 'remedies' in other cultural traditions would be something like 'liberation' (see Fernando 2002).

Spirituality

The term 'spirituality', like the term 'mental health', does not denote a precise concept but is used widely. Looked at cross-culturally, spirituality is basically about connectedness – of being, knowing and feeling that we are not just individuals but intimately connected in a variety of ways, not just with one another but with the world we inhabit, the earth we live on, the heavens above us, the universe around us. Some people may personify some or all of this as 'God' and various religions have been built around such personifications; but others, such as Buddhism and Taoism, do not go down that road. To make any further generalization about a cross-culturally applicable concept called 'spirituality' could be misleading. Admittedly, much more may be said *about* spirituality in poetry, music, art, and story telling, and perhaps in the 'scriptures' of various religions. However, in my view, the *experience* of spirituality is always in a communal setting linked to religion and culture.

I shall endeavor to explore mental health and spirituality across cultural traditions in two ways. First, I shall present some impressions – snapshots – of what 'spiritual' may mean vis-à-vis mental health in different cultural traditions, as they may be evident today. Then, I shall present as an example of spirituality some concepts within a particular tradition – the Buddhist tradition. Finally I shall try to draw some conclusions about spirituality and mental health applicable for the multi-cultural society in Britain today.

Snapshots of the spiritual

The 'I and I' principle of the Rastafarians 'expresses the oneness between two persons' (Cashmore 1979, p.135) – the personal and the 'other' being *the same*. This is a vivid exposition of spirituality as 'community spirit' – connectedness which strengthens feelings of belonging to one community as a part of religion. To Rastafarians, this connectedness does not stop there. It extends through the spirit of Ras Tafari across to Africa, from where their ancestors had been torn away. This separation from a spiritual base lies at the very heart of any psychological suffering they experience – the remedy being a spiritual restitution. In the worldview of the indigenous American, everything has a *spirit* or energy (Freke and Wa'Na'Nee'Che' 1996, p.69). Disharmony within oneself has its roots in the 'unseen' world inhabited by spirits or 'energies'. Since 'being out of balance with their own spirit' results from breaking of taboos such as telling lies about spirits, the restitution of the spirit comes about from appeasing the spirits, through medicines, magic, rituals, and so on (Freke and Wa'Na'Nee'Che' 1996, pp.68–70). Modern day Native American healers call themselves 'spiritual advisors' – for example, at a contemporary centre for healing in Toronto, Canada, called *Anishwabe* (personal observation).

In many cultural traditions, spirituality is woven into everyday life and an integral part of what constitutes 'culture'. Ross (1992) writes about indigenous Americans undergoing spiritual observance in preparing to embark on a task such as making a journey or venturing on a hunting expedition. Nobles (1986) believes that the integration of mind, body and spirit is characteristic of the worldviews derived from African thinking and Richards (1985) makes a case for this spirituality having survived the transatlantic slave trade to continue in an African-American spirituality. Indeed Du Bois in his classic *The Souls of Black Folk*, originally published in 1904, saw 'spiritual striving' as a characteristic of the cultural ideal of black African-Americans (Du Bois 1970). Ninety years later, bell hooks (1994) writing in *Outlaw Cultures*, regrets the 'spiritual loss' of modern African-American communities in the US and advocates the need for political movements that can effectively address the 'needs of the spirit' (hooks 1994, p.247). The Vedantic tradition (Hinduism) of the Indian subcontinent recognizes one supernatural spirit given different names, but recognizing 'no dualism of the natural and the supernatural...the spiritual is an emergent of the natural and is rooted in it' (Radhakrishnan 1980, p.88). Buddhism that came out of the Hindu tradition is discussed below.

Lack of spirituality may be experienced as an impoverishment of the spirit – for example, *susto* translated as 'soul-loss' (Logan 1979) in South America – in the sense of an emptiness similar to, if not identical with, that felt by people diagnosed in Western psychiatry as severely 'depressed'. Although *susto* appears to be a socially-based phenomenon, remedies for the 'illness' involve detailed re-telling of events leading to the condition (abreaction or catharsis), use of medicinal herbs (medication) and rituals (equivalent to psychotherapy) for returning the soul and replenishing the sense of 'loss'.

Buddhist spirituality

The term *bhavan*, a process of liberating the mind and realizing the ultimate truth (Yoshinori 1995), is the closest Sanskrit equivalent to spirituality in Buddhist writings. The earliest interpretations of the message of Buddhism is described by Pande as follows:

> Spiritual life consists in the effort to move away from ignorance to wisdom. This effort has two principal dimensions: the cultivation of serenity and the cultivation of insight. Ignorance is the mistaken belief in the selfhood of body and mind, which leads to involvement in egoism, passions, actions, and repeated birth and death. (Pande 1995, p.10)

Meditation is fundamental to Buddhism and generally the means by which spirituality is experienced in the search for wisdom or the ultimate truth (nirvana) – a wisdom characterized by no-self (*anatta*), impermanence (*anicca*) and suffering (*dukkha*). The variations of these characterizations, their elaborations and interpretations, have resulted in a variety of Buddhist traditions. Therefore, Buddhist spirituality may seem close to what in Western psychology would be seen as self-knowledge through introspection but with one important proviso. A fundamental teaching in Buddhism is the lack of a 'self' as something permanent – the 'non-selfhood of body and mind' (Pande 1995, p.10) – and the realization of 'self' as illusion is an integral part of liberation.

Conclusions

In this chapter, I have tried to explore the meaning of spirituality across cultures in relation to mental health. Whether in connectedness to one another (community spirit), to a land or environment (an ecological spirit), to the cosmos or creation itself ('God' or a pantheon of gods), the one thing we can discern across cultures is that spirituality is not a solitary person-centred, self-centred, *selfish* feeling, but one derived from connections and one harboured in religion and community. In some traditions, contact with the spirit world or 'spirits' as non-physical beings with human characteristics resemble some aspects of Western psychological theories of 'forces' exerted by unseen entities such as the 'ego' or 'id'. Sometimes, activities such as the identification of particular entities as 'spirits' with meaning, and communication with spirits during séances, is bound up with the sense of connectedness that characterizes spirituality in a wider sense. Although spirituality is not necessarily the same as adherence to an organized religion with a specific dogma given or interpreted by a hierarchy, 'being religious' and 'being spiritual' are similar and may well be identical in some instances in some places.

The thoughts and impressions presented here may provide a sense of what spirituality means across cultural traditions. I believe that contrasting cultures provides an impression of how spirituality should permeate our thinking about mental health, Western psychology and Western psychiatry. But one word of warning. There is a view being expressed that psychiatry and Western psychology should incorporate a spiritual dimension, as a sort of add-on to therapy. My reading of how spirituality and mental health are associated across cultures would argue against such a move. If spirituality has any meaning, its significance comes from its religion–culture–community base. In my view, each of us would gain by being in touch with our spirituality, whether through organized religion or other communal activity. Surely this helps to make us better and more fulfilled people, but to make it into an entity detached from its roots is to debase and inactivate it. However, I can see how there can be a spiritual psychology, but that would be something fundamentally different from *Western* psychology – and I have started to discuss this elsewhere (Fernando 2004). For such a psychology to emerge there would have to be a major paradigm change in the thinking within Western psychology, and consequently psychiatry; a shift away from positivist thinking and objectivity that permeates these disciplines and, more importantly, a shift away from their reliance on mechanistic and reductionist approaches.

References

Carette, J. and King, R. (2005) *Selling Spirituality. The Silent Takeover of Religion.* London and New York: Routledge.

Cashmore, E. (1979) *Rastaman. The Rastafarian Movement in England.* London: Allen and Unwin.

Du Bois, W.E.B. (1970) *The Souls of Black Folk.* New York: Washington Square Press (first published by McClurg, Chicago 1903).

Fernando, S. (2002) *Mental Health, Race and Culture.* (2nd edn). Basingstoke: Palgrave.

Fernando, S. (2004) 'Spiritual psychology.' *Openmind 129*, 25.

Freke, T. and Wa'Na'Nee'Che' (Dennis Renault) (1996) *Native American Spirituality.* London and San Francisco: Thorsons (HarperCollins).

Fromm, E., Suzuki, D.T. and de Martino, R. (1960) *Zen Buddhism and Psychoanalysis.* London: Allen and Unwin.

Hammer, L. (1990) *Dragon rises, red bird flies. Psychology and Chinese Medicine.* New York: Station Hill Press.

hooks, b. (1994) *Outlaw Culture. Resisting Representations.* New York: Routledge.

Kakar, S. (1984) *Shamans, Mystics and Doctors. A Psychological Inquiry into India and its Healing Tradition.* London: Unwin Paperbacks.

Logan, M.H. (1979) 'Variations regarding Susto causality among the Cakchiquel of Guatemala.' *Culture, Medicine and Psychiatry 3*, 2, 153–66.

Nobles, W.W. (1986) 'Ancient Egyptian Thought and the Development of African (Black) Psychology.' In M. Karenga and J.C. Carruthers (eds) *Kemet and the African World View. Research Rescue and Restoration.* Los Angeles: University of Sankore Press.

Pande, G.C. (1995) 'The Message of Gotama Buddah and its Earliest Interpretations.' In T. Yoshinori (ed.) *Buddhist Spirituality.* Delhi: Motilal Banarsidass.

Radhakrishnan (1980) *The Hindu View of Life.* London: Unwin Paperbacks. (First published in Great Britain by Allen and Unwin 1927)

Richards, D. (1985) 'The Implications of African-American Spirituality.' In M.K. Asante and K.W. Asante (eds) *African Culture: The Rhythms of Unity.* Westport, CT: Greenwood Press.

Ross, R. (1992) *Dancing with a Ghost. Exploring Indian Reality.* Markham, Ontario: Reed Books.

Yoshinori, T. (1995) (ed.) 'Introduction.' In T. Yoshinori (ed.) *Buddhist Spirituality.* Delhi: Motilal Banarsidass.

For Bhen 'Aum Shanti Shanti'

Growing up, I constantly saw it in front of me,
My ancient Hindu Faith
Swirling bright colours, images with strong features,
Many armed gods
Holding us in, controlling us.
Dictating every aspect of our lives
What we did, the food we ate, how we thought and felt.

And we as children knew we dare not question
The time-honoured traditions of our family faith
Carrying out endless pujas and rituals
Repeating mantras that told us of our gods
And reminded us of our destiny –
The unending cycle, of birth and life and death.

Karma.

It always seemed so scary then to my childish mind,
Warning me of how my past had shaped my present,
And my present would determine my future.

Cautioning me to stay in check, restraining me
Stultifying my quest for independence
And freedom and autonomy.

But then I grew up and could do as I wanted
I distanced myself from my family
And lived an independent lifestyle
By-passing my Hinduism at every opportunity
Never realizing how deeply embedded
It lay in my soul.

Until last year when my sister died
And we came together in our grief,
To say prayers and sing bhajans, and carry out rituals
To help her on her journey into the next life.

And in those acts I realized
The Karma I had feared for so long
Was not about punishment from on high

But much more complex, acknowledging
The importance of interdependence
To which we could, and should, all contribute.

So on the third day, we dressed her in a fine new sari,
And anointed her with holy Ganges water
And placed a garland of flowers around her neck.
And in her coffin laid religious symbols
Ghee, coconuts, cunku, fresh flowers, powders
To take with her into the next life so she would never be in
want.

Then, in her right hand
Her eldest son placed a pind,
Representing the ancestors that had gone before
In that gesture creating a continuous interweave
Of generations and individual lives
Of past, and present and future.

Then we each circled the coffin and placed
Flowers at her feet, with each soft petal
Helping her soul to travel in peace
To a new life that would acknowledge and honour
The very many beautiful qualities
That we had so loved her for in this life.

And then, on the thirteenth day,
The last day her soul would inhabit the earth
We cried and laughed as we cooked
Her thirteen favourite foods and offered them to be blessed
Before they too would go with her into the next life
To feed her soul and sustain her spirit.

Then, with prayers and mantras,
Pinds representing the ancestors and my sister
Were joined together and placed before the Gods
And, one by one, we bowed to pay respect
To a bigger something, a tangible unity of generations
Rarely conscious in our earthly lives.

Then, her eldest son left the gathered family
And went to the river to place

Ashes, food, pinds and blessings into free-running water
To go with her on the next stage of her journey.
Tearfully leaving the river bank, resisting the urge to look back
Lest he stop his mother's soul leaving this earth.

And then, gathered together once more,
Our hearts ached and our tears flowed freely
As the pandit lit a holy fire to purify the air
And said some final prayers
Completing my sister's ceremony
Enabling her to move on.

This then was the final unbearable farewell
But with it for me came a surprising and overwhelming peace
That this was not the end, but another beginning
Not punishing Karma as I had thought for so long

But something more kindly, uniting and hopeful.
For Bhen and us – Aum Shanti, Shanti, Shanti.

Premila Trivedi

CHAPTER 4

LOSS AND GRIEF: SPIRITUAL ASPECTS

Neil Thompson

Introduction

Loss can be seen as a major existential challenge in our lives. It raises a range of important issues in relation to spirituality. This chapter therefore explains some of the main implications for both theory and practice. In doing so, it draws on existentialist philosophy for its theoretical foundations.

Morgan, in an important text relating to death and dying, defines spirituality as an 'existential quest for meaning' (1993, p.3). Spirituality can therefore be seen as a form of meaning making. A major loss in a person's life can seriously undermine this process and the meanings that we have developed that help us make sense of our lives and give us a sense of identity. The result of a major loss can therefore be the loss of 'ontological security' temporarily at least. Ontological security is an existentialist concept that refers to the sense of rootedness that each of us needs in order to maintain the coherent thread of meaning and identity in our lives in a context of constant change and potential threats to us.

A major loss can therefore be seen as a crisis of meaning. For example, in relation to religious beliefs, a major loss can result in polarized responses. At one extreme, many people lose faith, feeling that the intense pain and suffering that they are experiencing cannot be consistent with a beneficent god. At the other extreme, some people's religious faith can be strongly reaffirmed as a result of the major threat presented by such a challenging loss.

Death can be seen as a major feature of life, and so, when bereavement occurs, death becomes doubly significant in terms of both a reminder of our own mortality and the specific loss encountered in terms of the person who has died. However, it is also important to note that loss arises in a wide range

Case study: Bernadette

Bernadette had been brought up in a Catholic family but, after working in a hospice for some time, she began to question her faith, wondering: how can God allow so much suffering and pain in this world? Over time she wavered, sometimes having her faith reaffirmed, as she saw not only suffering, but also the overcoming of suffering, sometimes finding it difficult to reconcile the pain she saw with the idea of a caring God. What was also significant was that she saw the same issues reflected in the lives of the people she was seeking to help at the hospice – the patients and their loved ones. She saw some people lose their faith, while others had their faith reaffirmed – or, in some cases, became believers for the first time. These issues applied to people from a variety of religious backgrounds, not just Catholics like herself. She realized that the relationship between loss and grief on the one hand and religious faith and spirituality on the other was a very complex one.

of contexts that are not necessarily related to a death (Thompson 2002a). The focus of this chapter will include death-related losses, but will not be restricted to them, as both sets of loss can generate intense feelings of grief that have very significant implications in terms of spirituality.

I shall begin by discussing a range of issues relating to life and death in general. This will lead on to a discussion of bereavement in particular, followed by an account of other non-death-related losses. This will set the scene for, first, a discussion of developing theory in this area and, finally, developing the practice implications.

Life and death

A common misconception of existentialism is that it is a morbid philosophy preoccupied with the negative aspects of life, primarily that of death. However, the reality is that existentialism is a philosophy of *realism*, in the sense that it recognizes the immense joys that can be part of human experience, but is not naïve enough to pretend that human existence is not also characterized by considerable problems, pain and suffering. It is therefore not true to say that existentialism is preoccupied with death, but it would be entirely accurate to recognize that death is a significant feature of the philosophy, insofar as the existence of death as a phenomenon emphasizes the finite nature of human existence, and it is this finitude that proves to be so significant. See the discussion of Heidegger below.

Existentialism is often perceived as an atheistic philosophy, and may therefore be dismissed by some people of faith. However, there are religious forms of existentialism (e.g. Tillich 2000) and, as Sartre argued, while he personally wrote from an atheistic perspective, the existence of God would make no difference to the philosophy, as we would still face the same existential challenges – as reflected in the work of Kierkegaard (1996).

Recognizing that we are finite beings can be a challenge of meaning in its own right. Albert Camus, an absurdist writer whose thoughts have much in common with existentialism, asks the basic question of: why do we go on? Why do we not end it here and now – that is, commit suicide? (Camus 2005). This was not a plea of despair but, rather, a recognition that part of human experience is the challenge of finding meaning. If we cannot find meaning, what is there left except death?

This is closely linked to the Buddhist notion of 'impermanence' that is also a feature of other Eastern philosophies. The idea of impermanence is not to be a source of despair, but rather of celebration. The recognition that, because our lifetime is of a limited duration, we need to make sure that we make the best use of it while we can, that we do not waste the precious resources of life and humanity that are available to us. Clearly, this has spiritual implications.

Within existentialist thought, these ideas can be found to feature strongly in the works of one of the earliest existentialists, namely Friedrich Nietzsche, and more recently, in the work of Cioran (see Wicks 2003). Again, the emphasis on death and finitude is not intended to be negative, but rather to be part of a philosophy of realism, recognizing that human existence is characterized by both great joy and great suffering. Existentialism helps us to recognize that there is a very strong tendency for many people to distance themselves from death, to make the mistake of living each day as if they were immortal. Wicks provides helpful comment when he argues that:

> With regard to the conception of one's own death, Heidegger points out that the public conception of death – the conception forced upon us by the public at large, or by 'them', or 'the They' [das Man] – tends to hide the reality of our own death from us. In an obvious sense, the public conception is misleading, for it conveys the message that death always happens to someone else; death appears as a well-known event in the mass media, and as something which, at present, does not have much to do with those who are still living. Heidegger says that the public conception 'provides a continual comforting about death' and 'does not allow to arise, the courage for

anxiety in the face of death'. In short, the way the public, or 'the they', obscures the reality of our eventual death from us, precludes a proper contemplation of it, and provides us with a false understanding of death. (2003, p.196)

Here we can make an important link with the existentialist concept of authenticity. To be authentic means to avoid bad faith – that is, to avoid failing to face up to the responsibilities we have for ourselves and others within our finite lifetimes. Golomb captures the point well:

> What is authentic must be finite since one cannot *own* and grasp an infinite process or entity. Death enters life to conclude it, making possible its adequate explication. Hence, only Being-towards-death can be *fully* meaningful and authentic. Each time we entertain the possibility of dying we undertake an assessment of our Being. In our anticipation we define our existence. (1995, p.107)

The concept of 'Being-toward-death' mentioned here is one introduced by another important existentialist writer, Martin Heidegger (1962) who has already been quoted. What he meant by this term is that it is necessary to recognize that life cannot be separated from death in the sense that: (i) death is an ever-present possibility; and (ii) death makes life finite and therefore precious.

Bereavement

The loss of a person important to us can be a major source of pain and suffering, a devastating blow that can be both very detrimental and very disorientating. The significance of bereavement has not been lost on us over the years, as it is a subject that has been studied in great detail. However, one thing that has held back the development of our understanding of this important aspect of human experience is that, for a very long time, there has been an acceptance of received wisdom to the effect that bereavement results in grief that is experienced in stages. Based on the work of Kübler-Ross (1969), Parkes (2004) and others, the idea that grieving happens as part of a process that unfolds in stages has become so well-established as to have become common knowledge, both within the human services and in the general public at large. However, despite the immense influence of this conception of grief, empirical evidence to support it is very thin on the ground, and we have seen wave after wave of theoretical critique of the premises on which this perspective is based (see, for example, Stroebe and Schut 1999). It is now clearly no longer feasible to maintain the view that people grieve in stages, although there is evidence that, given the influence of this dominant mode of thinking, many bereaved people try to grieve within a stage frame-work, as doing so offers them some degree of structure and possible onto-logical security (see, for example, the work of Walter 1994).

One of the theoretical perspectives that have helped us to move away from the problems of an uncritical acceptance of the stages approach is that of *meaning reconstruction theory* (Neimeyer 2001a, b; Neimeyer and Anderson 2002). The basic idea underpinning meaning reconstruction theory is that, when we experience a major loss, we lose not only the person or thing that was dear to us, we also lose a constellation of meaning. That is, we have to face up to the loss of what the person or thing meant to us, and this can be a very slow and painful process. On this basis, one of the implications of meaning reconstruction theory is that a narrative therapy approach can be a helpful response to helping people who are grieving. We shall return to this topic below.

Richards (2001) makes the important point that: 'Providing care to a dying person, witnessing death, losing a loved one – all can open us to exis-tential issues and spiritual experiences that refocus our lives' (p.173). Bereavement therefore clearly has distinct spiritual implications. Attig takes this a step further by focusing on what he calls 'spiritual pain'.

> I use *spirit* to refer to that within us that reaches beyond present cir-cumstances, soars in extraordinary experiences, strives for excellence and a better life, struggles to overcome adversity, and searches for meaning and transcendent understanding. When we suffer spiritual pain, we lose that motivation. We feel dispirited, joyless, hopeless. Life seems drained of meaning. We wonder whether we have the courage and motivation to face the challenges of daily life, much less relearning the world we now experience. (2001, pp.37–8)

Attig's earlier work on this subject offers very helpful insights into this area (Attig 1996, 2000).

Anyone working in a field that involves helping people cope with bereavement (and this can mean any area of human services) is therefore charged with engaging in a process of helping people respond to a very sig-nificant challenge of spirituality.

Other losses

The point was made earlier that loss is not simply related to death. There is a very wide range of situations in which people can experience major losses that do not directly involve a death. Examples would include divorce or breakdown of relationships in general, redundancy or unemployment, becoming disabled, losing status or a position of respect, and so on. Indeed, we can go so far as to say that grief is part of life and not something that only arises on the occasion of a person's death.

The field of mental health is a good example of how a wide range of losses that are not necessarily death-related can nonetheless prove very significant. People with mental health problems are often stigmatized and discriminated against, and this can result in (or exacerbate) a range of losses: status and self-esteem, relationships, access to housing and employment and so on.

An important aspect of losses that is often neglected is the fact that some forms of grief can be disenfranchised (Doka 2002). What this refers to is that grief can sometimes not be recognized or socially sanctioned. This can be where the loss is in some way stigmatized (for example, in gay relationships in a homophobic society). It can also arise where the griever is disenfranchised – that is, where there are discriminatory stereotypes that deny the validity of some people's grieving (for example, the ageist stereotype that older people do not grieve because, by that age, they are used to grieving). Also, the loss itself can be disenfranchised, in the sense that, for example, if someone dies as the result of suicide, there can be a degree of stigma that prevents the grieving persons from receiving the social support that would otherwise be available to them. Clearly, the concept of disenfranchised grief raises significant issues in terms of spirituality and the meaning making involved in trying to come to terms with a major loss. For example, a key part of the meaning reconstruction processes associated with loss is rituals, but it is often the case that, in circumstances of disenfranchised grief, such rituals are not carried out (because of the lack of a social sanction to support them).

This is just one example of how losses in a person's life and spirituality can be seen to be closely intertwined. If we want to understand spirituality, we need to have a good understanding of loss, certainly far more than an uncritical reliance on the simplistic notion of grieving in stages.

Developing theory

Thompson (2002a) provides a useful summary of some of the key developments in loss theory and is therefore a useful starting point. However, in terms of linking loss and spirituality at a theoretical level more broadly, there are some important issues to consider.

First, it is worth revisiting the notion of meaning reconstruction that was mentioned earlier. Work on this topic has developed quite markedly in recent years and we now have a significant body of helpful literature. The stages model of grieving implies that there is a relatively standardized way of grieving rooted in biology. Meaning reconstruction theory, by contrast, helps us to understand that the 'one size fits all' approach is far from adequate. Different people will respond to losses in different ways, because the meanings they have lost in the process will be different for each person. Therefore, the help that people may need will also be different. We cannot assume that people will follow the same process, as much will depend on their frameworks of meaning and their social circumstances.

Another strong criticism of traditional approaches to loss and grief is that they are predominantly psychological in their focus. While there are clearly strong psychological implications in terms of the experience of loss and grief, there is also a sociological dimension to consider, although, sadly, this is often neglected. Losses and grief reactions to them do not take place in a social vacuum. People grieve in the context of cultural formations and structural relations. To try to understand grief without taking account of this wider social context is to rely on a far from adequate understanding of the complexities involved. Similarly, when it comes to drawing links between grief and spirituality, it is essential that we take account of the social context. This is because an individual's sense of meaning and identity will, in large part, have its roots in the wider cultural sphere and in terms of structural factors, such as social divisions, power relations, the experience of discrimination and oppression, and so on.

While clearly spirituality is an individualized matter in terms of the uniqueness of each person's worldview, that uniqueness needs to be seen within a broader social context. That is, each one of us is indeed a unique individual in life generally and in terms of our experiences of loss and grief, but we also have to recognize that we are unique individuals *in a social context*. Both sides of the coin have to be taken into consideration if we are to develop our theoretical understanding of these complex and demanding issues.

A further point to consider in terms of developing theory in this area is the notion of 'transformational grief'. Both death and grief need to be seen as primary features of life and not simply as exceptional events. The point was made earlier that problems can arise when people fail to recognize the significance of death and try to live as if impermanence were not a feature of human existence. An alternative to this inauthentic existence arises for many people when they experience a transformational mode of grief. This refers to the way in which a major loss or trauma in a person's life can result in the individual concerned becoming stronger and more resilient as a result of that experience. This should not be oversimplified as if to suggest that grief is a positive experience; it most certainly is not. However, we should also not fail to recognize that, within the immense pain and suffering of grief, there can be a silver lining. For example, Calhoun and Tedeschi (1999, 2001) have written extensively on how loss and trauma in people's lives can lead to developments in three areas:

- *A changed sense of self:* People who have gone through the process of transformational grief report that they have a stronger sense of who they are, a greater degree of ontological security, as it were.

- *Changed relationships:* An increased sense of connectedness to other people can be one positive result of a grief experience.

- *Existential and spiritual growth:* While some people can be devastated by significant losses and never recover, for some people the result can be more positive with an increased understanding and awareness of human experience.

Calhoun and Tedeschi (1999) argue that the transformative dimension of loss can be seen as a process in which the lives of some people are imbued with an enhanced sense of meaning and purpose – that is, an intensified level of spirituality.

Developing practice

In order to develop the practice implications of an increased level of understanding of the relationship between loss and grief and spirituality, we need to undertake two significant changes. First, we need to update our understanding of loss theory and make sure that professional education and practice are based on more sophisticated understandings of the complexities of loss and grief than the stages approach permits. One example of this, namely meaning reconstruction theory, has already been given, but there are many others that can be drawn upon – for example, dual process theory (Stroebe and Schut 1999). Second, we need to incorporate more fully a spiritual dimension into our understandings of not only loss and grief, but also of professional practice more broadly. As Moss (2005) points out, there has been a strong tendency to neglect these issues over the years. Clearly, this cannot continue if we are to develop a more adequate understanding of the relationship between grief and spirituality. Spirituality involves maintaining and developing a coherent thread of meaning and identity. Grief can seriously challenge that thread. Spirituality also involves a sense of connectedness to other people, both individuals and humanity more broadly. Grief can challenge our sense of connectedness and, in some cases, actually destroy it.

Third, spirituality involves a sense of direction or focus in our lives. Grief can destroy that too, temporarily at least. Any adequate attempt to understand spirituality must therefore incorporate an understanding of grief. This chapter has not only presented the case for that particular point, but has also argued that our understanding of grief needs to be at a far more sophisticated level than commonly applies for many professionals practising in the human services. This is not a criticism directly of those professionals, but rather a reflection of the sad reality that an unhelpful and discredited approach to understanding loss and grief has become such an uncritically established part of received wisdom. Clearly, an important step in terms of developing our understanding is to move away from any previous adherence to such an oversimplified approach.

References

Attig, T. (1996) *How We Grieve: Relearning the World.* New York: Oxford: University Press.

Attig, T. (2000) *The Heart of Grief: Death and the Search for Lasting Love.* New York: Oxford University Press.

Attig, T. (2001) 'Relearning the World: Making and Finding Meanings.' In R.A. Neimeyer: *Meaning Reconstruction and the Experience of Loss.* Washington DC: American Psychological Association.

Calhoun, L.G. and Tedeschi, R.G. (1999) *Facilitating Posttraumatic Growth: A Clinician's Guide.* Mahwah, NJ: Lawrence Erlbaum Associates.

Calhoun, L.G. and Tedeschi, R.G. (2001) 'Posttraumatic growth: The Positive Lessons of Loss.' In R.A. Neimeyer: *Meaning Reconstruction and the Experience of Loss.* Washington DC: American Psychological Association.

Camus, A. (2005) *The Myth of Sisyphus.* London: Penguin (originally published in 1942).

Doka, K. (ed.) (2002) *Disenfranchised Grief: New Directions, Challenges, and Strategies for Practice.* Champaign, Ill: Research Press.

Doka, K.J. and Morgan, J.D. (eds) (1993) *Death and Spirituality.* Amityville, NY: Baywood.

Golomb, J. (1995) *In Search of Authenticity: From Kierkegaard to Camus.* London: Routledge.

Heidegger, M. (1962) *Being and Time.* Oxford: Blackwell.

Kierkegaard, S. (1996) *Papers and Journals: A Selection.* Harmondsworth: Penguin.

Kübler-Ross, E. (1969) *On Death and Dying.* New York: Springer.

Morgan, J.D. (1993) 'The Existential Quest for Meaning.' In K.J. Doka and J.D. Morgan (eds) (1993) *Death and Spirituality.* Amityville, NY: Baywood.

Moss, B. (2005) *Religion and Spirituality.* Lyme Regis: Russell House.

Neimeyer, R.A. (2001a) 'The Language of Loss: Grief Therapy as a Process of Meaning Reconstruction.' In R.A. Neimeyer *Meaning Reconstruction and the Experience of Loss.* Washington DC: American Psychological Association.

Neimeyer, R.A. (ed.) (2001b) *Meaning Reconstruction and the Experience of Loss.* Washington DC: American Psychological Association.

Neimeyer, R.A. and Anderson, A. (2002) 'Meaning Reconstruction Theory.' In N. Thompson: *Loss and Grief: A Guide for Human Services Practitioners.* Basingstoke: Palgrave Macmillan.

Parkes, C.M. (2004) *Bereavement: Studies of Grief in Adult Life* (3rd edn). Harmondsworth: Penguin.

Richards, T.A. (2001) 'Spiritual Resources Following a Partner's Death from AIDS.' In R.A. Neimeyer: *Meaning Reconstruction and the Experience of Loss.* Washington DC: American Psychological Association.

Stroebe, M. and Schut, H. (1999) 'The dual process model of coping with bereavement: Rationale and description.' *Death Studies 23*, 7, 197–224.

Tillich, P. (2000) *The Courage to Be.* London and New Haven, CT: Yale University Press (originally published in 1952).

Thompson, N. (2002a) 'Introduction.' In N. Thompson: *Loss and Grief: A Guide for Human Services Practitioners.* Basingstoke: Palgrave Macmillan.

Thompson, N. (ed.) (2002b) *Loss and Grief: A Guide for Human Services Practitioners.* Basingstoke: Palgrave Macmillan.

Walter, T. (1994) *The Revival of Death.* London: Routledge.

Wicks, R. (2003) *Modern French Philosophy: From Existentialism to Postmodernism.* Oxford: One World Publications.

The Well of Grief

Those who will not slip beneath
the still surface on the well of grief

turning downward through its black water
to the place we cannot breathe

will never know the source from which we drink,
the secret water, cold and clear,

nor find in the darkness glimmering
the small round coins
thrown by those who wished for something else.

David Whyte, 1990

Wild wind

These tears of searing pain
Are at the same time
Jewels of surging joy.
The sparkle of dew
On soft grass
Can look as cold
As a cutting edge.
In death life exposes
Its deeper meaning.
In this white washed garden
Of lucid solitude
I feel you closer than ever.
And faith rides full sail high
On this wild wind of change,
Which I pray is whirling
Around your travelling light
In extravagant farewell,
And will know its own way home.

Rose Snow

Me

Through the darkness a light shone through
The voices of my past, now but a distant
memory

I no longer hold on to the labels and names
attached to me
I no longer belong to the 'unknown'
I no longer feel weak and helpless
I no longer acquire their food for my thoughts
I no longer play 'ball' to their games...

My heart illuminated by Islam
My faith carried me to my abode
For once I tasted sweet joy
The joy of success, freedom and enlightenment

I am no longer patient 'X'
I am ME and whatever I want that to be.

Fozia Sarwar

SECTION B
Diverse Perspectives

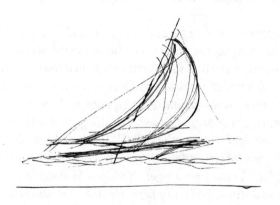

CHAPTER 5

THROUGH A GLASS DARKLY: LOOKING FOR MY OWN REFLECTION

Sarah Carr

On 4 October 2005 I was admitted to a psychiatric ward and I didn't see myself again for several days. This wasn't just due to my state of mind. There are things you gradually notice about a place, first obliquely, then more clearly, as if waking slowly from sleep, eyes adjusting and brain processing your surroundings. You steadily enumerate instances, until a trend becomes a truth.

I had been admitted late at night and it wasn't until the next day that I slowly began to take in my surroundings. As I did so I saw that along the corridors, in the bedrooms, in the bathrooms and communal rooms there was an absence. It was the absence of reflective surfaces to show me myself; where mirrors once were there were gaping grey squares with screw holes still evident in each corner. These bare walls were speaking: 'you are no one'; 'you are nothing'; 'you are lost'; 'you are invisible'. It seemed like the external reinforcement of my loss of self and my internal fragmentation into nothingness seemed complete. I could no longer check my features to see if I still physically existed as a whole body. My face, my hands. In an alien environment a mirror gives you a point of space that is familiar – your own reflection: 'Here I am'. But I couldn't even locate myself as an object in the room.

Physical self-scrutiny seemed forbidden and yet I was constantly under scrutiny. I was positioned by the gaze of others: the suicide watch. I began to ask myself, 'Why are there no mirrors here?'

> Depersonalisation: a recognition of self breaks down. When a
> person suffers from the disorder (or symptoms associated with it) he

or she finds that when looking in the mirror, his or her face is not familiar…the self is felt to be unreal.[1]

Most of my belongings had been taken from me, sealed in a bag and put out of harm's way, while I was put out of harm's way. With my belongings I had also signed away my right to assail my own body to try to relieve the pain in my mind. Among them was a powder compact with a mirror, the shattered shards of which I could have used to slice myself back into being. When I looked in my little mirror it could have reflected back a stranger, an archangel, a vampire (a void) or myself. Perhaps in my state of mind I was like the figure in the song who 'stepped into the hall of mirrors, where she discovered a reflection of herself. Sometimes she saw her real face, and sometimes a stranger in her place.'[2] So there may be a simple explanation for the lack of mirrors: to stop the insane from fashioning weapons; to stop us from arming ourselves with swords of silvered glass. And perhaps there is a kindness also: to stop us from seeing ourselves and not seeing ourselves; to stop us from seeing familiar faces in such pain. Are mirrors confiscated for safety then?

In her poem, Mirror, Sylvia Plath wrote that the looking glass is 'just as it is, unmisted by love or dislike. I am not cruel, only truthful – The eye of a little god, four-cornered.'[3] The mirror has had great symbolic power in religion and myth and has subsequently been used as a psychoanalytic metaphor. A reflection sealed the fate of Narcissus and the mirror shield of Perseus ensured the death of Medusa. The Lady of Shallot's cracked mirror released a curse and Alice fell through a looking glass into a strange land.

The psychoanalyst Jacques Lacan seems to posit the mirror as a deceiver and a curse. His theory, 'the mirror stage' (Lacan 1977), suggests that when an infant sees herself in a mirror she gets an external, unified image of her body. On identifying with this image she is deceived. Before this false revelation of selfhood in the mirror, she perceived her physical self as fragmented. The unified person in the mirror does not correspond with her actual vulnerability, and so she develops a false ideal of herself that she will perpetually strive for all her life. In many cultures children are prevented from seeing themselves in mirrors.

The Hebrew practice of covering mirrors or turning them to the wall after the death of a member of a household later passed into Christian tradition. Reflective surfaces are covered to remind the bereaved to look to others for sympathy and support, rather than to be a tower of self-reliance. In Judaism the mourning period of 'shiva is a time to look inward at the deepest parts that hurt, when superficial answers and the mirror's reassurance "you look like you're holding up well" do not help'.[5] By having no reflective surfaces in which to see their face the mourner is no longer distracted by their physical reality and is able to concentrate on their soul or inner self. This soul or self may be fragmented in times of grief or madness and even if the mirror's reflection isn't something or someone the beholder recognizes it can also be deceptive, showing a wholeness that isn't felt inside. But the absence of a mirror can also symbolize the need to turn to others or to God instead of suffering alone, as these lyrics suggest:.

> You found the ladder in the pattern on your wrist,
> You've seen and you've marked horizons.
> Mother was difficult, she made you cry,
> Cover the mirror, look to the sky.[4]

I had reached a stage of madness where it seemed like a matter of life or death. I had to let someone in or die. I could no longer rely on myself and I wasn't safe with myself. As in mourning, the absence of mirrors in the psychiatric ward now symbolize for me the need to turn to others or (in doing so?) to God. So I opened up to trusted friends who, in my utter worthlessness showed me great kindness and reflected back to me some of the self that was lost. Through this, I now feel I know myself better than if I had been alone in a room with madness and my own reflection. And I now realize that the eyes of others are also reflective surfaces.

> For now we see through a glass, darkly; but then face to face: now I know in part; but then shall I know even also as I am known.

> *(New English Bible, 1 Corinthians 13:12)*

Acknowledgement

This piece is dedicated to Kelly, Dettie, Nataly and Melanie.

Notes

1   See http://en.wikipedia.org/wiki/Depersonalisation
2   Siouxsie and the Banshees (1986) 'Hall of Mirrors', from *Through the Looking Glass* (Geffen Records).
3   Sylvia Plath (1971) 'Mirror', in *Crystal Gazer and Other Poems*. London: Rainbow Press.
4   REM (2001) 'Saturn Return', from *Reveal* (Warner Bros, WEA).
5   See www.mazornet.com/deathandmourning/OrthodoxFinal.html

References

Berman, R.C. 'Death and mourning in judaism.' Available at www.mazornet.com/deathandmourning/OrthodoxFinal.html (accessed 20 September 2007).

Lacan, J. (1977) *Écrits: A Selection*. New York: W.W. Norton.

New English Bible. (1970) Oxford: Oxford University Press.

Plath, S. (1971) 'Mirror'. In S. Plath: *The Crystal Gazer and Other Poems.* London: Rainbow Press.

Survivor

Etched upon a tired heart
A void of wasted noxious years
Where flailing limbs respect the chore
Embedded in a sea of guilt
And drown in our own tears
Licentious deeds in toy boxed halls
Where children play with dolls and drums
A play thing for the adult world
A wound up toy when duty comes
Where trust can mortify and scar
The core of every kid in chains
Who searches all its adult life
To make some sense of what remains
Where hairy hands like cumfry spread
To smother what was really you
And prod you like a piece of meat
Abandoned as too tough to chew
Where night time is for pillows wet
And throbbing pains you can't forget
And mornings just a punishment for being born
The victim serves the sentence for a crime that's never seen
And corridors of silence mark the places we have been
Where echoed screams and slamming doors
And visitors on squeaky floors
All talk about the weather and the Christmas tree at home
As hurt grows deeper by the day
A pain that will not go away
You find it hard conversing
But you hate to be alone
A diadem of heavy thorns press deep into the head of me
And thrust them deeper still in flesh
For every hurt that's come to be
The long and lonely winters nights
Left soiled and defiled
Are nailed to my memory
Like the raping of a child.

Ju Blencowe

CHAPTER 6

A JOURNEY – WITH FAITH: COMPLEX TRAVELS WITH ISLAM THROUGH THE MENTAL HEALTH SYSTEM

Mariyam Maule, Premila Trivedi, Andrew Wilson and Veronica Dewan

Premila, writing in 2006

It was 2003 and Mariyam and I had been asked by Andrew Wilson (Chaplain in Croydon at the South London and Maudsley Trust) to give a presentation at the Touching Lives, Healing Souls Conference he was organizing for World Mental Health Day (WMHD). Both Mariyam (a practising Muslim) and I (a Hindu) knew from personal experience how religious faith could manifest itself in troubling ways when we were at our most distressed, but also how that very same faith could also enable and sustain our recovery. We therefore decided to base our presentation for WMHD on this and Mariyam suggested we use her most recent hospital admission as an example, focusing particularly on how expression of her Muslim faith was so seriously and damagingly misinterpreted. At the time of writing in 2006, when any outward manifestation of Islamic belief seems to arouse so much fear, suspicion and hostility and when Muslims throughout the world are being demonized, it seems particularly pertinent to include the script of that presentation in this book.

I remember us sitting on the floor in 2003 in my flat eating Chinese takeaway, clarifying exactly what we would say in our presentation. Mariyam was clear and articulate as she dictated what she wanted to say about some of her most personal and painful experiences. I was more hesitant and at times found myself feeling frankly uncomfortable, and several times stopped Mariyam to check out if she was really going to be OK with being so honest in front of so many people. But she had no doubt – she wanted people to know how important her faith was to her, how challenging that could sometimes be and how damaging misinterpretation of her expressions of faith could be. In her typical way, she did not seek to apportion blame but rather to inform so that there could be increased knowledge and understanding. That was so Mariyam, not afraid to be honest, not shying away from difficult issues, always urging you to look below the surface…

The Presentation in 2003

Assalamu Alilkum Wa Rahmatulah Wa Barakatuh (peace, mercy, and blessings be upon you).

Between the mystical insights of human experience and the numinous confusions of psychosis, there are some shared experiences. Joseph Campbell has said that the mystic and the psychotic share the same ocean, but whereas the mystic swims, the psychotic may drown (Campbell 1972).

We would like to illustrate this by telling you about some of Mariyam's experiences during one of her hospital admissions when she was very severely depressed. At the time, Mariyam believed Iblis the devil had killed off Mariyam and taken over her whole personality. In her nihilistic delusions, Mariyam asked nursing staff to call her Iblis. The nurses (for whatever reason) complied, greeting Mariyam as Iblis and even writing Iblis rather than Mariyam on the nurse/patient allocation board in the day room. Not surprisingly, these actions reinforced Mariyam's negative view of herself and confirmed to her that she was inherently evil and had irrevocably become Iblis.

Also at this time, Mariyam was not able to sleep in her bed, believing it was infested with evil jinn.[1] The nurses, not knowing what jinn were, did not understand why Mariyam insisted on sleeping on a blanket on the floor or the deep and terrifying fear she was experiencing. Their impatience with what they perceived as her 'attention-seeking' behaviour and their subsequent silence towards Mariyam only served to increase her distress and exacerbate her 'psychosis'. It was only when the hospital Imam (Muslim Chaplain) and a Muslim nurse bridged their gap of ignorance that ward staff

---

1   The word jinn comes from an Arabic root meaning 'hidden from sight'. Jinn are supernatural, invisible beings made from fire. They are not angels or fallen angels. They can be good or bad and are capable of looking like humans or animals.

were able to appreciate to any degree how distressed Mariyam actually was and the massive internal battles she was struggling with.

A Possession Coveted by the Beast

The shadow of wickedness
Consumes my very soul
Foreboding, bleak, birthright stolen
Elusive, the self bartered for a lie
Steeped in deception,
Deceit sustained by whispering, my father
The masquerading angel, appears
Flutters, darts about surreptitiously
Conspiring to claim my origins
As he tries to assume my entire identity
An experiment conducted by hate
Oversees my destiny
Suicidal desires seal my fate.

Mariyam Maule, 2000

Religious belief clearly then shaped Mariyam's feelings about herself and the ways in which she was expressing her distress. However, ignorance and misunderstanding of these connections, and insistence on seeing Mariyam's behaviours simply as manifestations of a medical illness devoid of any meaning, only increased her sense of isolation and extreme vulnerability. Knowledge of Islam and how its tenets may become subverted during times of distress would have helped ward staff greatly in understanding what was going on for Mariyam. Skills of how to work with spiritual beliefs would have enabled staff to communicate more effectively with Mariyam and reach out to her, rather than judging and isolating her. But most importantly, attitudes of acceptance and a fundamental belief in there being a meaning behind people's expressions of distress would have enabled staff to hear, acknowledge and validate Mariyam rather than judge, ignore and pathologize her.

We acknowledge that such attitudes are not easy to acquire and require complex ethical and moral understandings. But without these, the spiritual dimensions of our mental 'illnesses' will never be recognized and mental health staff will continue to judge and treat complex human issues in simple reductionist ways. Furthermore, those who do have the courage to recognize and work within a spiritual context will be likely to be marginalized and the vital role they play in our recovery never recognized.

For Mariyam, it was the hospital Imam who recognized the spiritual significance of Mariyam's 'psychiatric symptoms'. His fundamental acceptance of Mariyam as a person, his ability to engage and his consistent belief in her enabled Mariyam to gradually get back in touch with her true sense of self and regain a positive relationship with her Muslim faith. This faith, wise and well-established with its systems of thought, belief and practice, gave Mariyam contexts to interpret her experience in a way that supported and encouraged her as the person she was and generated hope for recovery. As she slowly came out of her severe depressive psychosis, Mariyam wrote the following poem to describe how she felt about her faith and its intangible sacred core, the soul.

The Soul

The soul, a magnetic field
Connected to North, bonded with the Creator
Resonating His mercy through canals of love
Radiating warmth and tranquillity
The core of the reactor generating cosmic energy
The nucleus of our very existence.

Perceptions of the Ultimate Good collide harmoniously
Causing great friction and life itself
Emotions fall and rise
As the tides come in and out to greet the body of land in its midst
The soul, a Divine union, as One
A unified whole in balance
The ear registering moods, attitudes
Through electrical currents
Blinded but with wilful insight and awareness
Heightened by a gravitational pull to be truly complete.

Conducted by an all knowing, telling wavelength
Controlling the physical reality
Perfectly tuned into Allah's radio broadcast to the entire cosmos.

Conscious, constantly picking up its vibrations
A secret communication with the Maker of all that is
Coming directly into His sphere of influence.

The soul, the domain, the lynchpin of His grand design
A force manipulated by an overarching Supreme Authority,
discipline
Left to positive and negative stimuli affecting our very being
The soul, creation in its entirety.

The soul, encapsulated in a physical plane
Where internal reality is projected outwardly
Completely in touch with every sense
Faced with interpreting, sometimes conflicting
With the external complexity of things.

The soul, in conjunction with all Divine attributes
As peace, knowledge and understanding neutralises acid to water
The soul yearns for, needs purification.

Mariyam Maule, 2000

So it seems imperative that an understanding of our mental health problems includes an understanding and acceptance of our spiritual dimensions. Such dimensions may arise from traditional faiths or from no particular faith, but all exist side by side and should be a resource to enrich our knowledge and understanding of the world and the people in it. But we live in an age when economics, a hunger for power and the agendas of political leaders mean religion is often used to cloak insidious motives and wars are waged in the name of fundamental beliefs. So faith becomes distorted and the essential goodness we see at the heart of every (and no) world religion gets somehow forgotten. Surely it would be better if individuals, communities and nations worked together to create a world in which religious difference could be accepted and valued, with the courage and capacity to encourage unity in diversity? Surely individuals, groups and societies can function so we all benefit, with a clear acknowledgement of similarities as well as differences within a wider common context of humanity (Brown 2000, 391–419)?

The Peacemaker

I come as one, but many
With one voice
One truth
One vision
One destiny.

I come in peace
To show that we are many
And all are chosen
The same, one.

I come in peace
To bring together and
Break bread at the table.

I come in peace
To heal the wounds which
Inflicted the soul to bleed.

I come in peace
An arbiter of spiritual harmony.

I come in peace
To witness the divine union

I come in peace
To honour the glorious matrimony
Between black and white
Between all mankind.

I come as one, but many
I come in peace.

Mariyam Maule, 2000

Andrew, writing in 2006

We had arranged a celebration for World Mental Health Day which would acknowledge the depths of wisdom and creativity our varying faiths and cultures afford us, and which, as Mariyam reminded us that day, are the wellspring and core of our life.

Perhaps people thought that the poems Mariyam would offer us might bring a gentle relief after much talk, but the moment she started we began to realize that here was a woman of prophecy. Mariyam, and her writing could catch us up in her energy, challenging us with her vision of how the world should be; the place of justice, mercy and respect for all comers. And yet this intense energy was held within someone of great fragility and pain. She refused to be satisfied with half truths no matter what struggles or journeys this might involve her in. Her final poem that afternoon stripped bare all the illusions and defences we construct to maintain our self-interest and complacency. There was a full and searching silence when she finished. May her courage and her craft still speak to us.

Veronica, writing in 2006

Mariyam, our beautiful, affectionate, compassionate, feisty, funny, fiercely intelligent friend and sister died in hospital on 7 May 2005, aged 32.

As a baby, Mariyam was transracially adopted into a loving Scottish family and raised in the Christian faith. Those of us who knew Mariyam in the last 10 years of her life were aware of how separation from her birth mother and from her Egyptian cultural roots, growing up in a white environment of daily racist taunts, plus two major bereavements in 1994 shortly before completing a degree in African History, led to a sense of deep despair. After graduating from London University's School of Oriental and African Studies, Mariyam became suicidally depressed and was admitted to the Maudsley Hospital. She would return to the Maudsley as an inpatient on numerous occasions over the following 11 years, and in that time would very rarely receive understanding of her experiences of loss and desperate search for belonging.

Among the professionals at the Maudsley Hospital was the Imam, under whose guidance Mariyam would reconnect with the Muslim faith heritage from which she was severed as a baby. Her faith provided her with sustenance and a sense of belonging as she tried to unravel the painful and confusing story of her abandonment. Cruelly, the effects of electroconvulsive therapy (ECT) damaged Mariyam's memory and she was distraught that she could not remember how to recite the Islamic prayers that provided her with such solace and the strength to retain her strong sense of self and challenge injustice.

For more than half her young life Mariyam campaigned against discrimination and injustice and, as a founder member of SIMBA (Share in Maudsley Black Action), she was committed to influencing psychiatric services to provide more thoughtful care and support not only for herself but for black service users as a whole. Mariyam had a vibrant and engaging personality, and would communicate powerful ideas and feelings through her words and poetry at numerous presentations and training of mental health workers.

The poems included in this chapter form part of a bigger, profoundly moving manuscript: Mariyam left a legacy of more than 100 poems. It was her greatest wish that her poems would one day be published so that she might continue to inspire other service users to express unspoken feelings and for professionals to understand and become more accepting and supportive of service users, including those whose religious and spiritual beliefs have been fundamental in their lives. She would have been incredibly proud to know that the spiritual experience she shared so that others might learn has been included in this anthology.

This chapter would not have been published without the generous consent and ongoing support of Mariyam's father, Eric Maule. Mr Maule's understanding of the importance of his daughter's human rights writing continues to enable greater access to her prophetic legacy and carries on the activism that was such a significant part of her young life.

Acknowledgement

This chapter was adapted from a presentation given at a WMHD event in Croydon organized by SLaM chaplain Andrew Wilson – Touching Lives, Healing Souls Conference 10 October 2003.

References

Brown, D.G. (1998) 'Foulkes's Basic Law of Group Dynamics 50 years on: abnormality, injustice and the renewal of ethics.' *Group Analysis 1998, 31*, 391–419.

Campbell, J. (1972) *Myths to Live By.* New York: Bantam.

Reflection: *Sehnsucht Cinema*
Sarah Carr

> And sometimes at the cinema, in the midst of its immense dexterity
> and enormous technical proficiency, the curtain parts and we behold,
> far off, some unknown and unexpected beauty. (Virginia Woolf
> 1926)

> When I am ill, cinema can be like a womb, a dark safe space where I
> can temporarily retreat into another reality while my own is too
> painful to bear. When I am disintegrating and feeling dependent it
> gives me a sense of autonomy and containment. When I am too agi-
> tated to read, it teaches me and tells me stories. When my mind is
> assailed by intrusive thoughts and voices, it gives me other images,
> other words, some familiar and some unfamiliar. When I am with-
> drawn and afraid of humankind, it keeps me in touch with humanity.
> (Carr 2007, p.55)

Certain films can do even more than this for me. There are a few, the nature
of which evoke in me a feeling that has no name in the English language.
This feeling is something I associate closely with my mental pain and my
longing to be at peace, to have a quiet mind. In German this feeling is called
Sehnsucht and it can be understood as a deep longing of the soul. The
German Romantics of the 19th century wrote of a longing for home and a
longing for what is far off. They said it is a yearning without greed. It can
also be understood as 'a close relationship between ardent longing or yearning (das Sehen) and addiction (die Sucht) that lurks behind each longing,
waiting to turn the feeling into a destructive, self-defeating force'. For some
of us who have experienced the kinds of madness that drive us to harm or to
try and kill ourselves, this description of Sehnsucht may make great sense.

Another feature of Sehnsucht is that it is 'so deeply personal that it does
not occur to the one feeling it that others would have similar experiences and
so is rarely communicated verbally'. But in its early days Virginia Woolf recognized that cinema can be freed from the restrictions of verbal expression:

> All this, which is accessible to words, and to words alone, the cinema
> must avoid. Yet if so much of our thinking and feeling is connected
> with seeing, some residue of visual emotion which is of no use to
> either painter or to poet may still await the cinema... Then, indeed,
> when some new symbol for expressing thought is found, the
> film-maker has enormous riches at his command. The exactitude of
> reality and its surprising power of suggestion are to be had for the
> asking. (Woolf 1926)

For me something of Sehnsucht can be communicated by what has been called 'visionary' or 'devotional' cinema by the filmmaker and philosopher Nathaniel Dorsky. He says that 'viewing a film has tremendous mystical implications; it can be, at its best, a way of approaching and manifesting the ineffable'. The particular film I want to talk about here has helped me approach this ineffable thing, which I'd like to call Sehnsucht. Perhaps unsurprisingly the film is German and was released in England under the title *The Enigma of Kaspar Hauser* in 1974. Its title in German is *Jeder für sich und Gott gegen alle*, which translates as *Every Man for Himself and God Against All*. It was directed by Werner Herzog who is revisiting the true story of a feral boy named Kaspar Hauser who was found in the market square at Nuremburg in 1828, having lived for the first 17 years of his life in a cellar devoid of human contact except for that of an unseen stranger who feeds him.

The real Kaspar Hauser appeared during the German romantic period when 'he embodied the mourned for loss of youthful vision, sinking back from the rapt pinnacle of childhood into the light of common day'. Film critics have recognized that 'German romanticism, with its respect for the incalculable mysteries of life and its deep suspicion of the "civilized" world' strongly influenced Werner Herzog not only in his choice of story, but in the way he and his crew told it. So it is not only the film's subject but the way the story is told, the film is directed, photographed and edited, the screenplay is written and delivered and the soundtrack used – for me, everything about the film evokes Sehnsucht and as a consequence I have found it moving and healing.

Nathaniel Dorsky has described this power:

> When a film is fully manifest it may serve as a corrective mirror that realigns our psyches and opens up appreciation and humility. The more we are open to ourselves and are willing to touch the depths of our own being, the more we are participating in devotion. Similarly, the more film expresses itself in a manner intrinsic to its own true nature, the more it can reveal to us. (Dorsky 2005)

When the film was first released in America, the critic Richard Eder wrote:

> It is impossible to know why these things move us, or why they prepare us for an experience out of the ordinary. Throughout 'Every Man for Himself and God Against All' there are moments when we drift a bit outside of ourselves, in a kind of detached gratefulness that the person occupying our seat is being given so much. (Eder 1975)

The Enigma of Kaspar Hauser is a devastatingly moving and strange story of alienation and the struggle to survive in a world where, as Kaspar says, 'people are like wolves'. Kaspar's vulnerability is something with which I can closely identify. Herzog and Bruno S (the man who plays the lead role) – an untrained actor who had himself been a psychiatric patient – beautifully portray Kaspar's sense of otherness, confusion and alienation. I feel that in doing so cinematic art is used to reveal Sehnsucht to the viewer, or at least to this viewer. In one scene Kaspar tells his guardian, the kindly lawyer Herr Daumer, 'it seems to me that my coming into this world was a terrible fall'. In the kitchen of the family who first take him in he stands rocking the cradle of a crying baby. The baby stops crying and grasps his finger. The baby's mother comes into the room and puts the baby into Kaspar's arms. He is then seen standing still, silently crying as he is so overwhelmed, eventually saying, 'Mother, I have been so far away from everything.' In these scenes Kaspar is lost and longing, but in later and closing scenes he glimpses his longed for place of peace.

After his discovery Kaspar is subjected to tests by theologians, philosophers, lawyers and logicians, all of whom are concerned with what they want him to be and not with what he is. By his very nature, Kaspar innately defies their attempts to classify him. For someone who has been subject to diagnosis and classification in the psychiatric system, this is a resonant theme in the film. While the external, rational world tries to force Kaspar into modes of thinking and behaviour to which he cannot conform, he retreats into trances and finds comfort in visions – his mind drifts into states of Sehnsucht.

Towards the end of the film, Kaspar is attacked by an unknown assailant but survives only to be eventually murdered by a stranger. After the first attack his visions of a longed for land intensify. The cinema screen fills with painterly, dimly flickering visions of an archaic landscape; the mountains and plains of the Caucasus. Is Kaspar glimpsing home, the home for which his soul is longing, the home he cannot find in a world that misunderstands him so? Then, as he lies dying, theologians ask if anything is burdening him. Kaspar tells them about a mystical dream of a caravan in the Sahara, whereupon the film cuts to glimmering shots of Berbers crossing the desert. His dying preoccupation is with journeying and being lost:

> I see a great caravan coming through the desert over the sand. And this caravan is being led by an old Berber. And this old man is blind. The caravan stops because some of them believe they are lost. They see mountains before them. They check their compass but they are no wiser. Then their blind leader picks up a handful of sand and tastes it, as though it were food. 'My sons,' the blind man says, 'you

were wrong. Those are not mountains you see. It's only your imagi-nation. We must continue northwards.' They follow the old man's advice and they reach the city in the north where the story takes place. But how the story goes after they reach the city, I do not know. (Herzog 1974, p.99)

He then thanks the theologians for listening to him. 'I'm tired now,' he says, and he dies. Historical records show that Kaspar Hauser's final words were, 'I am tired, very tired, and I have a long way yet to go.' Knowing this only deepens the force of Sehnsucht in the story for me. Perhaps Kaspar senses that his death in this world is not the end of his journey towards a longed for place of peace and final belonging. Is there an end to Sehnsucht? Is there an end to the deep longing of the soul for its 'own far off country'?

In *The Problem of Pain*, C.S. Lewis wrote of Sehnsucht:

> All the things that have deeply possessed your soul have been but hints of it – tantalizing glimpses, promises never quite fulfilled, echoes that died away just as they caught your ear. But if it should really become manifest – if there ever came an echo that did not die away but swelled into the sound itself – you would know it. Beyond all possibility of doubt you would say 'Here at last is the thing I was made for'. We cannot tell each other about it. It is the secret signature of each soul, the incommunicable and unappeasable want…which we shall still desire on our deathbeds… Your place in heaven will seem to be made for you and you alone, because you were made for it – made for it stitch by stitch as a glove is made for a hand. (Lewis 1940)

Although we may not be able to fully communicate Sehnsucht to one another, as a piece of 'devotional cinema' Werner Herzog's *The Enigma of Kaspar Hauser* allows me to hear a faint echo and to take comfort in its sound-ing. At least, it makes me feel less alone in my longing.

> And God shall wipe away all tears from their eyes; and there shall be no more death, neither sorrow, nor crying, neither shall there be any more pain: for the former things are passed away. (The New English Bible, Revelation 21:4)

References

Carr, S. (2007) 'The Cinema Cure'. In P. Lehmann and P. Stastny (eds) *Alternatives Beyond Psychiatry*. Shrewsbury: Peter Lehmann.

Dorsky, N. (2005) *Devotional Cinema*. Berkeley: Tuumba Press.

Eder, R. (1975) 'Herzog's "Every Man for Himself" Is Stunning Fable Full of Universals.' In: *New York Times*, 28 September 1975. Available at www.moxie.com/fpstage/fpvideo2005/pages/hauser.html (accessed 20 September 2007).

Herzog, W. (1977) *Screenplays of Aguirre and Kaspar Hauser*. Munich: Skellig Edition.

Lewis C.S. (1940) *The Problem of Pain*. Available at http://en.wikipedia.org/wiki/Sehnsucht_%28C._S._Lewis%29 (accessed 20 September 2007).

Lewis C.S. (1942) *The Weight of Glory*. Available at www.doxaweb.com/assets/doxa.pdf (accessed 20 September 2007).

Malcolm, D. (1999) *Werner Herzog: The Enigma of Kaspar Hauser*. Available at http://film.guardian.co.uk/Century_Of_Films/Story/0,4135,96504,00.html (accessed 3 January 2007)

Newton, M. (2003) *Savage Girls and Wild Boys: A History of Feral Children*. London: Faber.

New English Bible (1970). Oxford: Oxford University Press.

Woolf, V. (1926) 'The Cinema.' In *Arts*, June 1926. Available at www.film-philosophy.com/portal/writings/woolf (accessed 3 January 2007)

CHAPTER 7

CONNECTING PAST AND PRESENT: A SURVIVOR REFLECTS ON SPIRITUALITY AND MENTAL HEALTH

Vicky Nicholls

Waking up

There we were, Dad and I, pulling ourselves out of the vehicle and stumbling onto the path. There were choices of ways to go. The landscape was rich and varied – there was some enormous area of mud we would have to negotiate, somewhere in the distance – directly ahead was an entanglement of briars and two paths.

The path to the right was apparently the one to take. It was starkly divided into sunlight and shadow. In the shadows it was icily cold and I was tempted to move into the sunlight. I shivered and asked Dad for a coat. I think he began to suggest we should move into the warmth. But I knew that if we took ourselves out of the shadows, we would not be able to see the magical snow sculptures that punctuated the briar-entangled gloom. Looking to the left now, we could make out the most beautiful of all the carvings, a whole butterfly delicately chiselled out of snow, as high as a human, her glittering wings displayed. What were we to do, other than hold our breath in awe and *wonder*? (Nicholls 2001a)

★ ★ ★

This vision was a dream. They aren't always. Neither are they always so beautiful or affirming. Reading the description of my dream immediately after experiencing it, I was still immersed in the wonder and the emotions of it. Looking at it from a growing distance, questions immediately begin to form themselves in my mind. Who was the creator and who the observer here? What was the meaning of the dream?

> It seems to me it was about the survivor in me, learning to follow my own wisdom whilst remaining connected to my creator, learning to respect the awesomeness, beauty and fragility of other survivors' souls. (Nicholls n.d.)

The sorts of wonderings that come to me are influenced by who I am, by the forces and events that have shaped me. The awakening brings the potential of risk, and danger, and healing.

Dreams can of course be an important vehicle for messages from the subconscious; some means of expressing aspects of our experiences that do not always emerge in our waking hours. They can give significant clues to the deeper meanings of everyday events. However, it is all too often the experience of people using mental health services that our dreams are hijacked by outsiders who pull open our fragile wings and analyse their patterns using questions framed by particular – often medical – approaches that have little to do with our personal consciousness or identity. In Western medicalized approaches our experiences can then be squeezed into theoretical models that force rationality onto the uncertain and often chaotic flight-path of the butterfly. Perhaps this sometimes comes from the professional's fear of facing their own inner chaos, or of admitting that there are no easy answers.

Whatever the cause, such rational analysis can lead to a devaluing of the direct experience: 'As I walked into the hospital I said, "For God's sake somebody get me a Bible", and they looked at me with horror in their eyes and no-one would get me a Bible' (interviewee, Somerset Spirituality Project, 2002). The well-known survivor Sally Clay has said that:

> We who have experienced mental illness have all learned the same thing, whether our extreme mental states were inspiring or frightening. We know that we have reached the bare bones of spirit and of what it means to be human. (Barker, Campbell and Davidson 1999, p.35)

The shaping of services

As people who have lived through extremes of mental and emotional distress, we are tired of being categorized and feared, worn down by being voices in the wilderness – voices that cry out for a humane and holistic understanding of who we are, that embraces physical and spiritual as well as psychological and emotional well-being. After all, we carry everything that has ever happened to us in our bodies (Webster 2002), and many of us know only too well the spirit-breaking nature of some mental health services (Pat Deegan, cited in Barker and Buchanan-Barker 2003, p.60).

How is it that services which are meant to be there to support people in pain are on the whole so boxed in, and so unable to nurture the spirit at times of distress? There is an oppressive positioning of distress that locates the problem entirely within the person and fails to recognize the full impact of external influences.

Economic circumstances – poverty and deprivation in particular – are of course hugely influential. Social conditions such as poor housing or problems with housing, education, family dynamics, experiences of abuse, violence and substance misuse are well known to play a part in the development of distress. Political conditions such as benefits systems that make people feel worthless and guilty and trap people in particular roles can have an enormous influence too. Cultural influences also have a significant role, as do prejudice, stigma and discrimination based on gender, race, sexuality or mental health status. Religious prejudice, particularly Islamophobia, has unfortunately increased since the September 11 bombings and in the current 'war against terrorism' climate, although it is also important to remember the many who are working to raise awareness of the diversity of beliefs that exist and to strive towards peace.

Any or all of these can play an oppressive role in needling down an internalized stigma, a negative self-image which can be reinforced by dismissive or neglectful experiences in mental health services. What is needed is for services to believe in people, in every individual's intrinsic self-worth and capacity to heal and recover, such that services become about supporting and nurturing people's well-being (see Chapter 20).

History

Psychiatry has grown up in the context of a separation from religion that has deep historical roots. While of course these two institutions do not represent the whole picture of either mental health or spirituality, they can be seen as external manifestations of or structural responses to individual depths of experience in both areas. Each has taken its turn in bearing responsibility for areas of medical care.

While for several hundred years the Church was in charge of medical care, when the Church lost this control a separation developed between religion and medicine (see Koenig, McCullough and Larson 2001). This has been attributed by some to the influence of scientific discovery and the accompanying loss of acceptance of scriptural truths: in this volume, for example, Andrew Powell (Chapter 12) points out that Newton's research into the properties of physical matter was taken to mean that God as the prime mover had to be located elsewhere, beyond a mechanistic universe, and was thus unlikely to have a significant influence on the workings of the human body, or mind, except by means of occasional healing. In psychiatry, the hostility of Freud and others towards religion may have contributed to this schism (Kroll and Erickson 2002).

The legacy of this division is that, commonly, questions of the soul are seen to be the responsibility of religion while matters of the mind belong to psychiatry. This seems somewhat ironic, given that the root of the word psychiatry is 'psyche' or 'soul', and sadly, it has been many people's experience that there is a lack of care of the soul within both.

Many who have experience of psychological, emotional and spiritual distress would argue that framing such experiences solely within a medical paradigm is at best inadequate and at worst positively damaging, and that neither religion nor medicine can provide the whole answers to people's complex and ongoing struggles.

Where is the spiritual in our struggles?

The realm of the spiritual is subtle and difficult to define. Nonetheless, definitions of spirituality abound and we are sometimes in danger of cheapening this word through casual use (see, for example, the popular press's current fad for shortcuts to 'spiritual well-being'). Sometimes it seems there is a perception of spirituality that it is all about being nice, kind and caring, or drinking the right kind of herbal tea. David Brandon – the well-known survivor who sadly died in 2002 – eloquently expressed the danger here:

> Just because we don't like the shadows in Plato's ancient and draughty cave [of science] doesn't mean we want to rent out rooms in Disneyworld. (Brandon 1998, p.3)

Shallow versions of spirituality leave out the crucial truth that for many people their spirituality is intensely painful, harrowing, a source of torment, and that for some it is a matter of life and death.

What do I mean by spirituality here? I am thinking of that something in us that strives for inspiration, for reverence, for meaning and purpose, even in those who do not believe in God (Swinton 2001). This does not necessarily mean that we find these things! For many who have survived periods of chaos, confusion and profound distress the following definition may feel particularly resonant:

> Religion is for those who are afraid of hell: spirituality is for those who have been there. (Source unknown)

The dark night of the soul, experienced as a stage on a spiritual journey that then moves on for many, is a landscape that can remain home, or non-home, for people whose access to internal and external sources of hope and renewal is blocked or just not enough to pull them out of the abyss.

Manifestations of spirituality

There is now a vast diversity of religious and spiritual belief systems and practices in the West, including traditions ranging from the mystical to the conservative within all of the major world religions – Christianity, Islam, Judaism, Hinduism, and Buddhism. Latest Census figures show that 78 per cent of the UK population consider themselves to have some form of religious affiliation (Office for National Statistics 2003). In Christianity this includes evangelical and charismatic approaches that are growing in popularity and often dominant in Black African and Caribbean churches. Other systems of belief and practice include traditional beliefs in, for example, voodoo; shamanism with roots in eastern Europe and south America; paganism and earth spirituality; energy medicine; spiritualism; the occult and esoteric spirituality; and many cults or New Religious Movements to which people may be drawn at times of particular vulnerability (see, for example, Barker 1997).

There has been positive campaigning by those whose traditions and practices have affirmed them in their belief in the importance of faith, given them an honest and open relationship with personal and collective history, and buffered them against life's storms with a sense of hope in the future. This campaigning, often by people from black and minority ethnic communities, combined with governmental recognition of the increasing diversity and importance of religious and spiritual belief and practice, has forced those in powerful positions in mental health and social policy formation and service commissioning, to look for ways to improve practice to include a greater understanding of religious and spiritual issues.

Research into spirituality and mental health

Research, meanwhile, has expanded exponentially over the past 10–15 years, and there is now a significant body of research evidence concerning the interface between religion, spirituality and mental health. In particular there is evidence to suggest that spirituality has the potential to support people to cope or move towards recovery (Larson, cited by Powell 2002).

Until recently much of the research was based in the US and was about religion and mental health, primarily about the external manifestations of Christianity such as membership of a church community. In the late 1990s, however, several developments in the UK fostered increasing recognition of the importance of both religion and spirituality in relation to mental health, and opportunities for further exploration of these areas: notably, the establishment of a specific *Mental Health, Religion and Culture* journal (published by Blackwell); John Swinton's seminal work (Swinton 2001); and, from service users' and survivors' own perspectives, the Strategies for Living Project (2000) based at the Mental Health Foundation and all that flowed from it.

The development of transpersonal psychology and more recent developments such as Isabel Clarke's innovative explorations of the interface between psychosis and spirituality (Clarke 2001), have also opened up avenues for exploring this sacred and complex territory which, as an area not readily lending itself to measurement, had often been left out of mental health research.

Most recently the Mental Health Foundation undertook a comprehensive literature review which found that research to date tends to display shortcomings, including an over-reliance on quantitative, observable measures of religious or spiritual activity such as church, temple, synagogue or mosque attendance (Mental Health Foundation 2006, p.6; Swinton in this volume, Chapter 22). The review looked at mechanisms or mediating factors between spirituality and mental health and reported that a collaborative approach to religious coping is associated with the greatest improvement in mental health (ibid, p.3); and that spiritual or religious support can be a valuable source of self-esteem, companionship and practical help (ibid, p.3; Foskett and Roberts in this volume, Chapter 23). It called for further research combining methods and seeking out ways to reflect the diversity of spiritual beliefs and practices in the UK.

This review also reported on findings that people with a diagnosis of schizophrenia find hope, meaning and comfort in spiritual beliefs and practices; that religion can play a central role in the process of reconstructing a sense of self and recovery (ibid, p.15); and unwrapped some of the research, including Swinton's, examining the importance of having a meaning or purpose in life and how central the loss and rediscovery of this can be in mental distress, particularly depression.

During the last few years user and survivor-led research has seriously taken off, and the perspectives of those of us starting from our own experience are being given much more credibility in the broader world of social research. The Strategies for Living initiative has been a key development here, carrying out and supporting a wide range of user and survivor-led research that included work either starting from or exploring religious and spiritual viewpoints.[1] In this we tried to be true to the many service users and survivors who explained to the Project how crucial their spirituality was to them. This research has provided further evidence of the significance of spirituality and religious and spiritual beliefs in helping to give people a sense of meaning and purpose. In Chapter 23 in this volume John Foskett and Anne Roberts give an illuminating account of the Somerset Spirituality Project, linked to one of these strands.

From the UK-wide *Strategies for Living* research and the other strands of work of the Strategies for Living Project, several positive aspects of holding religious and spiritual beliefs are identifiable:

- meaning and purpose
- peace and comfort
- prayer
- presence of God
- sense of belonging and community
- support of others
- a reason for living.

There are of course negative aspects to people's experiences of religious and spiritual beliefs and practices too. Some of these include:

- exclusion and rejection
- damaging teachings
- deliverance ministry.

This last point, deliverance ministry, is complex, but some find it helpful. On the other hand some find it damaging and detrimental, and it needs to be approached with great care (Faulkner and Layzell 2000; Nicholls 2000; Mental Health Foundation 2002).

---

1   See Mental Health Foundation 1997; Faulkner and Layzell 2000; Mental Health Foundation 1999; Mental Health Foundation 2002.

Our voices

As powerful and important as the research with which some of us have been engaged, have been our own steps as individual survivors and groups of survivors towards deeper mutual understanding, compassion, integrity, support and respect. Time and again it is through *our* retelling of our own stories that we learn and grow – whether through speaking or writing, prose or poetry, words, images, music or other forms of expression.[2]

> On the wings of butterflies and the backs of bees
> Ride infinite ideas and ideas of infinity. (Nicholls 2002a)

I have personally been involved in a survivor spirituality support group in which sharing our stories has been a powerful and deeply spiritual way of connecting, of being in relationship. The experience of this respectful and honouring shared space has had a profound influence on my own journey and my understanding of others. Comparable groups are taking shape around the UK, such as in Oxford where a group of survivors meets regularly to talk about particular themes relating to members' spirituality and experiences.

How does it all fit together?

Many people who experience distress may feel particularly sensitive to events and atmospheres in the world around us. Perhaps this is partly because individuals' own torment has made them more empathetic to the suffering of others; partly an awareness of the connectedness of all living beings and the potential that exists in each of us to commit great acts of love and kindness, but also of hatred and destruction.

Many people coming into contact with mental health services bring with them a legacy of damaging childhood experiences that include religious teachings expressed in a misdemeanour-and-punishment framework that is sometimes internalized to lead to a disproportionate sense of guilt and responsibility. The experiences of people who were abused as children can become hostile and vindictive voices; the boundaries between what is here and now, and there and then, blurred and sometimes indistinguishable.

> The shadow of envy in the crows on the wire
> Gives fuel to my vices and insistence to my fire. (Nicholls 2002b)

2   See, for example, Barker, Campbell and Davidson 1999; Survivors' Poetry 1996; Mental Health
     Foundation 1999, 2001.

However, maybe there is hope in some developments in mental health care. Postmodern psychiatry is part of a new paradigm which, as Phil Thomas has pointed out (Thomas 2000) gives priority to meaning and interpretation, which are to be explored and illuminated but not explained. Thus while the experience of hearing voices, for example, may be understood to be internally generated, it can have metaphorical significance and relate to past events.

For others, their voices may be experienced and understood as externally generated, and the boundaries between mystical and psychotic experience are not always clear. MacMin, for example, (Mental Health Foundation 2002) has highlighted that if Jesus and Mary were around now they would probably be sectioned. If Joan of Arc had not heeded her voices there would have been no liberation for France, and Socrates' daemon is well documented. Joseph Campbell famously described the 'schizophrenic' as 'drowning in the same waters in which the mystic swims in delight', and the Ark of the Covenant was borne by a people trusting entirely in the visions of their leader Moses.

There can be no doubt that the true essence of the divine nature of humanity is all too often obscured by strata of suffering and unhealed wounds:

> The forked tongue of deceit and slavery
> The oppression of the spirit. (Nicholls 2001b)

The experience of crisis can be an opportunity for transformation. Laing (1970) called madness the birthpangs of a higher consciousness, and while many of us may try and see ourselves as being on a journey of healing and growth following crises, it is not always possible or desirable to put back on the lid.

In his Tidal Model of mental health care Phil Barker describes how we all live on an 'ocean of experience' of which mental health crisis is only one thing among many that threatens to drown people. Many in distress are seeking meaning. The developmental journey is a risky one not adequately explained by mapping human experience onto psychological or biological templates which leave little room for appreciating the mystery or awe of human experience (Barker and Buchanan-Barker 2004).

> I arrive at a meeting of psychiatrists at the Royal Society of Medicine
> – all potentially overwhelming doors, badges and smart suits – in a
> cloud of butterflies and a deep pink silk blouse and wonder who can
> see what. I hear many profound words that speak of the soul; life in
> cloistered corridors and life in the prison of the mind; the journey

into self and the 'true' spiritual journey to obliterate the self; chaos and the construction of meaning; the Spirit and the spirits and who they are. (Nicholls 2002b)

For me and for many others the presence of spirits can be comforting, guiding and encouraging; voices and guidance can be nurturing and life-enhancing as well as destructive and oppressive, and may be evidence of particular gifts or knowledge such as speaking in tongues or shamanism.

I look at my black star jet ring and picture Tobermory where I bought it, to remind myself of my Granny – the peaceful harbour, the still waters. I picture myself under the water. It is cool, and quiet, and deep. I look now at my other Granny's engagement ring I was given when she died. And I know I am connected to her beyond death and that she guides me. And I am grateful to have learned to be true to myself and my experiences of Spirit and spirits, and I pray to be guided to nurture the truth of others. (ibid.)

References

Barker E. (1997) 'New Religions and Mental Health.' In D. Bhugra (ed.) *Psychiatry and Religion – Context, Consensus and Controversies* (paperback edition). London: Routledge.

Barker, P. and Buchanan-Barker, P. (2004) *The Tidal Model: a Guide for Mental Health Professionals*. London: Brunner-Routledge.

Barker, P. and Buchanan-Barker, P. (eds) (2003) *Spirituality and Mental Health: Breakthrough*. London: Whurr.

Barker, P., Campbell, P. and Davidson, B. (eds) (1999) *From the Ashes of Experience*. London: Whurr.

Bhugra, D. (1997) (ed.) *Psychiatry and Religion – Context, Consensus and Controversies* (paperback edition). London: Routledge.

Brandon, D. (1998) *Speaking Truth to Power*. London: British Association of Social Workers.

Clarke, I. (2001) *Psychosis and Spirituality: Exploring the New Frontier*. London: Whurr.

Faulkner, A. and Layzell, S. (2000) *Strategies for Living*. London: Mental Health Foundation.

Koenig, H.G., McCullough M.E. and Larson, D. (2001) *Handbook of Religion and Health*. Oxford: Oxford University Press.

Kroll, J. and Erickson, P. (2002) 'Religion and psychiatry.' *Current Opinion in Psychiatry 15*, 549–54.

Laing, R.D. (1970) *The Politics of Experience*. London: Penguin.

Mental Health Foundation (1997) *Knowing our own Minds*. London: Mental Health Foundation.

Mental Health Foundation (1999) *The Courage to Bare Our Souls*. London: Mental Health Foundation.

Mental Health Foundation (2001) *Something Inside so Strong*. London: Mental Health Foundation.

Mental Health Foundation/Nicholls, V. (ed.) (2002) *Taken Seriously: The Somerset Spirituality Project*. London: Mental Health Foundation.

Nicholls, V. (n.d.) Unpublished personal reflection.

Nicholls, V. (2000) *Doing Research Ourselves*. London: Mental Health Foundation.

Nicholls, V. (2001a) Unpublished diary entry.

Nicholls, V. (2001b) Unpublished personal reflection.

Nicholls, V. (2002a) Unpublished poem.

Nicholls, V. (2002b) Unpublished diary entry.

Office for National Statistics (2003) *2001 Census*. London: HMSO.

Powell, A. (2002) *Spirituality and Mental Health*. In 'December 2002 newsletter of Royal College of Psychiatrists Spirituality Special Interest Group'. Available at www.rcpsych.ac.uk/pdf/nl10_nine.pdf (accessed 20 September 2007).

Swinton, J. (2001) *Spirituality and Mental Health Care: Rediscovering a Forgotten Dimension*. London: Jessica Kingsley Publishers.

Survivors' Poetry (1996) *Under the Asylum Tree*. London: Survivor Press.

Thomas, P. (2000) Psychiatry and Philosophy Biennial Conference 2000 presentation (unpublished).

Webster, A. (2002) *Wellbeing*. Oxford: Society and Church: SCM Press.

Adam Forgets Himself

I'd like to claim that I made you,
shaped with a seeing thumb your big bones,
fisted their ends into blunt flowers,
strung them tight with purple tendons.

That *I* had scooped those secret places
which give you always the option of wings
and cunningly slung the counterpoise
of your breasts.

That *I* held you tight till you cracked
open, where I wanted you to open
and with hasty inspiration
adorned all those holes
with palmed dabs of jewels,
hatching, gathered shreds,
improvised folds.

That *my* deft palps had printed
the rouge of your fugitive bruises,
the dents and scallops
where I've tried to live.

But, in the evidence of the light,
I hold up a hand unemptied.
At the end of more than the day
I was found in the gloom,
brooding over a growing rib –
so all of that would be saying too much.

Jim Green, November 2005

CHAPTER 8

WHO AM I? – THE SEARCH FOR SPIRITUALITY IN DEMENTIA. A FAMILY CARER'S PERSPECTIVE

Barbara Pointon

Who am I? What is it that makes each one of us unique? I suspect that most people, if asked to define the uniqueness of a friend, would come up with a haphazard mixture of notions, which might include physical attributes, occupation, where or how they live, possessions, hobbies, behaviour, morals, beliefs, sociability, personality…the list could go on. Or, we might start with Descartes' philosophy, 'Cogito, ergo sum' (*I think, therefore I am*) and place cognition as our first building block of essential selfhood. But what happens when dementia (or more aptly, brain failure) attacks not only cognition, but also normal functions, behaviour, communication and personality, until all that which usually defines a person's identity is stripped away? Does that make them less of a person, or does the stripping away of those 'outer' layers allow us to see more of their very essence hidden underneath? And what effect does this have on their main carer?

For 15 years, I have been caring for my husband, Malcolm, diagnosed with Alzheimer's when he was 51 and who is now in the very last stage of the illness. Throughout this time, I have been searching for what makes Malcolm unique – in other words, his spirituality. Is the severely mentally and physi-cally disabled Malcolm I see now essentially the same Malcolm I married 42 years ago and the Malcolm I remember before the illness struck? If so, where does his uniqueness lie? Should more attention have been paid to his essen-tial nature when Social and Health Care professionals devised packages of care over the last 15 years, and should I have cared for him differently? What is the relationship between spirituality and quality of life in dementia? To address some of these profound questions, I must begin at the beginning.

Who was Malcolm before the illness struck? Most people saw him first and foremost as the complete musician. He lectured in music at Homerton College, Cambridge, his talents manifold. As a performer (a brilliant pianist, organist or percussionist) he could turn his hand effortlessly to fiendish classical pieces, jazz or pop and also improvise on the piano in the style of any composer. His many compositions ranged from simple children's songs to film music and complex avant-garde pieces, sometimes using electronically generated sounds, for which he designed and constructed his own electronic equipment, long before synthesizers could be bought off-the-shelf. Previously, he had been employed by the BBC to write scripts for the then Third Programme (now Radio 3). His knowledge of music of all kinds was awesome, particularly of modern art music and the music of non-Western cultures. A good wordsmith and zany communicator, he could hold the attention of lethargic students or a class of fidgety 6-year-olds alike.

But he was not just a musician and teacher – he could speak several foreign languages and was also into astronomy, religions, philosophy, poetry, painting, history, physics and theatre. No ivory-towered academic, he could take on DIY, car maintenance and tough gardening. Despite all his knowledge, wisdom and skills, Malcolm wore his learning lightly – a very self-effacing and modest man. Serene and patient, generous to a fault, he was my rock and calm centre. Yet he had a mischievous sense of humour. An incorrigible mimic, and master of the swift witty remark, friends often said that he could make them laugh until their sides ached. I need to tell you all this, not to evoke sympathy, but so that you have a base-line – the 'Malcolm' as the world saw him – and can sense a measure of the 'losses'.

For, very gradually, but inexorably, Malcolm lost everything the world values, which in normal circumstances would define who he was. He had to give up his job, resulting in severe financial repercussions. All his knowledge and understanding vanished in the reverse order it was acquired: first to go was electronics, followed by foreign languages, then handling cash and arithmetic, spelling, writing, reading, drawing, naming objects, until by 1997 he was scoring zero on cognitive tests. Cogito ergo sum? Not a bit of it. Malcolm was no less of a person through loss of cognition. His spirit wasn't broken. I remember him being asked to count back from 100 in sevens (and who in their right mind wants to do this anyway?) and he faltered to a halt, smiled sweetly at the nurse who was testing him, and, without irony, asked, 'And can you play the piano?' For, despite some of the functions we take for granted also dwindling – the ability to wash, shave, dress or feed himself – and the first hints of loss of continence and incoherent speech appearing, amazingly, Malcolm retained his ability to improvise on the piano. With words faltering, it was through his improvisations that Malcolm could find expression for his feelings. Many pieces had an angry section, but most resolved into a tranquil resignation.

I learned my first important lesson at this point. It would have been easy to bemoan the losses, to catalogue what Malcolm could no longer do; I learned instead to celebrate what he could still do and enjoy. Apart from improvising and listening to recorded music, Malcolm seemed to gain a deep pleasure from nature – colours of flowers, textures of leaves, movement of water, shapes in the sunsets – and from simple things like taste of food, collecting stones, walks, holding hands, smiley faces. With cognition failing, and function dwindling, a new importance was being attached to the sensory and emotional. The essence of Malcolm began to be revealed.

This was the stage when Malcolm began going to daycare, mainly to give me a break. Often he was given a particular activity to do (e.g. artwork) because it was 'on' that day for everybody. But his severe visuo-spatial deficit, as shown by his tests and scans, made artwork a nightmare. I am amazed that information about the deficits in a patient's brain is not automatically conveyed to daycare providers so that they can avoid activities which are likely to produce frustration and anger. And I suppose that walking about, collecting stones and closely examining their colours and textures (which had become Malcolm's latest obsessive activity), is not usually on the menu. It raises questions about how to provide truly 'person-centred' care.

As the carer, I had been asked what Malcolm used to like doing – and painting came high on that list, so I am as much to blame as anyone. I also said he disliked dancing, explaining that it was as much as I could do to entice him onto the dance floor at PTA dances to saunter around for the last waltz. (Quote: 'Why would anyone compose a dance in three-time when you've only got two feet?'). But, one day, I arrived to pick him up from daycare to find him, with Alzheimer's having removed his inhibition, wiggling his bottom and disco dancing with the greatest of ease.

This was not the Malcolm I was accustomed to – but what a new delight and sensory pleasure for both of us! Perhaps the need to dance was always there, but his shyness prevented its expression? Who was the real Malcolm?

Then a dark shadow descended on this stage of the illness. Malcolm's speech became increasingly fractured and eventually collapsed into gobbledegook. His frustration and anger at not being able to communicate verbally his needs or wishes often erupted into physical violence. He broke windows, overturned furniture, pulled down curtains. I was seen as the author of all his problems; I had my hair pulled, face slapped, was held against a wall by my wrists in a vice-like grip or five fingernails dug into my arm, leaving bruises which lasted for weeks. For me, this was the most terrifying and shocking phase of the whole illness. Malcolm had always been gentle and peace-loving; he'd never laid a finger on me or the children. So where had the real Malcolm gone?

Was his dementia causing a fundamental change of personality? With 20/20 hindsight, I think not, for, as his insight receded further over three years, his usual patient, good-humoured nature returned. I believe his anger and violence came as a direct response to the inappropriate ways in which his professional caregivers sometimes treated him – those from an Agency who came to our home, some staff in daycare and respite – and I too was guilty. A very fine line exists between caring and controlling; not one of us would like to feel that we were losing our autonomy and that someone else was in control of our lives. But so often, carers of people with dementia take over and don't let the patient do things in their own time and in their own way; they can be bossy, talk patronizingly or loudly to them, make them do things they don't want to do. Down that road lies confrontation and loss of autonomy, respect and dignity. And if the patient can't find right words to protest, then challenging behaviour ensues. I learned eventually to Go With The Flow (e.g. not mind if he wanted to go to bed with his trousers on – there isn't a law against it), stop trying to make life 'normal', accept that things are never going to be the same again and if Malcolm could no longer enter our world, we had to enter his.

So this became another variation on 'Who is the real Malcolm?' Cognition gone, communication reduced to the non-verbal, aggressive responses, functions diminishing, those 'layers' were being stripped away and the emotional and sensory layers took on an even greater importance and intensity. Sounds (music, birdsong, voices and laughter), aromas, taste, colours and shapes (especially in nature), seeing smiley faces, touch (hugs, cuddles and holding hands – no political correctness here, thank goodness) and walking about became his whole world. His emotions were heightened – easily moved to laughter or tears, and, above all, he needed to feel safe.

It was at this point that going away to daycare or respite became a problem, for he always came back in a worse physical and psychological state than when he went away. We need to recognize that people with dementia reach a point (probably in this emotional/sensory phase) when they do not feel safe anywhere other than in the familiarity of their own home. Would you send your three-year-old to strangers for a week? That's what it must feel like for a person with moderate to severe dementia.

And there is a further consideration. Malcolm had never been a hearty joiner-in – he had preferred solitary pursuits, such as playing the piano or reading – so sending him away to unfamiliar environments and people (for no way would he remember that he'd been there the week before) to join in with communal activities created a double whammy. Again, the need for providers to take into account the psychological profile of a person becomes paramount. Yet I needed a break, and so argued at length with officialdom for respite at home with a familiar carer replacing me for a few days. This has worked superbly well for both of us – a good example of what is good for the patient being also good for the carer. Paying attention to the deeper, psychological needs of the patient – beyond the physical tasks – results in quality care. But is spirituality something even deeper than respecting the psychological, sensory and emotional layer?

Malcolm lost his mobility at the end of 2001, followed by a slow and inevitable further decline. He is now as helpless as a small baby. Mute (except for little whimpers) and unable to understand what is said to him, immobile, unable to process what he sees, doubly incontinent, subject to fits and myoclonic jerking (i.e. large involuntary movements of limbs), he is totally dependent on others to sustain and nurture him. All the autonomic functions we take for granted are also failing – such as temperature control, swallowing and peristalsis. It takes an hour to patiently feed him a small bowl of pureed food and a mug of thickened drink, a teaspoonful at a time. He is unable to smile or show emotion (except a little kicking when distressed) but that doesn't mean he can't feel the full range of emotions.

So, to return to the initial question: beneath all the disabilities of this ravaging illness, is the same Malcolm still in there? I believe the essential Malcolm is indeed still there. It can be seen in his patience and serenity, in his abiding passion for music (he turns his head slightly towards the source of the sound, and a tear will roll down his face when a favourite piece is played) and in his eyes when kindly people talk or touch his hands. Even his mischievous, subversive sense of humour will out: while being fed, he will lift an eyebrow, look his favourite carer straight in the eye and thwart her by clamping his teeth on the spoon for no good reason. But people who visit see only a man shattered, physically and mentally, and many gently ask why we strive to keep him alive.

When I asked his consultant why Malcolm is living way beyond all prognoses, he replied that it was continuity of care personnel (I no longer use agency carers, but choose and employ the team of carers directly), a tranquil environment and quality one-to-one physical and psychological care. Malcolm, above all, feels safe, has nothing to alarm him, so he can put all his energies into just living. While I would agree with that, as hallmarks of care to aim for in any setting, there is something else underpinning our care for him.

Malcolm is surrounded by love. We reach out to communicate with him at a profound level – often through eye contact and gentle whispering and touch – and from him there flows a deep childlike trust, luminosity and reciprocating love – as though it were his very self, the self he was born with, that we are privileged to glimpse. To me, and to close members of our family and the staff who help me care for him, it is beyond the solid physical world, beyond cognition, function, personality, senses and emotion, that the very essence of his being can be found. Does it matter what we call it – spirit, soul, inner self, essence, identity – so long as we have experienced it?

I have come to realize that despite all Malcolm's obvious mental and physical attrition, his spirit still shines through. Several of his carers have remarked upon Malcolm still 'being there'; we all lack the vocabulary to talk quasi-scientifically, or even anecdotally, about it, but it is strongly felt. So the search for spirituality and the real Malcolm ends here – in the revelation of his essential self because of the loving care he receives and the trust that it engenders.

As for me, it can only stiffen my determination to strive for quality of life and quality of dying for my husband. And amazingly, Malcolm is equally sensitive to me if I'm not feeling well, or trying to deal with a crisis – I can tell from his eyes and feel a psychic connection. To stand stripped of everything the world values and to see each other as we really are is a very precious and humbling experience, and one which I would never have encountered were it not for the ravages of dementia. Paradoxically, Malcolm's 'losses' have turned into 'gains'.

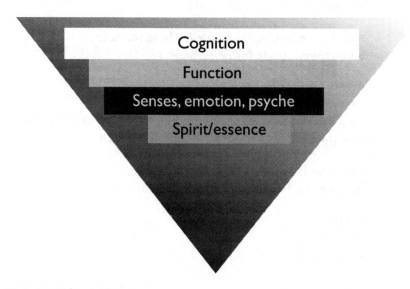

Figure 8.1 Who am I?

So I am left with an inverted pyramidal model to answer the question, 'Who am I?' (or it could be represented as layers of a cut onion, in concentric circles if I only knew how to do it on the computer!)

The top layers are the most complex layers of our selfhood, and as they peel away, changes take place in the person with dementia, gradually revealing the quintessential, simpler and deeper layers, until the essence of the person is reached.

A final thought. Is it possible to experience spirituality without a religious belief system? Malcolm and I began as fervent Christians (Methodists), but over the years learned about other religions and moved away from organized religion of any kind. Yet the one factor which unites all major religious beliefs is love. So where there is love (agape, compassion, empathy...) offered to the sick person by whoever cares for them, with or without a religious belief system, spirituality, in its broadest sense, may be recognized and nurtured. And that way leads to quality of care and quality of life for both the person with dementia and their family carer.

To Malcolm

You weren't always like this.

Your hands lie still and limp,
Yet once those fingers flew over the piano keys.

Your eyes stare vacantly ahead,
Yet once you saw pictures in the clouds.

Your legs twitch, dangling useless from the hoist,
Yet once you strode for miles, untiring.

Your voice is silenced.

Yet once, you handled words with mastery – for the BBC, for your students, for the drama group, ad infinitum.

Your arms have lost their strength,
Yet once you held me in passionate embraces.

But you
Are still you
And I will love you – always.

Barbara Pointon, 2004

CHAPTER 9

A CHAPLAIN'S OWN STORY

Paul Chapple

What am I?

'This baby's perished nurse; put it away'. So begins my own story at a hospital in northeast England during the second world war. I was 'put away' without washing or feeding. That could have been the end of my story except, for some reason, I was still alive some hours after my birth and was thus accepted by humankind as a person. Is this what constitutes a person – a collection of functioning organs bounded by skin as the defining organ?

> How we reflect upon and define ourselves is determined and constrained by the structures of knowing available to us. (Parker, Georgaca, Harper *et al.* 1995, cited in House 2001, p.110)

> We are the hollow men
> We are the stuffed men
> Leaning together
> Headpiece filled with straw.

> from '*The Hollow Men*', T.S. Eliot (1963):
> *Collected Poems 1909–1962.*

The composer of these lines had drawn from scenes in his own life (Gordon 1998, p.169) to write *The Waste Land* which he finished in 1922. While coping with the stress of an increasingly difficult marriage in England in the context of an unhappy family background in his native America, his father died in 1919. He then had to cope with the severe illness of his father-in-law in 1920 followed by his wife's breakdown.

My nerves are bad tonight. Yes bad. Stay with me.
Speak to me. Why do you never speak. Speak.

from 'The Waste Land', T.S. Eliot (1963): *Collected Poems 1909–1962.*

'Eliot began to see there would be no end to domestic crises' (Gordon (1998, p.168). According to this biographer Eliot experienced his own 'breakdown' in 1921 after a traumatic visit from his mother, sister, and brother (ibid, p.170). When contemporary commentators interpreted *The Waste Land* as a depiction of contemporary life in the wasteland of Western culture, 'Eliot was moved to issue a disclaimer of his poem as a social critique: "To me it was only the relief of a personal and wholly insignificant grouse against life"...a statement of the poet's self' (Schimmel 2002, p.388). Trosman (1974, p.712) reports that 'the predominant symptom complex was depression with exhaustion, indecisiveness, hypochondriasis, and a fear of psychosis'.

Eliot, although experiencing mental health problems, was already much acclaimed by the world at large as a poet. Which was his defining personality?

My personal experience of mental health problems occurred when I was aged about 30 and went through a period of depression. That this period was short and not repeated, I feel was through effective prescribing, a powerful application of the Judaeo/Christian scriptures, and through prayer, though not necessarily in that order! As a troubled teenager, during a time of acute anxiety I had urgently called on the name of Jesus and thus experienced a period of what I can only call absolute peace. The background fall-out from this experience has lived with me as I continue to trust him daily as God for life now and forever.

My own story centres on Jesus, but through my life I have enjoyed friendships with those I have valued from various faiths and, indeed none. Friends from other faiths were mainly colleagues working in hospitals further south; as one moves nearer the Scottish Border the population density generally reduces and the specific influence of Celtic Christianity still prevails! However, my colleagues and I have designed the chapel of our new hospital, which opened this year, to be without religious symbols, simply a space where anyone should feel comfortable to express their own spirituality.

Eliot consulted a neurologist (Schimmel 2002) or a nerve specialist (Gordon 1998) who made a diagnosis of 'nerves' and prescribed three months' rest. This prescription was dispensed over several weeks at Margate after which Eliot was no better and decided to see a psychiatrist, Dr Roger Vittoz of Lausanne, recommended by Julian Huxley (among others), an ex-patient of his. Eliot felt he was not suffering from 'nerves' or insanity but from 'psychological troubles' which, he felt, English doctors did not acknowledge (Gordon 1998).

From being very young I had a fear of hospitals and it came rather as a surprise to find myself working in a large city general hospital in 1964 as a pharmacy graduate, fulfilling my pre-registration training requirements before being accepted onto the register of the Royal Pharmaceutical Society of Great Britain. Is this how I would now define myself – as a pharmacist? As I began my career in 1965, T.S. Eliot finished his – or did he?

Where am I?

Shortly after my episode of depression I applied for the position of Chief Pharmacist in a specialist mental health hospital where I have now worked for 32 years. My own crisis experience had made me aware of the potential relationship between spirituality and recovery from mental health problems and I soon found opportunities for this to be demonstrated.

Because of my own experience I wondered if inpatients would be interested in being part of a self-help group where we could explore our spirituality in an informal, relaxed environment. This 'Hospital Christian Fellowship' has met regularly since then and many have claimed to be helped through the group meetings, some coming to faith in Jesus. Indeed medical and nursing colleagues and other professionals have seen improvements in their patients and often encourage them to attend.

The last part of The Waste Land – What the Thunder Said – was written in Lausanne at the end of 1921; here the thunder prompts the speaker to put a psychological waste behind him (Gordon 1998, p.185). This biographer records, however, that, despite a temporary calmness (Ackroyd 1984, cited in Schimmel 2002, p.391), when back in London in 1922 Eliot complained of being sick, miserable and excessively depressed (Gordon 1998, p.188). Between 1923 and 1925 when his marriage was in crisis, he began abusing alcohol, and one day Virginia Woolf and her sister found him in a state of collapse in his flat (Gordon 1998, p.207). In 1925 Eliot wrote The Hollow Men where he pictured himself as an effigy filled with straw:

> Shape without form, shade without colour,
> Paralysed force, gesture without motion.

> from 'The Hollow Men', T.S . Eliot (1963):
> Collected Poems 1909–1962.

At the Monday night meeting I met a man aged about 30 who introduced himself: 'I'm Robert; I'm schizophrenic.'

'Psychiatric patients, through the course of repeated assessments, come increasingly to define their experiences in accordance with a professional definition of "psychiatric illness"' (Parker *et al.* 1995, p89. cited in House 2001, p.110).

Robert further defined himself as a graduate computer programmer who had suffered his first episode of schizophrenia while experiencing a particular busy patch in his job and had been admitted to hospital under a section of the Mental Health Act.

What am I becoming?

'If a new life is to come into being the old must be washed, or more appropriately, burnt away' (Gordon 1998, p.210). Eliot's biographer sees the last part of *The Hollow Men* as a prologue to Eliot's religious conversion where he tries to pray but fails. This author believes that Eliot's entry into the Church of England in 1927 was brought about by rational progress:

> by rejection and elimination, until he finds a satisfactory explanation both for the disordered world without and the moral world within... It seems that at this time he felt no fervour, and was driven to the Church almost as a last resort. (Gordon 1998, p.211)

For Eliot, this drive began with 'a sense of "the disorder, the futility, the meaninglessness, the mystery of life and suffering"' (ibid p.64).

Eliot had been brought up in a church-going family but Gordon (1998) records that 'by the time he enrolled at Harvard he had become indifferent to the Church... With Unitarian scorn for evangelical enthusiasm, his grandfather said that educated, practical people reject "sudden miraculous conversion, wrought by divine power, independently of the human will"' (p.18).

Schimmel (2000) interprets Eliot's conversion as an attempt to 'shore up the ruin of himself' by 'the redemption and security offered in a relationship with the spiritual' (p.393). Trosman (1977, p.303, cited in Schimmel 2000) understood that Eliot 'turned more and more to a system of beliefs which would make intelligible his inner turmoil and provide the sense of unity he so sorely lacked.'

Until the day of his death in 1965 he remained committed to the church with its external ordinances but also to his very personal religion. '...he said that his religious life was "the whole of me, yet too many people think it is irrelevant"' (Gordon 1998).

Though I was practising pharmacy full-time from 1965, after I special-ized in psychiatric practise I often wished for time to spend with patients. The Monday meeting demonstrated the usefulness of the spiritual compo-nent to patients but when invited, I found it difficult to visit. In 2000, just before my 58th birthday, I welcomed the new millennium from my bed as I struggled with pneumonia. I was away from work for two weeks and had time to reassess my life and I found myself asking God to make the rest of my life really count for him. I was rather shocked when he seemed to be telling me to give up full-time pharmacy and become a Hospital Chaplain. I was not an ordained minister and I wondered where to start.

When I returned to work my secretary had dealt with the mail and left me the usual pile to work through. I began with the largest piece of mail, a portfolio of postgraduate courses from the University of Leeds. When I turned the pages at random I was amazed when the folder fell open first at a course entitled 'MA in Healthcare Chaplaincy'. I started there! I had every cooperation from my Trust Board of Directors and from the existing chap-laincy team at my own hospital. They were all clergy who were responsible for their own large churches in the community and found the chaplaincy work difficult to perform to their satisfaction. They very kindly welcomed me to the team and I became part-time resident chaplain and part-time pharmacist.

Am I alone?

I could now spend time with Robert. I found that he had been taken to church as a child as part of his upper middle-class background. His church attendance had lapsed while at public school and university but, now in hos-pital, he felt drawn to be part of the Christian group activity which was held from time to time on his ward. Activities included open discussion of spiritu-ality and prayer. I have found that while many people would not claim to be 'religious' many are happy to be prayed with or for.

One of the most ancient quotes concerning the association between mental health and religion must be that from the writings of the 16th-century mystic and monk St John of the Cross: 'He's just mad: take care of him and keep him safe in prayer' (Carr 2000).

All we know about this patient is that he was diagnosed 'mad' by St John. Religion in this case was good for the patient since it provided a place of refuge – a hospital – where he could receive care. It is worth noting that it was the safety of the patient that seemed paramount rather than that of the community. Finally, the importance accorded to prayer in this case should be noted.

I was asked to see Stephen, a newly admitted 19-year-old apparently experiencing a first episode of psychosis. He was anxious that he had been having increasing thoughts about 'God'. Being brought up in a hard-working family where the word did not have a religious meaning, Stephen had become convinced he was 'going mental'. After several sessions together, Stephen became open to the possibility of the existence of a transcendent 'higher power' who could also draw near to him. His anxiety appeared to be relieved and he was discharged.

'Success' in chaplaincy terms is hard to define. One weekend I was called in as a pharmacist to see a 30-year-old lady admitted on a complex medication regimen. Once a successful nurse, Tracy had been suffering from an organic syndrome for two years including muscle weakness and severe pain. She was admitted because she had become clinically depressed and had tried to take her own life; she asked me to continue seeing her but as chaplain. I soon discovered that she had a strict religious family background but had rejected the notion of 'God' after her father had died. Tracy laid down the ground rules: no God talk, no prayer, no religious stuff. She continued to want to see me for the whole of her stay since she did not regard me as a health professional; of all such she was consistently suspicious. Hardly ever leaving her room, her mood swung unpredictably, and all I could do was be there. Her consultant very reluctantly agreed to her discharge two years later when she went back to home alone. I received a very emotional letter of thanks from Tracy but she is one of many who need and accept support without tangible improvement.

As a pharmacist I do have some sympathy with the much-despised 'medical model'. I sometimes tell my colleagues practising in psychological therapies that, on occasions, before they can begin it may be necessary to use drug therapy to help a patient move to a more responsive position. This, to me, does not conflict with my belief in a God who hears and answers prayer. I sometimes pray that he would guide my medical colleagues to the choice of best treatment and I see this happening with my patients.

Over the course of two years Robert became well enough to be discharged to his own home where he now lives alone. Just prior to this he had requested to be part of a course being held in a nearby village where about 30 people were exploring the Christian faith. He became friendly with someone the course and on discharge began attending the Anglican church in that village. Robert is now once again active in the community using his IT skills.

Where am I going?

Barker (1999, p.89) looks back to Celtic monks 'who learned how to *be* with people in mental distress a thousand years ago' (his italics). He also refers to Frankl (1999, p.41) a Jewish Viennese psychiatrist who suffered in the Nazi concentration camps. Frankl defined spirituality as 'the meanings which people give to the experiences in their lives'. Can this be one of 'the structures of knowing' mentioned above?

   Barker submitted a research proposal which included asking mentally ill people to describe the human significance of their illness. His submission was rejected because 'we would likely only obtain people with religious fixations'. This upset Barker because he had used Frankl's definition to emphasize a secular view of spirituality. However, he acknowledges in his book (1999, p.42) that Frankl was at pains to emphasize his belief in God and was not another Freud, a 'godless Jew' (Frankl 1973).

   'Gold standard' evidence databases for the National Health Service in the UK are found in the Cochrane Library named after Professor Archie Cochrane (1909–1988), the Scottish medical researcher. He was a prisoner of war from 1941 to 1945, where as well as having to perform as doctor to his fellow prisoners he also had to act as priest. Having virtually no medicines and little clinical experience he eventually had to agree with the German commander who stated that 'doctors are superfluous'. He tells of the admission of a Soviet prisoner screaming in agony. He could neither speak with him or help him medically, but eventually simply took him in his arms whereupon the screaming stopped (Cochrane and Blythe 1989). Medical practice was of marginal benefit but the application of love worked.

   My own qualitative study was with a group of volunteers, all of whom had suffered from mental health problems for several years. Some had a religious faith (all Christian) and others had none. Several themes emerged from those with a faith in Jesus:

- 'When you feel at a low ebb, the first thing you do is pray' – prayer to God was central to this group. It was purely individual and expressed a personal reliance on God. Feelings of the nearness of God varied, sometimes with mood, but to believe he was available was important and this was a main means of promoting mental health.

- 'I walk hand in hand with God' – the concept of being on a journey was important. Even if prayer was difficult the sense of his presence was valued. The companionship, through mental illness, of someone each called 'God' was valued and seemed integral to health.

- 'My faith goes on just the same, even though a bit ragged when I'm ill' – a personal faith was important to all. This was not expressed in any stereotypical way. Sometimes it was the result of an experience: 'Having that experience I couldn't doubt God at all, but when I was going through terrible experiences... I wondered what it was all about.' This faith or trust in God was something intrinsic to each interviewee and seemed vital to their psychic survival.

- 'I have a God... And a warm, loving God'. This was the kind of God experienced generally by the group even though they had all suffered greatly in their lives. Interviewees did not blame God for their illness, but depended on a relationship with him to experience a deep, healing love.

- 'I occasionally have a little chat. I just ask him for simple things and remember to thank him afterwards. It's that leper story isn't it?' – The quality of the faith of the group is in evidence here: it is never deeply theological but very practical – 'My belief in God has helped in every way all the time' – it is profound but accessible. Each one expected God to help and claimed to receive his help.

The conditions of my study included complete confidentiality and I discovered that despite the value placed upon a personal faith not one interviewee felt able to discuss it with other people, not even a partner, and certainly not with a health professional. One of the group confided: 'I do remember the social worker I have at the moment saying "It's a load of rubbish!" so I don't mention it to anyone now. It's such a fundamental thing to people – the soul and heart of people.' One hospital patient told me that the stigma that came with mental illness was bad enough without being branded a religious nut!

Maybe this is one reason for the growth of Buddhism in the West – a way of life independent of religious faith. Carly followed the Buddhist way. She had become mentally unwell and was admitted to hospital. With a Buddhist acceptance of suffering, physical and mental, she was uncomplaining but withdrawn. However, she was drawn into the Monday evening fellowship by the sound of music (as I would learn later Carly loved singing). I discovered over the two years she was an inpatient that she had been satisfied with her Buddhist tradition, but she now wanted to explore the Christian faith.

In my work, although I am committed personally to Jesus Christ, I undertake not to impose my beliefs on those of other faiths or none. In the time leading up to Carly's discharge I therefore instructed her only in the direct teaching of Jesus as recorded in the accounts of the gospel writers in the Bible, rather than my own interpretation and understanding of the faith. She appreciated our sessions and claimed that they had helped her.

What is my story?

T.S. Eliot's biographer describes Eliot's religion as involving 'a God of pain, whose punishment until the last eight years (when he remarried), was almost the only sign of the absolute paternal care' (Gordon 1998, p.534).

If this is the case, the biographer for some reason ceases to continue to emphasize Eliot's mental suffering as he had done prior to his conversion. The sudden lack of this emphasis would appear to indicate that Eliot's quality of life changed at that point. His marriage and other relationships continued to cause him major difficulties but the symptoms of mental illness seem to have all but disappeared.

Gordon concedes that 'He certainly knew, after his conversion, moments of bliss; he did, late in life, meet the comforting face of his faith' (ibid p.535).

> Because I cannot hope to turn again
> Consequently I rejoice, having to construct something
> Upon which to rejoice
> And pray to God to have mercy upon us
> And I pray that I may forget
> These matters that with myself I too much discuss
> Too much explain
> Because I do not hope to turn again.

These lines from *Ash-Wednesday* (Eliot 1963), written in 1930, demonstrate the hope that he has found in his new-found religion. When Eliot married again 30 years after his conversion this was 'the second turning point' (Schimmel 2002, p.396), leading to 'the last eight years' of his life.

Recently some chaplaincy colleagues and I have been spending some time publicizing the training resource *Promoting Mental Health: A Resource for Spiritual and Pastoral Care* published jointly by The Church of England, the charity Mentality, and the National Institute for Mental Health in England (C of E, Mentality, and NIMHE 2004). I have found the resource useful myself in local churches where I have found knowledge of mental health matters to be on a par with that of the general population. Because of the evidence from many studies, including those carried out by the Mental Health Foundation (2000 and 2002), as well as my own, I am convinced there is a positive link between a person's spirituality and her/his good mental health. I believe, therefore, that faith communities need training on mental health issues. When I have provided the training myself, Robert has sometimes accompanied me and been able to effectively field questions from course members.

So, how to define Robert, T.S. Eliot, and myself? As the obstetrician was verbally signing my death certificate 65 years ago, Eliot was completing his third quartet:

> The hint half guessed, the gift half understood, is Incarnation.
> Here the impossible union
> Of spheres of existence is actual,
> Here the past and future
> Are conquered, and reconciled.

The Dry Salvages (Eliot 1963) expresses our faith in 'The God he (Eliot) needed, on whom he could lean his whole weight, … God who had become man, an infinitely gentle, infinitely suffering incarnate thing, recognizably human, unknowably divine' (Matthews 1974).

We surely emerge as persons in our own right without an identity crisis. We have come to know that our creator God revealed in Jesus loves us just as we are and this fulfils our humanity. Restored to his image, we are free to use our renewed self-will to make choices. These choices and their results may lead us into stressful situations maybe issuing in mental health problems, but these need not have overwhelming pathological consequences. I am not 'a depressive'. Robert should not be labelled 'a schizophrenic'. T.S. Eliot will always be celebrated as a poet but, should the value of his work ever be assessed negatively he, with us, will still have made his mark on this earth. 'God has accepted him. Who are you to judge someone else's servant? To his own master he stands or falls. And he will stand, for the Lord is able to make him stand' (The Holy Bible, New International Version, Romans 14: 3–4).

References

Ackroyd, P. (1984) *T.S. Eliot.* London: Hamish Hamilton.

Barker, P.J. (1999) *The Philosophy and Practice of Psychiatric Nursing.* Edinburgh: Churchill.

Carr, W. (2000) 'Some reflections on spirituality, religion, and mental health.' *Mental Health, Religion, and Culture 3*, 1, 1–12.

Church of England, Mentality, and the National Institute for Mental Health in England (2004) *Promoting Mental Health: A Resource for Spiritual and Pastoral Care.* Available at www.mentality.org.uk, www.nimhe.org.uk and www.cofe.anglican.org (accessed 20 September 2007).

Cochrane, A.L. and Blythe, M. (1989) 'One man's medicine.' *Why the Cochrane Collaboration?* London: British Medical Journal Memoir Club. Available at www.cochrane.org/cochrane/archieco.htm (accessed 4 October 2007).

Eliot, T.S. (1963) *Collected Poems 1909–1962.* London: Faber and Faber Limited.

Frankl, V. (1973) *The Doctor and the Soul: From Psychotherapy to Logotherapy.* Harmondsworth: Pelican.

Gordon, L. (1998) *T.S. Eliot: An Imperfect Life.* London: Vintage.

Holy Bible, New International Version. Copyright © 1973, 1978, 1984 by International Bible Society, Guildford.

House, R. (2001) 'Psychopathology, Psychosis and the Kundalini: Postmodern Perspectives on Unusual Subjective Experience.' In I. Clarke (ed.) *Psychosis and Spirituality – Exploring the New Frontier.* London: Whurr.

Matthews, T.S. (1974) *Great Tom – Notes Towards the Definition of T.S. Eliot.* London: Weidenfeld and Nicolson.

Mental Health Foundation (2000) *Strategies for Living.* London: Mental Health Foundation.

Mental Health Foundation (2002) *Taken Seriously: The Somerset Spirituality Project.* London: Mental Health Foundation.

Parker, I., Georgaca, E. and Harper, D. *et al.* (1995) *Deconstructing Psychopathology.* London: Sage.

Schimmel, P. (2002) '"In my end is my beginning": T.S. Eliot's The Waste Land and After.' *British Journal of Psychotherapy 18,* 3, 381–99.

Trosman, H. (1974) 'T.S. Eliot and The Waste Land: psychopathological antecedents and transformations.' *Archives of General Psychiatry 30,* 5, 709–717.

Trosman, H. (1977) 'After The Waste Land: psychological factors in the religious conversion of T.S. Eliot.' *International Review of Psycho-Analysis 4,* 295–304.

Reflection: Rituals and Recovery – Sacrament and Smoking Room in a Mental Health Acute Unit
Christopher Newell

I have recently spent time as a patient in an acute mental health unit. When I am well, I work as a mental health chaplain both in the community and in acute units so I have had the opportunity, over a number of years of exploring the uncertain boundaries between psychosis and spirituality, madness and sanity, the sacred and the profane. One of the most fascinating areas of this personal exploration is how important the experience of private and communal rituals is in the way we confront and manage our mental health issues and problems and in the way we re-integrate them into our sense of personal self and common humanity.

We can easily make the mistake of relegating the idea of ritual behaviour purely to the religious realm. The very activity of being human and engaging both individually and corporately in the myriad human activities involve the actions of unique rituals, the way of doing things, of establishing patterns and rhythms special to that particular activity, that particular social group. There are rituals in family relationships in the way we engage in sport and cultural activities, even in the way we shop. Just look at a supermarket car park on a Sunday morning; the social ritual of the weekly family shop has largely, for many, replaced the sacramental ritual of church attendance.

I must add, however, that the experience of receiving Holy Communion while I was in hospital was one of the most deeply moving encounters with a religious act which offered, for me, a way of communicating with the transcendent truths at a time when I was finding it hard to be in touch with myself. So, I am not in any way seeking to devalue the religious significance of rituals in hospital that offer such encounters.

We can also make the mistake of seeing social rituals as having largely replaced the idea of the sacred, an idea that remains implicit in activities beyond the narrow definition of the religious, of an act of reflection and communion that makes sense of who we are in relationship to the world around us, to the people we love, to those deeper, transcendent truths I mentioned earlier. This is the area I wish to briefly explore in relationship to the sacrament of the smoking room and how, in the laudable interests of health, we might be in danger of losing something rather special and irreplaceable.

Consider the act of rolling a cigarette. What do you need? Well you require a comfortable place to sit, a place to put the paraphernalia of the rolling baccy process: the baccy itself, the ciggy papers, the filters (an optional extra), and the lighter (if you are allowed one). The other important ingredient, particularly if your hands are unsteady, through the anxiety or the effects of medication, is a helping hand, a friend to participate in the ritual. Indeed, if you have not been able to leave the ward, the gift of some baccy itself may be needed.

So here are the elements of a ritualistic process which has within it its own regular determined pattern, its own symbolism and imagery, its own need to take place at particular times. How often, after what has felt like a gruelling ward round or particular times of stress and anxiety, there has been the overwhelming desire to enter the 'sacred' room and perform the 'sacred' act and, in the process, share, in contemplation, with yourself or with others, your own thoughts and reflections. How often, when sleep has been hard to find at 3 a.m., do we find fellow travellers in that smoking room and share cups of tea and the rolling of a fag and in that sharing rediscover a little of ourselves.

At times like these, there is no other place to be and nothing more important to do. It feels like, it looks like, it is an act of the deepest communion. Burnt cigarette marks on the carpet, and stray strands of tobacco and scattered cigarette paper packets reveal the purpose of this 'sacred space' as profoundly as icons and candles do a chapel. The ritual of the act of rolling a ciggy can, like the most sacramental of religious rituals, be deeply nurturing an act of profound significance and meaning. It can, for a few contemplative seconds, seek to make sense, both personally and communally, of a human life lived for a time in the context of an acute mental health unit, a context which, often, finds it hard to provide such moments of reflection, meditation and contemplation. This can be particularly true of psychiatric intensive care and forensic units. It can do what all ritual practices help us do, provide a deep, transcendent sense of our personal and communal humanity, a humanity which is sometimes hard to discover in ourselves and others when we find ourselves in profound emotional and mental crisis.

The smoking room, however, for the best of health reasons, is a doomed space in our mental health hospitals as it has become in our general hospitals. The unit at which recently I was a patient, provided the smallest of 'pods' at the end of each bay, barely large enough for two people to sit. The only other alternative was to brave the freezing weather and smoke outside in the garden, reducing the act of smoking to its barest essentials. I say all this as a committed former smoker who finds himself approving of the soon to be enforced ban on smoking in public places but, at the same time, deeply worried about the implications for those who find themselves needing to stay in a mental health unit, where, it is said, over 70 per cent of patients may be smokers. As I have tried to explain, it is the nurturing, self-motivated, reflective ritual of a particular practice of smoking, the process of rolling your own, or rolling someone else's own, which we are in danger of losing and I am not sure any other human act could replace it.

So I make perhaps a forlorn plea for those concerned with the holistic care of people in our mental health units, concerned with their spirituality and humanity, not to dismiss the value of the smoking space, a value often unseen and unregarded, but profoundly sacred in the strangest, mysterious but most human of ways.

CHAPTER 10

KEEP UP YOUR SPIRITS: RUN FOR YOUR LIFE! A VIEW OF RUNNING AS A SPIRITUAL EXPERIENCE

Peter Gilbert

Breathing in, breathing out, air into the lungs, breath of life; feet, legs, body frame, eyes, mind, spirit, heart and body, all connected. I notice the sights, smells, sounds, sensations of my surroundings as I run, with a group of companions, down the Worcester Canal; round Diglis canal basin and its sign displaying the locks to Tewkesbury and Birmingham; over the bridge, past the imposing 13th-century Cathedral of St Oswald; and up towards the Old Bridge where a rowing eight is shooting the arches, scattering swans as it goes. We double back to the tail-enders, as the proud boast of Worcester Joggers is that 'we don't leave anybody behind', and I look into the faces of my community: Ruth, Ali, Mike, Vicki, Charlie, Jo and others. Some are wearing shirts displaying the races they have run as badges of honour: Pat with his bright 'Sodbury Slog' emblem, and Teri with her 'Race the Horse' (don't ask!).

I feel inspirited by the physical sensation of running, the connection with nature and the buildings of an ancient city, and the company. I am also inspired by old friends and new ones, the telling of jokes, mutual support, the sharing of news and problems, the encouragement to push oneself that bit further, and also the non-talking, the ability to run with people but to be within one's own head and thoughts and feelings – solitary, but not lonely. As we pause to cross the bridge, I mention this article to 'Gary', who tells me that he had depression, when work pressures, moving house and the birth of a new child pushed him into an unfamiliar zone, where a combination of a sympathetic GP, anti-depressants, good friends and running kept him going, and eventually lifted him again. I am constantly stirred by the number of runners who say to me that they have experienced an episode(s) of mental distress at some stage of their lives, and that running has helped them to recover and thrive.

As we run over the bridge, down the Riverside Promenade, with its flower baskets and towards the park, a group of youngsters remark that we must be '****ing mad!' Of course, a few years ago, that's exactly what I was, but I need to go back a bit.

I had an idyllic childhood, growing up on the island of Jersey. A major turning point in my life came when I was sent away to boarding school at the age of eight. I can't think of much good that came out of it except that it gave me, when I was a Childcare Social Worker, an empathy with kids who were removed from home. One of the problems that remains from those years, is the little voice that comes into my head when things get tough, and tells me what the teachers at that boarding school used to say: 'You'll never achieve anything.'

Talking with a variety of people over the years, I realize just how prevalent the problems caused by these childhood voices are. One of the benefits of any strenuous exercise is that it clears your head of pressures, and negative thoughts, and tends to refresh you. As a Social Worker with 13 years' direct practice, I found running a great release. Speaking with a new runner this week, she remarked simply: 'Running keeps me sane.'

Now, from preserving sanity to recovering from mental illness. In 1997 I went from Staffordshire to Worcestershire to become Director of Social Services of a new (post local government reorganization) department. I had been warned that there would be problems with particular people, and that it had gone through a series of financial crises over at least the last 10 years. Having to take 7 per cent in the first year, out of a budget which was already a 'busted flush', created inevitable problems three years down the line. What happened left me with an abiding sense of what ethical, value-based leadership is and what it isn't (Gilbert 2005). I found that trying to do the impossible meant I got into a pattern of sleeping about 2 hours a night, losing 2 lb a day, and finally ending up in my GP's surgery. Her response was human, direct and very reassuring: 'This is shit!', she proclaimed angrily, 'they are using you as a scapegoat.' I spent six months off sick with depression and I feel myself very fortunate to have survived, and even more fortunate to be in a valued work role again.

What helped me were a number of factors. Firstly, I had a good GP, who, while she recommended anti-depressants, gave me some measure of control. Initially I was very reluctant to accept her prescription, but, I have to say that it was extremely helpful, had minimal side effects, and certainly assisted my recovery. I was also fortunate to have a place of spiritual asylum – Worth Abbey (BBC2's *The Monastery*, May 2005); a friend who was able to absorb both my sadness and my anger (because I was certainly 'mad' in a different way!); *real* leaders, like Professor Antony Sheehan, who welcomed me back into the world of work; a friend who had been through a similar experience and *understood*; and my running club, Worcester Joggers.[1]

In 2005 The Mental Health Foundation brought out its report on the benefits of exercise in mental health: *Up and Running?* (MHF 2005). The research found that 55 per cent of GPs commonly prescribed anti-depressants as their first treatment response to mild or moderate depression, while only 35 per cent believed that this was the most effective strategy (p.18). The Foundation points out that there are many advantages of exercise therapy, and these can act in four main ways:

- *Biological / chemical* – through the increased release of endorphins and encephalins (Burfoot 2005).

- *Social* – exercise enables people to build new social networks.

- *Esteem boosting* – the learning of new skills and achieving goals.

- *Distraction / flow* – moving away from the preoccupation with negative thoughts, and creating a more positive state of mind. (MHF 2005, pp.26–7).

The report makes the case for advantages flowing from the factors above: exercise is cost-effective; it has co-incidental benefits, and fewer potential side-effects than those of anti-depressants; it is an active, sustainable, recovery choice; and it is a 'normalizing' experience (see also Wolpert 2006).

There are inspiring stories, e.g. Laura Boswel (*Runner's World*, August 2004, pp.77–8): 'I'd liken it [depression] to a Victorian ghost story; you know something bad is lurking, but you don't know what. You just have a creeping dread.' Training for the London Marathon – she ran even though there were days 'when…I could hardly clean my teeth'. This accords very much with my experience, where I felt I was literally running to save my life. Although the Lofepramine helped enormously, there were days in the 'chasm' when I couldn't do anything, but would still get out and run.

Worcester Joggers (now an affiliated club: Black Pear Joggers) has existed as a relatively informal group of runners for many years, but in the last seven it has grown from about 20 to 100+ members. This seems to be partly due to people's desire to run as a social group. Because we found that

---

1   NB: Worcester Joggers are now an affiliated club, Black Pear Joggers, but retain their ethos of sociability and solidarity. They can be found at: www.blackpearjoggers.org.uk

so many people had experienced some form of mental distress, I conducted a small survey, and people were very open about what caused them distress:

'Stress caused by life!' as one put it. Many people had indeed experienced extreme mental unhappiness, and they explained how running helped. Bereavement, childhood experiences, relationship breakdown, children leaving home, stress from work, were all cited, in very moving ways:

> It was a celebration of life and good health. I was just so grateful my body worked. (Having cared for their partner who died from cancer)

> I became depressed and got to the point where I didn't want any contact with the outside world... I continued to run and became quite competitive, as this was my way of dealing with my anger. (After the break-up of a relationship)

> When I was extremely stressed at work and under a lot of pressure, running helped to make me forget work.

Running helped, especially running in a community, because as Professor Peter Beresford (2005) has remarked: 'The thing I fear most is still loneliness.' This was also outlined in the comments:

> Running puts people at the same level, irrespective of their professional status or standard of living. The club is like an extended family, sharing experiences and ideas, achievements and disappointments.

> It's preventative medicine.

> As a Christian, running seems to bring together the spiritual, mental and physical aspects of life. It is a wonderful way to enjoy God's creation.

> It can give you that space between a problem and a solution.

Interestingly, at least one person spoke of the wider issue of social responsibility:

> It is also extremely fulfilling when running to raise sponsorship money, as you feel you are putting something back into the world.

Yet again, for some people, it was just simply the sheer exhilaration of running:

> Running helps me connect with Nature. I enjoy MUD and lots of it, it's a kind of adventure!!

A recognition of the spiritual dimension of each individual is becoming increasingly prevalent in Western societies, despite the increased secularization and materialism. People often feel that they are just one more commodity, and that their value as human beings is often based purely on their financial ability to consume (see Moss 2005; Cox, Campbell and Fulford 2007; Mind in Croydon 2005; Gilbert 2006).

Spirituality and religion are not identical. As Stephen Wright puts it:

> Everybody is spiritual, but not everybody is religious. We all seek meaning, purpose, relationship and connectedness in life, but not everybody chooses to channel that quest through the more formal structure and belief system of a religion. (2005, p.3)

There are a huge number of definitions of spirituality, but these might involve: the essence of our humanness as unique individuals within a common humanity; what is deepest in us, inspiring us and giving us direction, especially at times of crisis; the human quest for meaning, purpose, identity, meaningful relationships, and a sense of the holy (see NIMHE/ MHF 2003, and Swinton 2001). Running as a spiritual experience can provide a sense of well-being; bring one closer to nature; stimulate a sense of beauty; and fosters community and solidarity. As the Joggers commented:

> Running helps me connect with myself when running on my own, or silently.

> As a group, running helps me make and connect with new friends and existing friends, as it gives me a common interest.

> It is a good reminder of what we are doing – living, rather than living to work.

Is it stretching a point too far to say that being a member of a running club has some aspects of religion? A definition of religion might be that it encompasses aspects of spirituality, usually in the context of belief in a transcendent being or beings. Religious faiths can provide a 'worldview', which is acted out in narrative, creeds, symbols, rites, rituals, sacraments and gatherings; and the promotion of ties of mutual obligation. It creates a framework within which people seek to understand and interpret and make sense of themselves, their lives and daily experiences – it provides a sense of identity.

It could be said that runners have a set of beliefs. There are a number of 'birth' runners, who started running on the beach with their parents; while there are also 'born again' runners, who only came to the activity late in the day, a 'Damascene experience' brought on by seeing oneself in the mirror (!), or hitting a crisis of health or meaning.

Club runners certainly have rituals. They gather on the club nights, and the gathering can seem like a church congregation, especially when the Chair of the Club welcomes people to the gathering, gives out the notices, and praises 'Sister Emma' and 'Brother Jim', who ran some muddy cross-country in some remote part of Worcestershire! The Joggers also head off for a monthly Club meal – usually at a Worcester Balti house.

We also have a strange coded language, while sacramental institutions may involve rites of passage, sharing a meal and also awards and prizes. Those who have dropped out through injury or lethargy, are welcomed back like those who repenteth!

My comments about the religious nature of running are only partly serious. However, there is no doubt that running not only has physical benefits, but the spiritual experience is one of being inspirited, solidarity with others, a sense of the sacred in nature and in people, and as one person put it, 'a sense of belonging'.

Acknowledgement

Reprinted by kind permission of *Openmind*.

References

Beresford, P. (2005) 'Solitary confinement.' *Community Care* June 2005, 16–22.

Burfoot, A. (2005) 'Does Runner's High exist?' *Runner's World*, May 2005.

Cox, J., Campbell, A. and Fulford, K.W.M. (2007) *Medicine of the Person: Faith, Values and Science in Health Care Provision*. London: Jessica Kingsley Publishers.

Gilbert, P. (2005) *Leadership: Being Effective and Remaining Human*. Lyme Regis: Russell House.

Gilbert, P. (2006) 'Breathing Space.' *Community Care* 19–25 January, 2006.

Hard to Believe, DVD, directed by Ben Hole. London: Mind in Croydon, 2005.

Mental Health Foundation (2005) *Up and Running: Exercise Therapy and the Treatment of Mild or Moderate Depression in Primary Care*. London: MHF.

Moss, B. (2005) *Religion and Spirituality*. Lyme Regis: Russell House.

NIMHE/The Mental Health Foundation (Gilbert, P. and Nicholls, V.) (2003) *Inspiring Hope*. Leeds: NIMHE.

Swinton, J. (2001) *Spirituality in Mental Health Care: Re-discovering a Forgotten Dimension*. London: Jessica Kingsley Publishers.

Wolpert, L. (2006) *Malignant Sadness: The Anatomy of Depression* (3rd edn) London: Faber and Faber.

Wright, S.G. (2005) *Reflections on Spirituality and Health*. London: Whurr.

The Guru's Prayer

Our Therapist, who writes self-help books,
Hallowed be thy bank balance.

Thy wisdom come, thy will be done
In our lives as it is in your imagination.

Give us this day our daily behaviour therapy
And forgive us our self-defeating behaviour patterns,
As we forgive those whom we try to blame
For all our problems.

Lead us not into introspection
But deliver us from denial.

For thine is the moral high ground,
The recognition
And the last word on all our lives
For ever and ever.

Same time next week then?

William Burt, February 2002

SECTION C
Good Practice

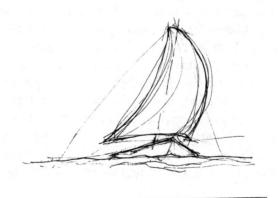

CHAPTER 11

SPIRITUAL ASSESSMENT – NARRATIVES AND RESPONSES

Wendy Edwards and Peter Gilbert

Wendy Edwards: Listen...

As a young child I became aware of the universal presence of God through nature and silence. I sometimes used to creep downstairs during the night and experience God pulsating through the cosmos. The vastness of the night sky filled with billions of stars would fill me with wonder and awe.

Like many children I went to Sunday school, although my parents did not go to church. At the age of seven I decided that Sunday school was a bit tame and I announced to my mother that I wanted to go to church. So, I started to attend the local Anglican Church. I was disappointed that I didn't experience God in the powerful way that I was used to. However, what I did find was an accepting congregation. Soon I was invited to join the choir and I was singing at both the morning and evening services every Sunday. I also joined the church youth club and learned bell ringing. I continued to seek out God in the countryside around me, the open spaces of the downs and the night sky.

My life wasn't completely dominated by church activities and I pursued other interests. I played hockey for the school from the age of 12, and also for a ladies team in a nearby town. I did actually play hockey for the local Methodist church! Being a sporty person I spent a lot of time on the playing fields, and on walking expeditions with the school rambling club. However, my relationship with God and my membership of the local church continued to be important, and when I left home for college and then employment, my Christian faith and membership of faith communities were central to my life.

As a teenager I felt called to the Religious Life which posed a problem for me as I didn't know that there were Anglican religious sisters (or men for that matter), and I knew that I couldn't become a Roman Catholic. I spoke with the local vicar about this and learned that there were actually quite a number of Anglican Religious Communities. However, I didn't think about it too much, but it kept niggling away. Also, as a teenager, I experienced moments of depression and suicidal feelings. In retrospect I think that the support of my church community and Christian teachers protected me from spiralling into a major mental health problem at that time of my life.

Eventually, I ended up in an Anglican religious community where I spent seven years. As a Novice, and when a sister in first vows, I worked in a number of parishes and found that I was an effective communicator. This led to invitations to lead retreats, speak to groups of all ages, but particularly teenagers, and preaching engagements. I also found myself being asked to put together liturgies for particular groups and occasions. Together with this I also led the life of a Religious with the round of five Offices, a daily Eucharist, private prayer and intercession, and spiritual reading. Then there was the cleaning, cooking, washing up and gardening duties. A busy life!

Increasingly, I was torn between a very active ministry and being led more and more into contemplation and intercession – time for the latter having to be found outside my community commitments and the time-consuming preparation for my 'outside' work. It was also a time of change in the Church, with feminist theology and the introduction of inclusive language, and the debate about the ordination of women to the priesthood. This cause tensions within the community, which also had to make a decision about leaving the huge 19th-century convent after around 100 years. There was a lot of turmoil going on. All of this was taking its toll on my spiritual and mental health. I knew something was very wrong, but I didn't know what. However, I was sure that the community was where God wanted me, and this was confirmed with my election to Life Profession.

A few weeks before I was due to make my Life Vows I had an accident. I went through a red light on my moped and collided with a car. Although I escaped with few injuries, except for the traumatic loss of a front tooth, I proceeded to have a complete breakdown. This led to me being asked to leave the community, which was heartbreaking. I was ill and couldn't understand what was happening to me, and I had lost my home, my sisters and friends, and my vocation. I didn't understand for many years that it was as much a spiritual breakdown as a mental one.

Since leaving the community, problems with my mental health persisted, as did my sense of dislocation from God and the Church. After well over 30 years of a God-filled life, God was absent. I was unable to go to church as it was too painful, and what was the point? I had periods of severe depression, which became prolonged, numerous suicide attempts and multiple admissions to a psychiatric hospital. My first overdose led to the loss of both my employment and my home, and I was discharged from my first hospital admission on to the streets, still not well.

Obviously, I have had many psychiatric assessments, *but nobody ever tried to listen to my story*. It was a matter of describing symptoms and ticking diagnostic boxes. I found inpatient psychiatric care dehumanizing and traumatic. I was locked into a dark, confusing abyss, and there seemed to be no one who could provide the key to help me, despite an understanding GP and regular visits by a succession of nice community psychiatric nurses. All meaning and hope in my life had disappeared and the psychiatric system seemed to reinforce my growing sense of hopelessness. I felt assigned to the scrap heap of society with no value whatsoever.

After a few years I was able to identify that I had spiritual issues that needed to be addressed, and a couple of years ago started to see a female chaplain, recently employed by the local Mental Health Trust, and I was able to begin to address some of these needs. I am gradually coming to terms with the rejection of the community and an unfulfilled vocation there. I have also found a local church, although there are still times when it is too painful to attend, and I have found peace and reconciliation with my former community. My relationship with the chaplain has helped me to feel more valued as a person, and I don't feel that I am being defined by my illness. It is not an easy journey; I still experience periods of depression and despair, and I still need the medication. It may not be the only key to my recovery, but it has been an important and effective one. I have someone who can accompany me, at least for now, somebody who sits alongside me and *listens*.

★ ★ ★

Assessment as dialogue and responses

How can we assess someone's needs if we don't know who they are, where they are coming from and where they think they are going to? How arrogant we must be, if we think we can 'know' someone and what they need without *getting to know* them – going on a journey with them. As Professor Kamlesh Patel, Chair of the Mental Health Act Commission, put it recently:

> If you don't know who I am, how are you going to provide a package of care for me to deliver something? When you do not know how important my religion is to me, what language I speak, where I am coming from, how are you going to help me cope with my mental illness? (Mulholland 2005, p.5. See also Chapter 1 of this book)

Even then, can we ever 'know' someone else? We can only express the desire that understanding and attention is important to us. Also, I need to be at ease and in touch with *my own* identity before I can engage with others. There have been many concerns expressed over the past few years, that while 'scientific positivism' has created 'a mood of optimism ... concerning the benefits that the application of scientific methodology might bring to humanity' (Peacock and Nolan 2000, p.1066), across the Health and Social Care sector and among professional bodies, voices have been raised that technological progress is leaving a concern with humanity, and the foundations of care and caring, behind. The example of the care-lessness in a major Brighton general hospital (see Gilbert 2006a) where frail elderly patients were denied basic care, such as nutrition and hydration, and the recent survey by Age Concern (Age Concern 2006) has raised similar issues of a 'care' system in a cul-de-sac.

Peacock and Nolan write that:

> There is a tension at the heart of modern healthcare ... it is about the increasing trend towards replacing caring with scientific technologies designed to meet the needs of populations rather than individuals. While such technologies have brought immense benefits ... too little attention is paid to 'care' as part of an ethical relationship and 'caring' as an expression of humanity. (Peacock and Nolan 2000)

Ray Jones, as a former long-serving Director of Social Services in Wiltshire, and Chair of the British Association of Social Workers (2006–2007) has expressed disquiet that social workers are being forced into a mode of working which is more technical than professional (conversation with the author, August 2006).

Mention the term 'assessment' to anyone using services, their informal carers, or a member of staff and, almost certainly, the image conjured up is one of a professional standing over an individual and divining their needs and aspirations through their own professional accomplishment, without any reference to the service user at all! In fact, the word 'assessment' derives from the Latin *assidere* – 'to sit beside'. The real concept is all to do with sitting with, communicating, walking with someone on a journey.

All the chapters in this book speak of the essential nature of an individual's spiritual dimension; about it being what makes people 'tick'; what is at the heart of them; their distinctiveness; what gives their life meaning, especially in the valley of shadows.

One of the ironies of assessment, is that it is often chance situations and informal conversations which lead to the most profound disclosures. Sometimes this discourse is with unqualified staff, or with professionals, but not in a face-to-face, one-to-one situation, but rather at a time when the masks are off and the guard is down and the chance remark, in a humane way, will spark a human response. Some of the most profound disclosures Peter has made and has listened to in others, have been initiated and ignited providentially and in informal settings, such as sometimes on a long run or a car journey (see Chapter 10).

'Zoë' was admitted to an Acute Unit with the diagnosis of bipolar disorder. Sunk in a depressive state, she happened to mention to an auxiliary nurse that she used to find exercise helpful in lifting her out of her depression. The auxiliary, 'Sandie', suggested that they go for a walk around the grounds. During this walk 'Zoë' confided that she felt she might not be able to ask for regular exercise in the Acute Unit, something which 'Sandie' was able to address with the Nurse Manager; but she also felt freed up to disclose that she felt it was a miscarriage, which had occurred several years previously, which was the underlying cause of her present mental distress and disconnection.

As a fabric designer, 'Zoë' saw herself as a very creative person, and her inability to carry a child to term, which she saw as the ultimate creative experience, had struck profoundly at her sense of personhood. She had never felt able to express this to any of the highly qualified professionals she had met, and it was 'Sandie', the auxiliary, on this long walk, who persuaded her that now might be the time to address this with somebody who could consider it in depth and long term with her.

The importance of spiritual assessment

Most service users wish, not only to find a way through the pain and trauma of mental distress, but also to understand the situation they are in and gain strength for the life ahead. As Wendy's story illustrates, people want both recovery and discovery. There is a well-rehearsed dissatisfaction from people who use services with a purely pharmacological approach to their experience (e.g. Escher et al. 2005; Mental Health Foundation 1999b, 2000). A switch, in a purely mechanistic way, to short-term cognitive approaches, however, may be just as dissatisfying. When Bradford Care Trust presented to the NIMHE Spirituality and Mental Health Pilot Sites Conference at Lincoln University on 3 May 2006, they spoke of the need for a culturally appropriate response (see www.nimhe.org.uk). There is sometimes a concern expressed by organizations that service users will demand too much. In fact, service users tend to say that what they want is:

- being seen as a whole person within their family and community environment
- having a relevant past, and hope and aspirations for the future
- being given time to tell their story in their own words
- attention to their emotional well-being
- working with, not doing to, to find solutions to practical issues
- being seen as having strengths as well as needs.

    (see Brandon 2000; Coyte 2007; Gilbert 2003).

Informal carers wish for all of the above, plus:

- to be seen as individuals, with their own life role, rather than just 'a carer'
- to be seen as having expertise
- to be worked with as partners.

Service users do wish to be seen as having expertise in their own life and condition:

> We are all primary experts on our own mental health and what works for us…we can and should value the coping strategies we have developed for ourselves…' (Mental Health Foundation November 1999 quoted in Gilbert 2003, p.27)

It is vitally important that spirituality does not become another area which professionals 'colonize' in an hegemonistic manner. Working with a service user recently, he stated:

> My spirituality is intensely personal and one of the few things I can really call my own. I fear professionals invading my personal space. It is important that those who are meant to care for me *do not take over aspects of my identity* (quoted in Social Perspectives Network 2006 Study Day Paper 9, pp.47–50).

However, they do not necessarily expect a professional to agree entirely with their perspective, just to acknowledge that it *is* their perspective. In the research in Westminster by McDonald and Sheldon (1997) a User remarked that the Social Worker did not necessarily agree with his voices, but accepted that they were real to him (Gilbert 2003, ch. 4). One of the best descriptions of the ongoing discourse between a service user and her psychiatrist, occurs in Kay Redfield Jamison's book *An Unquiet Mind* (1997) in which Jamison, herself a psychiatrist, works with her therapist during the highs and lows of a bipolar condition.

An increasing number of writers are stressing the importance of engaging with an individual's spiritual dimension. This is essential because:

- *If we are truly user-centred*, then we need to engage with the whole person and their deeper sense of motivation and meaning. As Hodge (2003) puts it: 'For many individuals, spirituality is central to their understanding of themselves and the world around them' (p.5).

- *Prognosis* – spirituality may well be a vital variable in predicting outcome.

- *Context* – we cannot really engage with an individual unless we have some understanding of their past and its impact on the present; current circumstances, and aspirations for the future. So often the past has laid a heavy burden on the person's shoulders, which they need to put down and look at with an empathic companion.

- *User self-determination* – if humankind's ultimate search is for meaning (Frankl 1959), then it is demeaning and undermining to the individual not to recognize the spiritual dimension.

- *Intervention* – the spirituality of the individual is likely to provide professionals with possible acceptable ways forward.

- *Attention to people's strengths* – with an increasing emphasis on recovery (Allott, Loganathion and Fulford 2002) and in strengths work generally (Healy 2005, ch. 8).

- *Outcomes* – working with people on a sustained and sustaining approach to life.

- *Ethical stipulations* – as put forward in professional codes of ethics, e.g. the North American Association of Social Work (NASW 1999) list four standards that explicitly mention religion as a category toward which social workers should strive to exhibit sensitivity (Hodge 2003; Robinson, Kendrick and Brown 2003).

As a simplistic approach to technological and technical improvement is seen to have its limits, and human and humane approaches make a comeback (Cox, Campbell and Fulford 2006; Furman 2007; Moss 2005). The NIMHE and Spirituality and Mental Health Project Pilot Site initiative has supported some profound initiatives from Mental Health organizations (Gilbert and

Watts 2006) where a number have produced excellent spiritual and religious care strategies (e.g. Sussex Partnership Trust 2006).

Bradford Care Trust (Bradford Social Services 2001), one of the Pilot Sites which presented at the National Conference in May 2006, works with one of the richest, diverse tapestries of ethnicity and language in the United Kingdom. They focus on the internal experience of the user, belief systems and religious practice. A significant number of Muslim service users have complained about possession, and Bradford has responded by introducing a project around this work, which has explicit, specific, liaison between services and accredited community practitioners.

Perhaps one of the major issues in assessment is that of 'travelling identity' (see Chapter 1), where people may leave a belief and practice early in life, but need to return to that belief system, or some aspects of it, at a later date.

It is important to note that spirituality is a vital element in the care of all ages and all conditions. Robinson *et al.* (2003) are especially sound in setting out the issues from childhood, to death and dying, and bereavement and grief (see also Holloway 2005; MacKinlay 2006; Puchalski and Romer 2000). Ruth Tanyi (2002) quotes a number of studies across a wide range of conditions, which 'revealed the participants found meaning in life and made sense of suffering when they embodied a sense of spiritual awareness'.

Dilemmas of spiritual assessment

An increasing number of professionals agree that an individual's spiritual dimension is of great importance (Furman 2007), but many people ask how it is to be done. McSherry and Ross (2002) have set out some of the dilemmas which relate to this:

- *Issues of definition:* For many people spirituality is still equated with religion; in other instances people find the term 'spirituality' too broad for them to grasp. Perhaps, what professional training schools need to ask staff, is the basic question as to what makes them 'tick', what keeps them going, what helps them through crises, and what gives their life meaning, so that they begin to grasp the importance of this issue for themselves, before they relate it to other people.

- *Motives for undertaking assessment:* The importance of ethnicity, and, in a post 9/11 world, the imperatives around faith means that, increasingly, these will be boxes which organizations and inspection bodies will wish to see ticked. While helpfully heightening the importance of these issues, the downside is that issues of meaning could be reduced to paper exercises.

- *'One-off' versus continuous assessment:* The meaning of people's lives cannot be elucidated in a single question or in a single meeting. At some stage this question, which many people find difficult to broach, has to be initiated; but, like life, the meaning of life and its discourse, has to be an ongoing process.

- *Direct questioning versus observation:* Direct questioning, such as 'do you have a religious belief?' can lead into a cul-de-sac, if an individual's spirituality does not connect with the question.

- *The practicalities of conducting an assessment:* As discussed above, people need time and space. Increasingly, some forward-thinking Mental Health organizations, a good example would be South Staffordshire Mental Health Trust (Shaw and Nolan 2006) are creating space, producing quiet rooms with a non-denominational ethos, which can also be used for faith gatherings, as appropriate.

- *Who should be involved in the assessment?* As spirituality becomes more 'fashionable', there may be competition between different professional groups, but in fact, as McSherry and Ross point out, 'all Health Care professionals' need to 'feel a sense of ownership' (p.483) and, again, the user needs to be in control.

- *Ethical issues:* As the quotation given above makes clear, 'spirituality is intensely personal', and that is at the heart of the ethical dilemma.

- *Who 'holds the hope'?* Some people may be at a stage when they do not wish or may temporarily have lost the energy to engage, and may need someone else to hold the candle of hope for them. That is a great privilege for the person in the holding role as they strive to avoid either snuffing out the flame or stoking it up.

The role of the chaplain

Chaplains have a vital role to play in the multi-disciplinary team and forward thinking Trusts recognize this (see Copsey 1997, 2001; Chapter 9). Unfortunately, less progressive Health and Social Care organizations talk about Whole Persons and Whole Systems approaches and then leave the chaplain out – one cash-strapped Acute Trust in 2006 wishes to axe its chaplaincy service, giving rise to questions in the House of Lords.

Both the Department of Health in England (DH 2003) and the Scottish Executive (2002) have policies on spiritual care and chaplaincy; and the Welsh Assembly Government, is working on a Spiritual Care Policy at present.

It is essential that there is a mutual understanding between Health and Social Care organizations and the diverse communities they serve. A project set up between the Church of England and NIMHE and written up by Mentality (Tidyman and Seymour 2004), attempts to explain Mental Health to parish communities and foster productive relationships between those communities and Mental Health services. The beautiful Mind in Croydon video *Hard to Believe* (2005) sets out in graphic form individuals' search for spirituality, the community context and the service response.

There is considerable debate around the role of the chaplain at present (see, for example, Mowat and Swinton 2005; South Yorkshire NHS Workforce Group 2003), but it is essential to see the chaplain as both a scarce and a specialist resource and also part of the team. In a sense, this sounds contradictory, but, as with all consultant staff, the chaplain needs to be so much of a presence that staff can call on the chaplain for specialist help when required. What is not helpful, but often happens, is when a service user mentions something which sounds like spirituality and/or religion, there is an immediate knee-jerk reaction of calling for the chaplain, rather than listening to the individual's human need.

In an increasingly complex cultural society the chaplain is a vital resource in direct care, consultancy, advice and support to staff, and building effective community networks (Khan 2006). Sometimes a chaplain is the only person who can break through the taboos which people in distress may erect against treatment and care. One chaplain recalls blessing a cup of water so a distressed youth could re-hydrate without thinking he was contaminating himself.

Guiding the assessment process

Just because spirituality is what makes one 'tick' doesn't mean it should be put in a tick-box! A further paradox is that, probably the first question around assessing somebody's spiritual needs, should not be a question at all, but the creation of a safe listening–responding space.

There are an increasing number of guides to assessment, but the essence is to keep it simple and start where the individual is. As we saw from Wendy's story, enquiries about spiritual needs can be intrusive, or simply come at the wrong time. The involvement of users of the service in devising methods of spiritual assessment is essential to provide the virtuous, rather than vicious, circle as shown below:

Dr Christina Puchalski (Puchalski and Romer 2000) produced an assessment remembered by the acronym FICA – touching on the domains of faith, importance, community and address. Some have found the following model a useful approach. It is based on four points, with the acronym HOPE:

H   sources of hope, meaning, comfort, strength, peace, love and connection

O   organized religion

P   personal spirituality and practices

E   effects on medical care and end-of-life issues

(Anandarajah and Hight 2001)

The Royal College of Psychiatrists (Culliford and Johnson 2003) have also produced guidance on the College's very informative website.

A number of Trusts, e.g. Sheffield Care Trust, South Downs Health NHS Trust (now Sussex Partnership Trust) have now produced very helpful, short, leaflets. Sheffield's focuses on questions such as people's sense of value and purpose in their lives; what makes them safe and secure; what helps them cope in hard times, and who do you talk to when having problems? Looking at a sophisticated and detailed approach, Phil Barker and Poppy Buchanan-Barker's (2005) 'Tidal Model' has a beautiful resonance, based around the idea that a mental/spiritual crisis can often feel 'like the appearance of shipwreck' (p.25). A less sophisticated model, but one that would also need time to be taken with an individual, might involve the following aspects:

- *Identity:* What are the components which make up an individual's identity, nurture and nature, ethnicity, values, belief systems (including possibly a religious faith); and how has that identity travelled and might still be travelling?

- *Belief and meaning:* What are the beliefs that give meaning and purpose to a person's life and the symbols that reflect them?

- *Sources of strength and hope:* Where does the individual derive their strength from and what gives them hope? Are these derived from individuals, groups, places, current or past experiences? What helps the individual draw strength and hope at a time of crisis?

Spiritual Assessment: Virtuous Circle

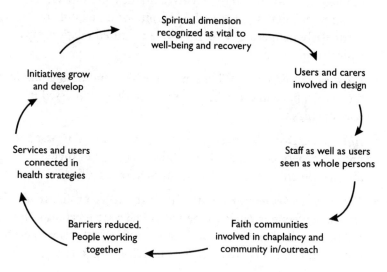

Figure 11.1 The virtuous circle

Spiritual Assessment: Vicious Circle

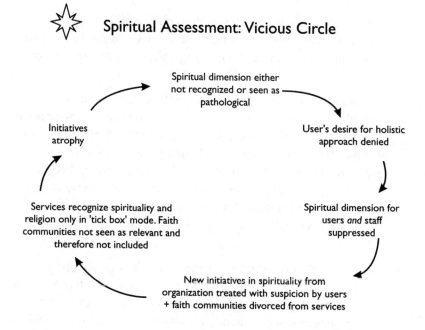

Figure 11.2 The vicious circle

- *Love and relatedness:* How does the individual relate to those intimate with them; family, relatives, friends and others? Assumptions that families will be helpful or unhelpful are particularly dangerous here. Are there fractured relationships which need healing?

- *Vocation and obligation:* What sense of calling and obligation does the person have in their life and how are these expressed in relationships?

- *Affirmation:* Does the individual feel affirmed by their past and present experiences and relationships? What gives them affirmation and can a vacuum of affirmation be filled?

- *Experience and emotion:* How does the experience of illness and the associated feelings relate to the individual's life meaning? How do the internal and external worlds of the individual relate to each other? How are 'negative' feelings handled? e.g. anxiety, guilt and anger.

- *Courage and growth:* This involves questions about how the person has coped with crises in the past and how adaptable are their views/beliefs now?

- *Transcendence:* What provides an individual with their sense of transcendence? This may or may not involve relating to a divine entity, but may be through an engagement with nature, art, sport, etc.

- *Rituals and practices:* Exploring the rituals which support the person's life meaning and how they are being used in the present situation. This will be relevant for people with religious faith, but also may be for those who have lapsed from their faith, and are re-discovering it, or may be of a purely secular variety. For some with a religious faith, the experience of mental distress and the arousal of some emotions, such as guilt, may make them feel cut off from prayer and sacraments and, therefore, deny them nurture and comfort.

- *Community:* How does the individual relate to their significant community? Is the service facilitating positive connection with the community, and how does it give meaning to her/him? There may be elements of community life which may be harmful, and the service may have to act as a conduit, but one with a filter, if a social group is reinforcing elements of 'punishment'.

- *Authority and guidance:* Where does the individual look for guidance about life meaning in moments of stress? Is this fixed or flexible? If there is a need for 'mediation', e.g. through an imam or priest, etc., is such a person available, e.g. through chaplaincy services?

(Adapted from Fitchett 1993; Narayanasamy 2001;

Robinson *et al.* 2003)

Conclusion

Increasingly, Government and professional guidance is emphasizing the importance of the spiritual and assessing people's spiritual needs; the latest guidance from the Chief Nursing Officer in the Review of Mental Health Nursing (DH 2006) emphasizes this again (para 5.47). But what we need to do is to create a language of the heart with individuals at the centre, in a state both of dialogue and presence, where we all learn to sit beside, listen to and then walk with people as they journey on.

Khan, in her article on multi-faith spiritual and cultural care (Khan 2006, p.26) quotes a poem by Guru Gobind Singh: 'All people have the same form; All people have the same soul.'

Our common humanity and our uniqueness are the watchlights of our journey together.

Bibliography

Age Concern (2006) *Hungry to be heard: the scandal of malnourished older people in hospital.* London: Age Concern.

Allott, P., Loganathion, I. and Fulford, K.W.M. (2002) 'Discovering hope for recovery from a British perspective: a review of a selection of recovery literature, implications for practice and systems change.' In S. Lurie *et al.* (eds) 'International innovations in community mental health' (special issue). *Canadian Journal of Community Mental Health 21,* 3.

Anandarajah, G. and Hight, E. (2001) 'Spirituality and Medical Practice: using the HOPE questions as a practical tool.' *American Family Physician 63,* 1, January 2001.

Anderson, R. (2003) *Spiritual Care Giving as a Secular Sacrament.* London: Jessica Kingsley Publishers.

Barker, P. and Buchanan-Barker, P. (2005) *The Tidal Model: A Guide for Mental Health Professionals.* Hove: Brunner-Routledge.

Bradford Social Services/Bradford Community Health NHS Trust/Bradford Inter-Faith Education Centre (2001) *Spiritual Well-being: Policy and Practice.* Bradford: Bradford Social Services.

Brandon, D. (2000) *Tao of Survival: Spirituality in Social Care and Counselling.* Birmingham: BASW/Venture Press.

Cassidy, S. (1988) *Sharing the Darkness: The Spirituality of Caring.* London: Darton, Longman and Todd.

Copsey, N. (1997) *Keeping Faith.* London: Sainsbury Centre for Mental Health.

Copsey, N. (2001) *Forward in Faith*. London: Sainsbury Centre for Mental Health.

Cox, J., Campbell, A., Fulford, K.W.M. (2006) *Medicine of the Person: Faith, Science and Values in Health Care Provision*. London: Jessica Kingsley Publishers.

Coyte, M.E. (2007) 'What service users want from faith communities.' In P. Gilbert and H. Kalaga: *Nurturing Heart and Spirit: Papers from a Multi-Faith Symposium*. Stafford: Staffordshire University Monograph.

Culliford, L. (2005) 'Healing from Within: Spirituality and Mental Health.' In M. McClure (ed.) *Partners in Care Resource Pack*. London: Gaskell.

Culliford, L. and Johnson, S. (2003) *Healing from Within: A Guide for Assessing the Religious and Spiritual Aspects of People's Lives*. Available at www.rcpsych.ac.uk/college/sig/spirit/index.htm (accessed 20 September 2007).

Department of Health (2003) *Meeting the Spiritual and Religious Needs of Patients and Staff: Guidance for Staff*. London: HMSO.

Department of Health (2006) *From Values to Action: The Chief Nursing Officer's Review of Mental Health Nursing*. London: DH, 20 April 2006.

Escher, S. *et al.* (2005) 'Learning to live with voices.' *Mental Health Today*, December 2005, pp.18–20.

Fitchett, G. (1993) *Assessing Spiritual Needs: A Guide for Care Givers*. Minneapolis: Augsburg Press.

Frankl, V.E. (1959) (first published 1946) *Man's Search for Meaning*. New York: Simon and Schuster.

Furman, L. (2007) 'Grief is a brutal but empowering teacher.' *Journal of Illness, Crisis and Loss* (special edition), Spring 2007.

Gilbert, P. (2003) *The Value of Everything: Social Work and its Importance in the Field of Mental Health*. Lyme Regis: Russell House.

Gilbert, P. (2006a) 'We need leaders at all levels with heart and guts.' *Open Mind* 138, March/April 2006, pp.16–17. (referring to *Panorama Special: Undercover Nurse*, BBC1, 20 July 2005.

Gilbert, P. (2006b) 'Assessing spiritual strengths and needs.' Presentation to Jersey Mental Health Services. May 2004.

Gilbert, P. and Watts, N. (2006) 'Don't mention God!' *A Life in the Day 10*, 3, August 2006.

Hard to Believe, DVD, directed by Ben Hole. London: Mind in Croydon, 2005.

Healy, K. (2005) *Social Work Theories in Context: Creating Frameworks for Practice*. London: Palgrave Macmillan.

Hodge, D.R. (2003) *Spiritual Assessment: Handbook for Helping Professionals*. Botsford: North American Association of Christians in Social Work.

Holloway, M. (2005) *In the Spirit of Things…Social Work, Spirituality and Contemporary Society*. Hull: University of Hull.

Jamison, K.R. (1997) *An Unquiet Mind: A Memoir of Moods and Madness*. London: Macmillan/Picador.

Khan, Q. (2006) 'Spiritual and cultural care in recovery.' *A Life in the Day 10*, 4, November 2006.

MacKinlay, E. (2006) *The Spiritual Dimension of Ageing* (2nd edn). London: Jessica Kingsley Publishers.

McDonald, G. and Sheldon, B. (1997) 'Community care services for the mentally ill: consumers' views.' *International Journal of Social Psychiatry 43*, 1, 35–55.

McSherry, W. (2000) *Making Sense of Spirituality in Nursing Practice: an Interactive Approach*. London: Churchill Livingstone.

McSherry, W. and Ross, L. (2002) 'Dilemmas of spiritual assessment: considerations for nursing practice.' *Journal of Advanced Nursing 38*, 5, 479–88.

Mental Health Foundation (1999a) *The Fundamental Facts.* London: Mental Health Foundation.

Mental Health Foundation (1999b) *The Courage to Bare Our Souls.* London: Mental Health Foundation.

Mental Health Foundation (2000) *Strategies for Living.* London: Mental Health Foundation.

Moss, B. (2005) *Religion and Spirituality.* Lyme Regis: Russell House.

Mowat, H. and Swinton, J. (2005) *What do Chaplains do?: The Role of the Chaplain in Meeting the Spiritual Needs of Patients.* Aberdeen: University of Aberdeen/Mowat research.

Mulholland, H. (2005) 'Counting on change.' *The Guardian,* 7 December 2005, p.5.

Narayanasamy, A. (2001) *Spiritual Care: a Practical Guide for Nurses and Health Care Practitioners.* Wiltshire: Quay Books.

Nash, M. and Stewart, B. (ed.) (2002) *Spirituality and Social Care: Contributing to Personal and Community Well-being.* London: Jessica Kingsley Publishers.

NASW (1999) *Code of Ethics.* Available at www.socialworkers.org/pubs/code/code.asp (accessed 4 October 2007)

Orchard, H. (ed.) (2001) *Spirituality in Healthcare Contexts.* London: Jessica Kingsley Publishers.

Peacock, J. and Nolan, P. (2000) 'Care under threat in the modern world.' *Journal of Advanced Nursing 32,* 5, 1066–70.

Penhale, B., Parker, J. and Kingston, P. (2000) *Elder Abuse: A Practitioner's Guide.* Birmingham: Venture Press/BASW.

Puchalski, C. and Romer, A.L. (2000) 'Taking a spiritual history allows clinicians to understand patients more fully.' *Journal of Palliative Medicine 3,* 1, 129–37.

Robinson, S., Kendrick, K. and Brown, A. (2003) *Spirituality and the Practice of Health Care.* Basingstoke: Palgrave Macmillan.

Royal College of Psychiatrists (2006) *A Short Guide to the Assessment of Spiritual Concerns in Mental Healthcare.* Available at www.rcpsych.ac.uk/college/sig/spirit/index.asp (accessed 20 September 2007).

Scottish Executive Health Department (2002) *Guidelines on Chaplaincy and Spiritual Care in the NHS in Scotland.* NHS HDL (2002) 76, 28 October 2002.

Shaw, K. and Nolan, P. (2006) *The Development of the Spiritual and Pastoral Care Centre at St George's.* Stafford: South Staffordshire Mental Health Trust.

Social Perspectives Network (2006) *Reaching the Spirit.* Social Perspectives Network Study Day Paper 9, pp.47–50. London: SPN.

South Yorkshire NHS Workforce Development Confederation (2003) *Caring for the Spirit: A Strategy for the Chaplaincy and Spiritual Care Workforce.* Available at http://nhs-chaplaincy-collboratives.com/resources_overview.htm (accessed 30 October 2007)..

Sussex Partnership NHS Trust (2006) *Spiritual and Religious Strategy,* May 2006. Available at www.sussexpartnership.nhs.uk (accessed 20 September 2007).

Tanyi, R. (2002) 'Towards clarification of the meaning of spirituality.' *Journal of Advanced Nursing 39,* 5, 500–509.

Tew, J. (ed.) (2005) *Social Perspectives in Mental Health: Developing Social Models to Understand and Work with Mental Distress.* London: Jessica Kingsley Publishers.

Tidyman, M. and Seymour, L. (2004) *Promoting Mental Health: A Resource for Spiritual and Pastoral Care* (a project between NIMHE/Church of England/Mentality).

Willows, D. and Swinton, J. (2000) *Spiritual Dimensions in Pastoral Care: Practical Theology in a Multi-Disciplinary Context.* London: Jessica Kingsley Publishers.

This poem owes its existence to Henry Reed's 'Today we have naming of parts'.

Today We Have Spiritual Assessment

Today we have spiritual assessment. Yesterday
We had medication and tomorrow morning
We shall have what to do after restraining. But today,
Today we have spiritual assessment. Wisdom
Glistens like fountains in all of the neighbouring viewpoints
And today we have spiritual assessment

This is the temporal lobe
And this is the frontal lobe, whose use you will see
When you are given your syringes. And this is the time to hear
people's stories
Which in your case you have not got. The branches
Hold in the gardens their silent, eloquent gestures
Which in our case we have not got

This is the safety catch, which is always released
By way of your heart connection. Please do not let me
See anyone using their heart connection. And this is the time to
take people out in the gardens. Which in your case you have not
got. The blossoms
Are fragile and motionless, always letting everyone see
Them using their heart connections

They call it spiritual assessment. It is perfectly easy
If you have any belief in the rule book: like the meds
And the TV; and nature and time and journey and acceptance
and trust and creativity and other holy moments and sacred
ceremonies
Which in our case we have not got.

Mary Ellen Coyte

CHAPTER 12

SPIRITUALITY AND PSYCHIATRY – CROSSING THE DIVIDE

Andrew Powell

Introduction

I would like to explain how I came to be involved in the field of mental health and spirituality. I want to do this not because I think there is anything so special about my case, but because it may encourage others in the healthcare professions to feel they can do the same. Although prejudice is still encountered in certain quarters, in recent years there has been an appreciable shift of opinion, enough to ensure that health professionals who declare their interest in the spiritual dimension will find themselves in good company.

Medicine as science of the body

After qualifying as a doctor in 1969, but before specializing in psychiatry, I worked for two years in acute hospital medicine. The experience lives vividly with me to this day. The technology of coronary care had just arrived, along with a whole raft of advances in the investigation and treatment of a wide range of disease. The medical model was highly mechanistic, as it continues to this day.

Following a paper chase of clues leading to a treatment that is specific and effective offers a great deal of intellectual satisfaction for the doctor, as well as the pleasure of seeing one's patient get better. I will confess that I was rather less taken with the task of supporting patients with chronic conditions, unlikely to recover and at best being maintained in status quo. There seemed to be less 'to do', and no one helped young doctors understand the art of 'being with'.

In those days, medical students learned to dissect dead bodies long before they were ever allowed to touch live patients. Later, when doing our obstetrics, we helped deliver babies under the watchful eye of the midwife. Even so, the miracle of birth took second place to the need to examine the baby, check for genetic abnormalities, listen to the heart, and so on. I remember a few years later trying to resuscitate a baby in casualty. It was a cot death and there was nothing we were able to do. I had to tell the mother. She was inconsolable, of course, and I felt wretched too. I couldn't think of what to say. Death, whether in the young or old, was invariably the great enemy of Life, and we had lost the battle.

I am not arguing in the least against medical technology. I needed a heart valve replacement some years back, and without it I would certainly have died! But I reflect on those early years as a doctor because of the difficulty in finding either the time or confidence to relate to the person rather than the disease.

Communication skills have now become part of the medical school curriculum but enormous problems remain; doctors still think there should be an answer to every question. It is not easy to say 'I don't know'. First, such an admission is not what the patient is hoping to hear. Second, it puts the doctor in the less assured position of being a fellow traveller on the unpredictable journey of life – the patient has to tolerate the pain of uncertainty and the doctor, whose customary role helps relieve him of personal anxiety of illness and death by naming the problem firmly in 'the other', becomes the more vulnerable.

Yet joining forces by reaching out to the patient's fear and pain brings the doctor a great opportunity for the medicine of healing, of 'making whole'. It is no less important than cure, but has a different function. Feeling whole does not promise cure, but it enables a person to make the best possible recovery and, when illness cannot be relieved, to continue life with an intact sense of meaning and purpose. How different it might be if we could truly live those words of Reinhold Niebuhr, 'God, give us grace to accept with serenity the things that cannot be changed, courage to change the things that should be changed, and wisdom to distinguish the one from the other'.

At this point, I had better say how I am using the term spirituality, since it is intrinsically bound up with wholeness. Among many definitions, it can be described as the experience of a deep-seated sense of meaning and purpose in life, a wholeness that brings with it the feeling of belonging, harmony and peace. It entails searching for answers about the infinite, and is particularly important in times of stress, illness, loss, bereavement and death. For some people, including those with religious beliefs, this sense of belonging is found explicitly in relation to God as the ultimate source of love.

To see why our medical care is so devoid of spirituality and so mechanical in orientation, we need to understand its roots in the Newtonian science of the last 300 years. It happens that Isaac Newton was both a great empirical scientist and a deeply religious man, but his research into the properties of physical matter were taken to mean that God as the prime mover had to be located elsewhere, beyond a mechanistic universe, and such a remote God could hardly be expected to influence the workings of the human body except by means of occasional miraculous (inexplicable) healing.

By the end of the 19th century, disease had become identified with organ pathology, and the subsequent discovery of bacterial infections, biochemical, degenerative and congenital disorders, cancer and other conditions all reinforced this materialist perspective. God was dismissed by science as irrelevant, with the Church ousted from medical care except for providing comfort, offering spiritual guidance to the afflicted and administering the last rites.

Psychiatry as science of the mind

Psychiatry was borne out of neurology in Europe at the end of the 19th century with this same emphasis on the physical basis of disease. For example, neurosyphilis had been demonstrated to cause mental changes resulting from damage to the brain, while porphyria and vitamin deficiencies were shown to affect mental functioning. Such evidence persuaded Emil Kraepelin, a pioneer in the history of psychiatry, to classify mental illness into the two main categories, schizophrenia and manic-depressive disorder, the assumption being that the underlying causes must be physical and in time would be elucidated.

These two major mental illnesses do indeed respond to pharmacological treatments and most psychiatrists believe that they have a basis in vulnerable brain chemistry, though the causes are as yet unknown. But this emphasis led many psychiatrists to treat the numerous and varied disturbances of mood and thought as being indicative of mental disorder similarly requiring medication. General practice too, has been influenced by this climate of opinion; all too often the prescription serves a ritual function, a poor substitute for the time needed by patients to talk, be heard and understood.

At the other extreme, what about Sigmund Freud's remarkable contribution to the study of the mind? Freud's early expectation that neurosis would similarly prove to be founded in brain dysfunction never materialized. Instead, psychoanalysis ran for a hundred years parallel to mainstream psychiatry. This epic approach to the study of the psyche elegantly charted the conscious and unconscious reaches of the human mind, but unfortunately it simply hasn't worked for serious mental illness.

In many departments of psychiatry today, in addition to physical treatments, a range of symptom-orientated psychological approaches is on offer. Psychoanalysis paved the way for shorter-term psychodynamic treatments; behaviourist psychology has led to cognitive-behavioural therapies; family therapy is largely based on systems theory. Yet with the exception of the transpersonal approach, to which I shall come later, such therapies rarely stray beyond the pragmatics of everyday life. The big questions about birth, life, death, what it is all for, why must we suffer, all those deep concerns that disquiet the troubled mind, generally have no place in which to find voice, and so don't get raised. Yet we know that such concerns frequently do come the way of the psychiatrist if only the interest is shown.

Psychiatry as science without soul

In drawing attention to the schism that shaped Western science, I have painted a bleak picture of medicine, and psychiatry too. Of course, there are countless physicians and surgeons who intuitively and compassionately care for the 'whole person'. But schisms, conscious or otherwise, are intrinsic to the reductive-analytic methods of Western science. These days, every specialist knows more and more about less and less. We know that the whole is always greater than the sum of the parts and yet the focus increasingly is on the parts.

From general medicine I moved to the renowned Maudsley hospital and Institute of Psychiatry in London. The academic and research base was first-class and the consultants were leaders in the field. But it seemed that the mind had got divorced from the body, which had been left somewhere behind. Liaison psychiatry was in its infancy and more or less confined to seeing patients with overdoses admitted to King's College Hospital across the road, or unexpected cases of delirium tremens on the medical and surgical wards. Psychosomatic medicine, too, seemed to have run out of steam, all this being prior to the discovery of psychoneuroimmunology.

As psychiatrists, we earnestly debated the finer points of diagnosis much along the same lines as in general medicine. But the mind is not the body, and I was struck how often this seemed to be about gleaning intellectual satisfaction from the work rather than of itself having much bearing on management and treatment, which was usually pretty obvious. If anything, the clinical environment had become more remote than ever – patients not so much got talked to as got talked about.

Psychiatry seemed to have no soul, although at the time it would not have occurred to me to put it that way. Instinctively, I turned to psychoanalysis. Aside from personal issues that I wanted to explore, the Maudsley psychotherapy department was the one place where enough time was given to sit with, and really 'be with', your patient. I realized at once that this was what I had come into psychiatry for.

The search for soul

Psychoanalysis, and subsequent training in group analysis, took up a lot of my time over the next few years. It was a love affair I remember with great affection. Sigmund Freud had an answer for just about everything that lay between birth and death, and it all made sense. My intellect was fired, while my admiration for Freud was unbounded. It served its purpose – I worked hard, became a consultant and was able to help a good number of patients. But later I came to see that Freud had for me been an irresistible father figure, and that had I remained obedient to his will, I would never have left home and made my own way in the world.

The work of Carl Jung barely got a mention at the Maudsley and I wondered why, until I read about his exile by Freud (if you go round Freud's house in Vienna, where the walls are lined with hundreds of photographs of Freud, his family, friends and colleagues, there is not one picture of Jung, the disciple who Freud had once seen as his natural successor). My curiosity aroused, I started to read Jung and I found myself engaged with a mind as profound as Freud's, with one great difference. Jung sought to understand man not only as the product of his childhood but endowed with an ineluctable spiritual birthright.

This opened a door for me. Patients had not infrequently brought to me what I would these days call spiritual concerns – deep searching questions about the whole meaning and purpose of life, especially of suffering. I had been inclined to interpret these in relation to problems that had been encountered in childhood and subsequent relationships difficulties and I was not always wrong. But sometimes I knew I had missed the boat, and it was no good ascribing it to 'resistance' on the part of the patient. I began to see that my need for an all-explanatory psychology of humankind was a defence against the unknown, not the small unknown of the human unconscious mind but the greater unknown that goes way beyond birth and death.

About this time, I began training in psychodrama. To my surprise, it found places in me that analytic therapy had never reached. Memories, dreams and reflections of my own erupted with full force, and could be dramatised without the constraints of having to sit or lie down (the golden rule of analytical therapy). The effect was to connect body with mind and to discover that the body has memories of its own, going back to the womb, let alone getting born! Rather than experiencing myself as an observer of life, I began to live more of it for myself – for psychodrama sees life as just that, a drama to be played out in which we each are protagonists in a script we simultaneously write, direct and watch.

When doing psychodrama, time is divided between enacting, as oneself, the scene of the memory, and role reversing with others whose perspective can add to an understanding of the situation being re-played. But the 'other' need not be of human form, as I found out in one of the first workshops I attended. I recall a woman had been deeply embittered by the loss of her son years before. In the session, she found herself back at the roadside scene of the car crash in which he had been killed. Weeping in despair, she cried out 'God, why have you done this to me?' The therapist instantly told her to reverse roles with God. At once this mother's face changed, becoming calm and composed, her sobbing ceased and as God she said with immense dignity, 'I have done nothing to you. Your son chose to die, so that he would not suffer any more. Be happy for him and thankful for his life which brought you joy.'

This involuntary utterance surprised the woman as much as it did us. She could see the meaning of it perfectly and began for the first time since her son's death to mourn without the bitterness that had held her captive for so long. She could at last start to heal.

I have detailed this event because it was a defining moment for me. I perceived that such deep wisdom brings with it the power to heal; I saw the harnessing of the strength and beauty of the soul and that without it, no amount of psychological insight alone can heal us of the traumas of life.

I began to ponder the limitations of dynamic psychotherapy. For instance, therapists talk a great deal about projection and splitting as pathological defences against psychic pain, while entrusting recovery to the resolution of the transference by way of interpretation.[1] This frame of reference is invariably one of patient as child and therapist as parent offering what has been called 'the corrective emotional experience'. Standing in loco parentis is no small undertaking, but more worrying still, the dependency needs of

---

1   The analytical method encourages the emergence of unresolved childhood emotions, which get unconsciously projected on to the therapist (a process called transference). The therapist remains as neutral as possible in order to be a 'blank screen' for such projections. By means of interpretation, the therapist endeavours to help the patient understand what is happening, and to own such feelings instead of splitting them off and projecting them onto himself and others. The process is often painful and good 'parenting' is required on the part of the therapist to enable the patient to feel sufficiently secure to cope with what is going on.

the patient too often result in the therapist being perceived as omnipotent, patently a God-like role. Yet therapists rarely respond to the deepest and most heartfelt questions of all, 'why am I here, what is it for, what happens when I die, why must I suffer?' Most will studiously avoid disclosing their own doubts and dilemmas in order to preserve the transference need for a wise and knowing parent. The tendency is rather to interpret these fundamental existential concerns according to the analytical method, along with everything else.

Healers, energy and consciousness

I have learned that in life nothing happens by chance. Around this time I met a number of healers and was struck by the good results they were having across a range of physical and emotional conditions. I decided to learn more and applied to train at the College of Healing where I met many healers and 'intuitives' who could directly perceive the human energy field or 'aura'. From a medical point of view, the therapeutic effects of hands-on healing are put down to the 'placebo effect', attributable to suggestibility. But what if the 'energies' being employed are real enough, but beyond the instrumentation of our current science to detect?

There is now very good empirical evidence that healing works. Double blind trials have excluded suggestibility as the mechanism. Quantum entanglement may hold the key; experimental physics is now challenging what was formerly regarded as the impenetrable limits of space-time. It is being argued that the ground substance of consciousness is non-local and that far from consciousness being generated by each brain, it is a unified field in which we are all immersed. Indeed, top-down theorists hold that matter is nothing less than precipitation of energy, which has (cosmic) intelligence inscribed in its very substance.

Such a cosmology describes a participative spiritual universe, fundamentally conscious in design, and very possibly evolving so as to know more of itself. If holographic theories of the universe are to be believed, the astonishing diversity of life on our little planet reflects a principle of differentiation manifested throughout the length and breadth of the cosmos, while our capacity for love likewise reflects the principle of unity, the oneness of all that is. The quantum image of wave and particle touches us because in it we discern the eternal dance of *yin* and *yang*, the emanation of a divine source of incomprehensible creativity.

We generally take the world of our ordinary sense perception for granted; after all, it comprises the 'consensus reality' of everyday life. But I began to see that there is actually no such thing as reality, in and of itself. All is perceived or construed in line with a person's subjective disposition. Most of us see and hear things the same way (in line with what quantum physicists call the collapse of the probability wave). But it is not always so, as the accumulated body of research into paranormal phenomena now demonstrates.

This raises another difficulty for psychiatry, for how then should we distinguish between mental illness and paranormal experiences, not least between psychosis and spiritual crisis? To make matters more complicated, there can be an overlap between the two.

One way is to postpone making a judgement about the status of a symptom while exploring what value it holds for the person and whether it stands to help the person find a more meaningful and purposeful life. Breakdown may yet turn into breakthrough.

This takes us away from the notion of disease, which is an objective measure, to that of illness, concerned more with the impact of physical or emotional adversity on how a person is functioning. This, again, is highly subjective, for people can be 'well' in themselves even as they are dying; wholeness of being and fulfilment of the moment can be of far greater importance than the disease process. How often we overlook the precious 'now' and instead worry about a future that must in any case, eventually bring death our way!

The life instinct is usually a strong one and the promise of cure is, of course, always welcome news. It restores, in the short term, a sense of immortality that distances us from that day of reckoning. But while death has aptly been described as the one appointment no one is in a hurry to keep, the materialist reality of our time makes the inevitable ending of life, including the loss of loved ones, a tragic and irreparable parting of the ways.

Loss as transition

The death of someone close is often the precipitant of breakdown in an already vulnerable person. Yet the belief that consciousness ends with death is merely one of cultural conditioning. We can appreciate the many benefits that 300 years of 'scientific realism' have conferred, without succumbing to its materialist ideology.

In any event, there continues to be intense speculation about life after death, and the many views articulated, both secular and religious, probably reflect nothing more than the very partial view we get from the embodied mind and the associated limitations of the human brain.

Bearing this in mind, spiritual psychiatry sets out to help a person value, trust and explore the authenticity of their own experience as fully as they can. It follows that the psychiatrist should avoid making assumptions or judgements, but instead to follow wholeheartedly the thoughts and emotions of his patient. No counter-culture proselytizing is required; this would be to replace one kind of conditioning with another. Fortunately, since our innate archetypes remain alive and well, it is only necessary to ask with genuine interest what a person would hope to be the case, and to give support to that possibility, for it cannot be disproved.

For example, when a bereaved patient entreats 'if only my mum were still here', it may be helpful to proceed by finding out what it is that person is most needing, and then to urge him[2] to take the chance of talking with mum, by asking him to close his eyes, to imagine her there in the room, and to go right ahead and speak with her out loud. When he has done so, the patient is asked to sit for a moment longer, eyes closed, and listen to, or simply experience, what may come back. Sometimes it is a verbal response, or it may be in silence, a loving embrace.

Crucial unfinished business can be completed this way, often with the farewell that had not been possible in life. Usually the person will have had a profound sense of the presence of the deceased, or even to have seen or heard them.

What does this actually say about life after death? It says everything and nothing, depending on your point of view. It can be understood on the psychological level, on the spiritual level, or both. Either way, it breaks the terrifying finality of death, because the mind has been helped to transcend the customary limits of space-time. And if there has already been a sighting of the deceased (known in psychiatry as a pseudo-hallucination), the spiritual affirmation will be all the more profound.

For some people, spirituality means finding the greatest depth of meaning and purpose in their existence without reference to other-dimensional realities. In my own case, however, my researches had led me to see the soul as a scintilla of eternal consciousness that chose to incarnate into this world in order to learn and grow. I was curious to find out more about my soul journey and it led me to the study of 'past life' regression, both academic and experiential.

The transpersonal perspective

Transpersonal phenomena arise in an 'altered' state of consciousness. But this does not have to be a trance state, or by taking psychoactive drugs. There are many subtle changes in consciousness, for instance in reverie, stilling of

---

2   Both the male and female gender is used interchangeably for the purpose of convenience.

the mind as in meditation and prayer and the hypnagogic state, when the bounds of space-time melt away. If someone brings an inexplicable symptom, such as a fear of suffocation, and after taking a history that gives no other clue, he is invited to close his eyes and to 'go into' that feeling of suffocation and describe what is happening, and if he suddenly finds himself in a burning house and cannot escape, a scene which ends in death, and if he then find himself leaving his body, just as described in the near-death literature, before returning to the here and now and is left with the vivid impression that the fear of suffocation is an imprint of a trauma from another place and time, and if he gets better as a result of having had such a realization, who is to say what has really happened? (I should add that such 'memories' arise equally often in people who have no thought of re-incarnation.) From the clinical perspective, the important thing is that the treatment worked.

The same principle applies to 'spirit release' therapy, in which the therapist engages with an 'entity' that has attached to the patient, and releases it into 'the light'. When a patient gives a history suggestive of such an attachment, it is not difficult to dialogue with the 'earthbound spirit', much as takes place in psychodrama or gestalt therapy. The patient finds herself speaking as the spirit, divulging how and when it came to be attached, and why it has got stuck. Such earthbound spirits are in general not so much malicious as lost or confused, often because their lives ended in violent death, or under the influence of drugs. This therapeutic intervention is a far cry from exorcism and calls instead for a compassionate understanding of the plight of both patient and attached spirit. The spirit is then guided on its way with love, and help from above.

Transpersonal therapy is open to abuse, just as any other form of treatment, and ethical considerations have to be high on the list. But while we may argue about the true nature of such soul-centred work, what we do know is crucial to the outcome is that the therapist must have a genuine and compassionate desire to help patients in need, and be fully willing to enter with them into their world.

The next step

In mental healthcare, treatment is largely pragmatic, based on the prevailing bio-psycho-social model of our times. It is a good working model yet spirituality, the highest function of the imaginal mind, has got left out. This is something of an irony since psyche means spirit or soul, and it is a lack that urgently needs putting right. Apart from the importance of encouraging patients to feel able fully to confide in their psychiatrists, research over the last 15 years has shown that spirituality is good for both mental and physical health. So we need to develop a 'bio-psycho-socio-spiritual' model of healthcare.

It struck me that we could make a start on this in the UK by setting up a spirituality and psychiatry special interest group in the Royal College of Psychiatrists.[3] Since 1999, we have attracted a membership of more than 1,200 psychiatrists. Our website is in the public domain and the subject of spirituality and mental health is now a stated concern of the College.[4]

None of this need be remote or esoteric stuff. A psychiatrist can easily include taking a spiritual history as part of the consultation process. Just a few questions asked with sincerity and interest will elicit a person's important beliefs, and how they affect the way he sees the world and the problems and challenges of life. And when a person is searching for answers that go beyond the limits of psychology, there are times when the psychiatrist may usefully go with his patient into the transpersonal realm. At all events, the psychiatrist who can be a caring confidant for his patient's soul-searching will be amply rewarded, for it is only required of him to be fully 'present'. The soul in its wisdom will find the place of healing and it is our privilege to be able to help give it the occasion.

For further reading, see Andrew Powell's publications on Spirituality and Psychiatry at: www.andrewpowell.name or go to: www.rcpsych.ac.uk/college/SIG/spirit/publications/index

3   See www.rcpsych.ac.uk/spirit
4   See www.rcpsych.ac.uk. The Royal College of Psychiatrists Homepage, Mental Health
     Information drop-down menu, 'Mental Health and Spirituality': leaflet available as pdf. download.
     Printed version available on request from the College, tel: 020 7235 2351 ext 259. e-mail:
     leaflets@rcpsych.ac.uk

Reflection: Guided by the Breath of God
Paul Grey

When I talk about spirituality I am talking about using the breath of God that is inside of me to do good. My spirituality is lived out in my Christianity – my developing relationship with Jesus. Some may ask the question, how could someone who has this dynamic relationship with the Almighty God experience mental distress for over ten years? Although the answer to this question is far from straightforward, the following verse in the Bible satisfies my yearnings. *'All things work together and are [fitting into a plan] for good to and for those who love God and are called according to [His] design and purpose.'* Holding onto the truth of the resurrection of Jesus Christ, gave me hope that I too would be resurrected from the despair of hospitals, medication and negative stigma.

The individuals that make up the church allowed themselves to be directed by the breath of God, in order to positively affect my life. Within my church people prayed for me, and encouraged me to dream, instead of calling my dreams 'grandiose ideas' as past psychiatrists did. As a black man it is very important for me to have a black spiritual mentor. My pastor at the time showed his faith in for me by mentoring me and recommending that I study to become a licensed minister; this was from a congregation of 450 people and only a few of us were put forward. Other friends took me into their homes and socialized with me, while I was unwell. Being a part of a loving community enabled me to heal sooner and boosted my self-esteem, which often took a beating in the cold, lifelessness of the mental health institutions.

The Bible gave me an endless stream of life-giving words to resurrect me from mental distress. *'I can do all things through Christ who strengthens me... I am...wonderfully made.'* The positive impact of speaking these words to myself day in and day out means that I am now able to take charge of my own mental health. Can something as simple as words really make such a difference? Most certainly. I have been able to use the same words that encouraged me to encourage other people who have experienced mental distress. One young man that I worked with passed his exams despite all the odds and he accredited his success to the words that I penned in a greeting card. *'You are more than a conqueror.'*

Where the mental health system fails, is in packaging every diagnosis, care plan and report in pessimism and negativity. The church provides hope, optimism and love. My life is an advertisement, that an injection of encouragement and love is intrinsically more powerful than medication.

Reverend Paul Grey is currently the senior pastor in the Nuneaton New Testament Church of God.

CHAPTER 13

SPIRITUAL COMPETENCE: MENTAL HEALTH AND PALLIATIVE CARE

Cameron Langlands, David Mitchell and Tom Gordon

Introduction

This chapter seeks to blend the examples and experience of providing spiritual care in palliative care with experience and reflection on mental healthcare. In recent years spiritual care in palliative care has seen considerable development through national and professional standards, guidelines and competencies (Association of Hospice and Palliative Care Chaplains (AHPCC) 2006a, 2006b; Clinical Standards Board for Scotland (CSBS) 2002; Marie Curie Cancer Care (MCCC) 2003; National Institute for Clinical Excellence (NICE) 2004).

Palliative care is about much more than caring for the dying, it is an 'approach' that is applicable from diagnosis and focuses on improving the quality of life for patients and their families through the assessment and treatment of physical, psychological, social and spiritual problems (World Health Organization 2003). Utilizing the skills and expertise of a multidisciplinary team, the focus of care is on the individual patient within the context of their family.

Chaplaincy standards in palliative care have shown that professional spiritual care provision can be defined and evidenced, and competencies for spiritual and religious care have demonstrated that individual healthcare professionals can be made aware of their skills and limitations in providing spiritual care (Gordon and Mitchell 2004; Mitchell and Hibberd 2004).

As will be seen from the practical examples in this chapter, all staff have the potential to provide spiritual care. However, chaplaincy has a particular role and expertise to offer patients, their families and all healthcare professionals (AHPCC 2006b; MCCC 2003).

Distinguishing spiritual care and religious care

The terms spiritual care and religious care are often used interchangeably, as two sides of the same coin, thus giving rise to much confusion. Some chaplains also fall into this trap by equating both spiritual and religious care within the context of a particular faith community. However, spiritual care and religious care are not the same, nor are they interchangeable: they are two distinct ways of caring for people.

The Scottish Executive through a Health Department Letter (HDL) has issued a helpful definition that clearly distinguishes the terms and sets them in a clear context:

- *Religious care* is given in the context of the shared religious beliefs, values, liturgies and lifestyle of a faith community.

- *Spiritual care* is usually given in a one-to-one relationship, is completely person-centred and makes no assumptions about personal conviction or life orientation.

- *Spiritual care* is not necessarily religious. Religious care, at its best, should always be spiritual.

(NHS HDL 76 2002)

Spiritual competence

To encourage and enable all healthcare professionals in their provision of spiritual care and religious care Marie Curie Cancer Care has published *Spiritual and Religious Care Competencies for Specialist Palliative Care* (MCCC 2003). These competencies use a format that encourages healthcare professionals to discern and consider the spiritual needs and religious needs of patients and their family/carers. The competencies are set out in a clear progressive format over four levels, with staff expected to be able to meet or be working towards the required level for their profession:

Level 1:   Staff with casual contact with patients and their families.

Level 2:   Staff whose duties require direct contact with patients, e.g. healthcare assistants.

Level 3: The multi-disciplinary team – doctors, nurses, physio-
therapists, occupational therapists, social workers.

Level 4: Chaplains – those whose primary responsibility is spiritual
and religious care.

It is fair to say that the role of the chaplain is regularly misunderstood by
healthcare professionals and aligned solely with religion. Level 4 of the
competencies clearly expresses the expertise and clinical experience required
of chaplains in the much broader areas of spiritual care and religious care.

At each level the knowledge, skills and actions required to evidence
competence in spiritual and religious care are distinguished. These include
the ability to discern and distinguish spiritual and religious needs, to assess
spiritual and religious needs, to recognize complex spiritual, religious and
ethical issues, to refer on to specialist spiritual care resources (chaplaincy)
and to document the assessment, referrals and interventions. A key element
in the competencies is the identification of education and training needs of
healthcare professionals in this area of care, alongside a clear recognition
of the individual professional's limitations and a referral pathway to the next
level.

As will be seen in the examples in this chapter, very often the catalyst for
discerning spiritual or religious distress comes from the health professionals
instinct and experience. It can be hard to put into words, but you know there
is something there. Our humanity alongside our professional and communication skills is a powerful tool. However, there is another side to healthcare
professionals' role in spiritual care and that is to be aware of our own spirituality and beliefs around life, illness, suffering, death and dying. If we are
unsure of what we think and believe we can very quickly feel out of our
depth with patients and their families/carers, and are more likely to say or
do something that is less than helpful.

With the example and analysis of patient scenarios the authors will now
consider the role of healthcare professionals working as a team with different levels of competency to deliver spiritual care and religious care.

Spiritual care and the healthcare team

The theologian Harry Vanstone (1982) wrote a book entitled *The Stature of
Waiting*. Most of us, especially in the procedure and protocol driven world of
health care, find waiting very difficult. Far from waiting being seen as something of 'stature', and, therefore of worth and value, it is so often viewed as a
'statue' activity, in other words, not a proper activity at all. 'Why don't you do
something?' 'Why don't you say something?' are often the cries which come

over the loudest, or the instructions we respond to first. For to appear to do or say nothing, or to wait until it is more appropriate to do or say something, is at best viewed with tacit suspicion, and at worse is openly criticized as failure.

Waiting

In an understanding of spiritual care, and as a competency through which good spiritual care can be delivered, waiting is to be seen as something of stature, and needs to be understood and worked on as a necessary offering of good care. Waiting is not a passive activity. If it takes places in a climate of sensitivity and awareness; if it is an attitude which avoids an overbearing or paternalistic approach – or what Purcell (1998) describes as 'spiritual terrorism' – if it is a product of an appropriate therapeutic relationship between the healthcare professional and the patient or carer (Hyland 2005); then it is the fertile ground in which good spiritual care can and does grow.

Case study: Patient scenario I

Edith was a 75-year-old long-term patient suffering from advanced dementia. Brian, the chaplain, knew Edith well, having spent many occasions in her company, holding her hand, and giving her gentle words of reassurance. But Edith never responded. There was no sign of recognition, animation or engagement. Each time Brian sat with her or walked her around the ward it was the same. Brian would ask himself 'What is the point of this?', or 'Where is spiritual care for Edith?'

One day as Brian and Edith walked around the ward in their usual silence, Brian turned to her and asked, 'Where are you, Edith?' He still doesn't know why he asked that particular question, it just seemed right at the time. And the response was what he described as a transforming experience. 'I'm on the farm,' Edith replied. Once he had caught his breath, Brian continued. 'What farm?' 'My grand-dad's farm,' was the reply, 'and I've got no shoes on.' 'What's the farm like?' 'It's warm, and there's a gentle breeze. I've to feed the chickens, and they've all come running round my pail. I like being on the farm. It makes me feel good. And I love the chickens.' And Edith smiled before lapsing once more into silence.

For a moment, Edith had been alive down on the farm. Deep within the recesses of her memory she was living again, happy and free, and those recesses had been unlocked by a simple question, asked after hours and days of waiting.

This essence of Brian and Edith's scenario is a spiritual issue, and the willingness to wait is an important aspect of competency in spiritual care. This was not a religions moment for Edith, nor a profound exploration of the meaning of life, or a sorting of end-of-life issues. It was simply allowing Edith to be Edith again, just for a moment. And it was the product of a climate which had been created by patience, sensitivity and the building of trust in a healthcare professional who did not impose or work to his own agenda.

There are three values to this approach. First, it recognizes the uniqueness of the individual with whom you are working and the context which informs their needs. Who knows why Brian asked his initial question? But what we do know is that it was a product of time spent getting to know Edith, picking up clues, concentrating on what is happening, living with a real person and not someone simply defined by a mental-health label.

In his times of waiting Brian had, perhaps unconsciously, become aware of a context, and it was within that context that he was able to allow Edith to live again down on the farm. On another occasion the context might be a faded photograph on a bedside locker, or a tune hummed in the bath, or a smile of recognition at a TV programme, or a glint in the eye when a joke is told. Time spent getting to know a person and their context, and, therefore, understanding the world they inhabit, is never wasted in the field of spiritual care.

The second is that it allows the spiritual to be seen as integral to the holistic care which is offered to the patient. It may well be that within a multi-disciplinary team (MDT) it has become clear that there is an area of a patient's well-being which, though identified, is not able to be handled by members of the team. There may not be the time, skills, patience, insight or knowledge in the whole team or in individuals within it to go further into the area of meaning and purpose which the patient requires. However, having identified the area of concern and need, and the MDT having gone as far within the levels of competency available in, for example, levels 1 to 3, are we to say that we can do no more, and leave this area of care unexplored? Or are we going to identify that there is an additional resource of a skilled practitioner operating a higher level of competency to whom such an area of care can be referred?

Given that Brian – with patience and awareness, and working with developed competencies of skill, knowledge and actions at competency level 4 – was able to help Edith be in touch with something which gave her life meaning, this did not mean that it was Brian's achievement alone or that the work of the team with Edith's spiritual welfare was complete. Brian represents the competency of the team at the highest level, and, as a result, Edith's spiritual care is owned, delivered and continues to be explored by the whole

MDT. And, indeed, with more patience and the sensitive response to further opportunities, would always be so.

The third value in this approach is that it is patient-centred, and allows for the territory to be mapped out by the patient and not the healthcare professional delivering the spiritual care. It is, if you like, the acceptance that patients can and do facilitate their own spiritual care, but what they need is someone to help make that happen. The task of spiritual care competencies is to help people 'articulate their longings' (Gordon 2001). Most people have no need for such articulation when life is fine and there are no crises to face or traumas to be overcome. And when they do need to articulate their longings, many find that they have no language, methodology or belief systems with which to operate. So the role of the spiritual carer is that of the companion, 'sometimes sitting empty-handed when you would rather run away' (Cassidy 1991).

In the procedure and protocol world of present-day healthcare, 'doing something' and 'saying something' may not always be the most appropriate ways to proceed. Good spiritual care does not fit neatly into procedures and protocols. But far from this being passive or 'opting out' approach, it provides both the healthcare professional and the patient with an appropriate underpinning for spiritual care. Such an underpinning, strengthened by the values of the uniqueness of the individual, the integration of spiritual care into a holistic approach, and the delivery of care being totally patient-centred, offers a firm platform from which carer and cared for can begin a journey of growth and wholeness.

Religious care and the healthcare team

> Even though I go through the deepest darkness…
>
> (Psalm 23:4)

When Marion was admitted to the ward it had quickly become apparent to the multi-disciplinary team that they were facing a situation that was outside their own area of expertise. Here was a lady that was uncooperative, shouting words of condemnation to all those around her and refusing even basic help from staff members. Marion was a religious person, she presented as such and the notes which came with her highlighted this fact. In addition to this, her language was punctuated with religious, and specifically Christian references. By using their instinct and experience, by discerning Marion's spiritual and religious needs and referring on appropriately, the multi-disciplinary team sought to bring in the member of the team who had that particular expertise.

Case study: Patient scenario 2

Marion was 80 years old and was refusing to both eat and take her medication in community. As her mental health started to deteriorate rapidly Marion was brought into the local psychiatric hospital as an emergency admission. Audrey, the chaplain, received a call from the Charge Nurse to say that Marion was refusing to eat, as well as take her medication, and that the staff were having difficulty in communicating with her. The Charge Nurse hoped someone non-medical might be able to find out why she was refusing both food and medication. The Charge Nurse also mentioned that Marion seemed very religious.

Audrey introduced herself to Marion as the chaplain. Looking at Audrey with a suspicious gaze, Marion wouldn't speak to her. 'Unless you come in His name, and look like a Chaplain then I won't be talking to you!' she said. Audrey went and put her clerical collar on and re-introduced herself to Marion. 'In whose name do you come?' Marion said. 'I come in the name of the Lord Jesus Christ,' Audrey replied. 'Well you had better sit down then.'

As the conversation continued over a couple of hours it became apparent that the reason Marion was refusing food and medication was that she was 'fasting for Christ'. The reason she hadn't told anyone on the ward was that she viewed everyone else as heathens. It was only in seeing the chaplain's collar, and the chaplain knowing the correct formula of words, that Marion felt secure enough to describe what she was doing. Audrey suggested to Marion that her fast be broken by celebrating Communion together. By doing this, Marion felt that she was honouring her Lord and also being true to her ideals. Through Audrey's patience, gently probing questions and an awareness of the importance of rites, rituals and dress to Marion, she was able to attend to her religious needs which, as a result, enabled Marion to eat and take her medication.

The initial visit that Audrey made to Marion highlighted the fact that the ward and staff were alien to her. The best way to describe her experience was as a stranger in a strange land. Marion was disorientated, didn't know where she was or why she was there. Although Marion had not seen the inside of a church for years due to an enduring mental illness combined with increasing frailty, she was holding on to the only thing that made sense to her, the thing that gave her life structure and meaning – her faith. Within this familiar world the staff were excluded; they were deemed to be heathen and so Marion was not going to contaminate herself by talking to them. Marion was fasting, keeping herself pure for her Lord, and so there was no way that she was going to allow 'them' to enter her world. By donning her clerical collar, by knowing and speaking the correct religious language, by reflecting back the language that Marion herself was using, Audrey managed to open the door to Marion's world for the wider healthcare team.

Through sharing Marion's values and understanding how they were working themselves out as part of her illness, in offering and taking part in a familiar liturgy when surrounded by the unfamiliar, by being seen to be part (and dressing the part) of the witnessing community, Audrey managed to deliver religious care that spoke to the heart of Marion's situation. Although there was still brokenness of mind, her intervention allowed the healing process to begin and enabled the other members of the healthcare team to use their skills and expertise in that on going process.

Conclusion

These two scenarios give a brief insight into the realm of competency in spiritual and religious care. It is evident that the holistic, multi-disciplinary approach of palliative care is applicable to other aspects of healthcare and especially so the speciality that is mental health.

All healthcare professionals have the potential, and it could be argued a duty, to discern, assess and address the needs of their patients. The competency model encourages healthcare professionals to use and develop their individual professional and human instincts and experience in order to raise awareness of their skills in spiritual and religious care. Just as important, however, is the raising of self-awareness and an understanding of our individual limitations.

It could be argued that by specifying different levels of competency and declaring an expertise in spiritual and religious care there is the potential to de-skill those who are already sensitive and proactive in assessing and addressing spiritual and religious care. The authors' experience is that the reverse is the case: by raising healthcare professionals' awareness to these competencies they can find they are affirmed and enabled to understand and gain confidence in the care they are already providing. In addition, by setting out a clear level of expertise and knowing that there is another level to refer on to actually encourages healthcare professionals to be more proactive in discerning and assessing spiritual and religious needs. There is a confidence to open the door and tentatively enter the patient's spiritual and religious world knowing that if you feel out of your depth, or it is clear the patient needs someone with specific skills, there is someone else on the team to whom you can refer.

If we are truly serious in making patients the focus of our care, if we are serious about multi-disciplinary team working, and serious about recognizing that spiritual needs and religious needs can be of real importance to patients, then we owe it to our patients to take spiritual and religious care competency seriously. Understanding the difference between spiritual and religious care, being self-aware of your own gifts, skills and limitations, and having the confidence to use your instinct and experience to refer on when appropriate, can be a liberating experience, and, therefore, considerably improve the spiritual and religious care for our patients and their carers.

References

AHPCC (2006a) *Guidelines for Hospice and Palliative Care Chaplaincy*. London: Association of Hospice and Palliative Care Chaplains.

AHPCC (2006b) *Standards for Hospice and Palliative Care Chaplaincy*. London: Association of Hospice and Palliative Care Chaplains.

Cassidy, S. (1991) *Sharing the Darkness: The Spirituality of Caring*. Maryknoll, NY: Orbis Books.

CSBS (2002) *Clinical Standards Specialist Palliative Care*. Edinburgh: (Formerly the Clinical Standards Board for Scotland) NHS Quality Improvement Scotland.

Gordon, T. (2001) *A Need for Living: Signposts on the Journey of Life and Beyond*. Glasgow: Wild Goose Publications.

Gordon, T. and Mitchell, D. (2004) 'A competency model for the assessment and delivery of spiritual care.' *Palliative Medicine 18*, 7, 646–51.

Hyland, M.E. (2005) 'A tale of two therapies: psychotherapy and complimentary and alternative medicine (CAM) *and the human effect*.' *Clinical Medicine 5*, 4, 361–7.

MCCC (2003) *Spiritual and Religious Care Competencies for Specialist Palliative Care*. London: Marie Curie Cancer Care.

Mitchell, D. and Hibberd, C. (2004) 'A Comparative Assessment of Hospice Chaplaincy Services.' *Scottish Journal of Healthcare Chaplaincy 7*, 1, 6–11.

NHS HDL 76 (2002) *Spiritual Care in NHS Scotland: Guidelines on Chaplaincy and Spiritual Care in the NHS in Scotland*. Edinburgh: Scottish Executive.

NICE (2004) *Improving Supportive and Palliative Care for Adults with Cancer Manual*. London: National Institute for Clinical Excellence.

Purcell, B.C. (1998) 'Spiritual terrorism.' *American Journal of Hospice and Palliative Care 15*, 3, 167–73.

Vanstone, V.H. (1982) *The Stature of Waiting*. London: Darton, Longman and Todd.

World Health Organization (2003) *WHO Definition of Palliative Care*. Available at www.who.int/cancer/palliative/definition/en/ (accessed 20 September 2007).

You Say You Have No Music?

For Stuart

And yet you have frequencies, daily,
Monthly, yearly and who knows more.
And the solemn dance of the beat of your
heart.
And the resonances of inner spaces,
The physical, spiritual, emotional and who
knows more,
And endless ocean of manifold tides,
And I swear your words raise tides on the
moon.
And how they sigh, those seawind sighs,
As they whirl and swoop and soar like
singing
And try to tell me you have no music?
While others gather to hear the singing,
And sigh and dance in turn, and forget,
That only the singer needs time to hear
What only the singer has power to tell.

Mark Bones

CHAPTER 14

WORKING WITH QI (CHI) TO HELP WITH MENTAL HEALTH PROBLEMS

Nigel Mills

For many years I have worked with people with mental health problems using strategies that encourage an awareness of the relationship between mind–body–spirit. These strategies are drawn from the ancient Taoist practice of Qigong (sometimes also written as Chi Gung). Central to this practice is the cultivation of an awareness of 'Qi'. We do not have a direct translation for Qi in English; the word 'energy' is sometimes used, but, to my mind, Qi has layers of meaning which go beyond just 'energy'.

Qi also refers to the sense of connection with the core of our being and that which gives us a sense of connection with the potential of the environment around us to nurture our being. It has been named in many cultures. Some of these names are Qi, Chi, Prana and Pneuma. Some might call it the life force or spirit. Or to put it another way:

> There must be some primal force,
> but it is impossible to locate.
> I believe it exists, but cannot see it.
> I see its results,
> I can even feel it
> But it has no form.

> (Zhuang Zi, Inner Chapters, Fourth Century BCE)

Qigong comes from the same tradition as Tai Chi. Qigong exercises cultivate an awareness of breath, of posture, of emotional holding, of connection with the earth and connection with others. The practice of Qigong predates the more structured format of Tai Chi and was being practised in ancient China many hundreds of years before Tai Chi. Qigong focuses directly on the awareness of 'energy' or Qi and does not involve the learning of sequential moves or 'forms' as are taught in Tai Chi.

It was through learning and valuing Qigong for myself that I began to consider its potential benefits for the service users I saw in my work as a Clinical Psychologist. I personally knew its value in allowing me to 'shake off' emotional tension and in helping me to feel grounded and more fully alive.

I had also noted, in my work as a Clinical Psychologist, that many people with long-term mental health problems were not able to engage with the usual verbal–intellectual approach to therapy. Verbal therapy sometimes seemed as useful as the application of a can opener to get inside a tank.

Weiner has described how: 'Language is only a representation, a second-ary experience of the primary experience... Primary experience exists apart from language and is often not accessible by it' (Weiner 1999).

Qigong provides one of the best ways I have come across of working directly with primary experience. Qigong deals directly with emotional experience and our way of being without having to become enmeshed in verbal analysis.

It is my belief that in the West, our education system and our culture, encourages us from a too-young age to become head-oriented. The fidgety six-year-old quickly learns that it is not safe to allow his Qi to flow through his body, he is told to 'sit still and listen' and so the flow of Qi becomes blocked and drawn to the head. We learn that it is not safe to allow our Qi to flow because reprimands follow. Similarly following emotional trauma, our culture encourages us 'to get on with things' or 'put a brave face on'.

It is my experience that people with mental health problems have often experienced some kind of trauma and have reacted to that trauma with a dis-tortion in the way in which they 'inhabit' their body. This distortion may take several forms, it could be a withdrawal of their Qi (just as a hedgehog withdraws under threat); it may be a thrusting out of their Qi (as a cat may arch its back to make it look bigger) or it may be experienced as a 'leaving' of the body in an attempt to escape the trauma, as described by Levine (1997). Levine compares and contrasts how animals and humans react to stress as follows:

> The duration of the immobility response in animals is normally time limited; they go in and they come out. The human immobility response does not easily resolve itself because the supercharged

energy locked in the nervous system is imprisoned by the emotions
of fear and terror…a vicious cycle of fear and immobility takes over,
preventing the response from completing naturally (p.101).

The process of Qigong provides a way for the fear to be released in a safe
controlled way so that it feels safe to drop the energy flow distortions, to
re-inhabit the body in a full way, and allow the Qi to flow harmoniously
again.

What does Qigong involve?

The typical image the person in the street may have of Tai Chi/Qigong is
one of Chinese people in a park moving their arms about in a funny way.
Why should they be doing this? Why on earth should moving your arms in a
funny way help your emotional state or state of mind?

It is not so much the outer movements which are important in achieving
peace of mind, it is rather the sense of inner movement. The inner movement
of awareness. In fact one can practise Qigong without moving at all. A lot of
the benefits of Qigong can be achieved though finding a different way of
sitting or standing. A way of sitting or standing which encourages a certain
way of being.

It is my experience that there are three phases in the use of Qigong to
help overcome mental health problems:

1.   Development of a sensation-based awareness of one's current way of
      being.

2.   A softening, a release, to allow that way of being to change.

3.   An 'opening' to allow 'something' to come in which can nurture.

DEVELOPMENT OF A SENSATION-BASED AWARENESS OF ONE'S CURRENT WAY OF BEING

Why should this be important? If we are not in touch with the sensations in
our body it can be very hard to gain any feedback as to how the way in which
we are holding ourself can be inhibiting our potential for self-healing.

As an example, if you stand with your knees locked and the legs straight
and rigid, notice what happens to your breathing. It becomes shallower, and
held. If you allow the knees to bend slightly so you are taking the weight of
your body more on the muscles of the thighs, then the weight of the body
can go down into the feet and your connection with the ground can be cultivated. The ground is a potential source of nourishment, as we will explore
later. If we cut ourselves off from the ground through a rigid posture, we cut
off a potential source of self-healing.

Secondly if the pelvis is pushed forwards or pushed backwards then this again creates a restriction and the sense of flow and connection between the upper body and the ground is disrupted. In Qigong we encourage a sense of the pelvis as being neither pushed forward nor pushed backwards but free to float in the middle.

A SOFTENING, A RELEASE, TO ALLOW THAT WAY OF BEING TO CHANGE

People with a tendency to anxiety and panic tend to hold their tension in the upper part of the body around the head and around the upper chest. People with a tendency to anxiety also tend to restrict their breathing. The breath becomes shallow and rapid, the shoulders often become tight and the neck also becomes tight, a sense of tension in head often accumulates.

Qigong provides a way of allow that tension to move and go down towards the floor and into the ground. Finding a pathway for the excess activity or 'Qi' of the head to flow to the ground can be a vitally important discovery.

Bruce Frantzis (1993) describes a Qigong exercise in which any sense of tension or tightness or something that doesn't feel quite right in the body can be allowed to flow down through the body until the tension melts away into the floor. This simple technique by itself can often be of considerable help to people who suffer from panic attacks or anxiety.

The way in which this exercise is taught is subtly, but very importantly, different from 'just relaxation'. Relaxation exercises are often used as a distraction from one's experience, somewhere else to place your attention instead of on the distressing experience. In Qigong the emphasis is not on distracting yourself from the distress, but rather *allowing* the distress to flow down through the body, so that it is no longer held in one place. Interestingly this is also the most recent recommendation of clinical psychologists who practice cognitive behaviour therapy. They describe how clients should be empowered to have the experience of 'surviving' their emotions rather than distracting themselves with relaxation or other 'safety behaviours' (Segal, Williams and Teasdale 2002).

Grounding

Our culture encourages a disconnection with the earth. We rush along in vehicles blocked from the grounding influence of the earth by rapidly rotating discs of rubber and steel; or we sit in armchairs watching flickering screens with our feet hovering above the floor. Jahnke (2002), in his excellent book on Qigong, describes how one can re-establish a connection with the earth by deliberately placing one's attention below one's feet. Imagining one's awareness being drawn to the very centre of the earth. Of course the connection with the earth can be encouraged not just through Qigong but through activities which remind us of our dependence on the earth like gardening or walking in the countryside. However, in the practice of Qigong you make this connection with the earth much more conscious, and you deliberately practise placing your attention below your feet. Sometimes it is useful to use the analogy of the roots of a tree. Imagining your awareness searching down, between the rocks, just as tree roots search for moisture and nutrients so our awareness can search for connection to the grounding influence of the planet beneath our feet.

When I work with people who suffer with anxiety, I generally recommend they practise this cultivation of connection with the earth on a daily basis, not to leave it until they are feeling anxious. The practice and skill need to be cultivated when one is feeling fairly calm and in a non-threatening environment. When the person has developed some skill in connection with the earth, then it is useful to test it out in an anxiety provoking situation. The task then is to allow the waves of anxiety to travel through the body and to pass into the earth, to allow the earth to soak up the anxiety.

Softening through breathing

It is my experience that people who suffer from mental health problems also suffer from a restricted breathing pattern. In the case of anxiety, this restricted breathing may serve a function of initially limiting the amount of anxiety that the sufferer has to experience. However, this limiting of the anxiety sensations is counterproductive as it holds the anxiety in the body and makes it last much, much longer than would be the case if it was allowed to run through the body and down to the earth.

It is not just anxiety which is accompanied by restricted breathing. In depression too, it sometimes feels that if one was to allow oneself to breathe fully then the emotions which would come up, whether of grief, of anger, or despair would be too great to withstand. Therefore many of us indulge in what cognitive behavioural therapists call a 'safety behaviour' of limiting the breath. It is as if we are saying to ourselves, 'If I was to breathe fully then the emotional distress that would be contacted would be too great for me to withstand; I must therefore restrict my breathing and so keep myself safe.'

An excellent guide to working therapeutically with the breath through Qigong has been written (and put on to audio and video formats) by Bruce Frantzis. Frantzis (1993, 1999) has made a lifelong study of the healing methods of Qigong including many years spent in China studying under renowned masters. He has described, for a Western audience, how the

Qigong approach to breathing can be used to enhance health, promote longevity and encourage a calm state of mind.

In this chapter I can only give a brief overview of some of the principles involved.

To release anxiety the emphasis is generally on the out-breath. If a full out-breath has been achieved, then the in-breath will follow naturally. This avoids a tendency to suck breath in or to pull breath in forcibly, which can in itself create a heightened state of tension and anxiety. Allowing a full out-breath, you can encourage a general sense of letting go and releasing.

In Qigong breathing, we allow the abdomen to expand and release one step further, and also bring our attention to the lower back. The whole cylinder of the lower torso can be encouraged to expand in all directions on the in-breath and to fall back on the out-breath.

In addition to increased oxygenation of the blood and the brain and calming of the autonomic nervous system, this relaxed abdominal breathing also has the effect of anchoring the awareness more fully into the body and away from the 'chatter' of the mind.

It should be noted here that some schools of Qigong and Yoga teach a 'forced breathing' technique. It is my experience that this can sometimes be counterproductive for people suffering with mental health problems as it sets up a situation where one part of the body is trying to do one thing and another is trying to do something else. So for self-healing we generally use words such as 'allowing' or 'giving permission to' or 'softening'. If this attitude of allowing and softening can be cultivated then the body will find its own fuller way of breathing without any battle having to be entered into.

It should be noted that when unhelpful patterns begin to release people can sometimes feel worse to start with. The holding-on has been for a reason, to shield ourselves from feeling, and we are now allowing ourselves to feel. The release can happen with waves of emotion which might be visibly expressed with crying, chuckling or laughter. The release allows something nurturing to enter, as described in the next section.

AN 'OPENING' TO ALLOW 'SOMETHING' TO COME IN WHICH CAN NURTURE

Initially, this is where the movement part of Qigong comes in. Although the movements of Qi Gong often have as their essence something which involves the arms coming up from the ground, palms up, to the level of the shoulders or above the head and them coming down again palms facing the earth, it is not really possible through the medium of the written word to describe Tai Chi or Qigong movements. They need to be observed and practised and the practitioner needs to be given feedback. In addition advanced practitioners of Qigong usually make very few movements. However, it is possible to use the written word to describe what one is aiming for, through carrying out these movements.

One of the main aims, to my mind, of the Qigong movements is to train the awareness to come through the body in a certain way and to create a pathway through which tension can be released and fresh QI absorbed. The movements are carried out with the intention of allowing 'something nurturing' (i.e. Qi/Chi/Prana/God's Love) to flow through the body in a calm nourishing way.

By carrying out the body movements of Qigong, it is my experience that people also find it much easier to root their attention in the intention of self-healing. It is as if the bodily movements can bring the mind into a certain relationship with the body, a relationship of self-nurturing.

However the nurturing is not just from the self to the self. The nurturing can also come from a much bigger system than our own. The ancient Chinese texts refer to the Qi we can absorb from 'Heaven' and from 'Earth'.

In Qigong many of the ancient writings refer to the tasks of human life as being to create a marriage between heaven and earth. In these Ancient Chinese writings, heaven and earth do not represent places, but rather qualities of energy. Thus the energy of the earth has the quality of being able to soak things up, to absorb and to root. The quality of heaven is more one of spaciousness, expansiveness, of light and love.

The ancient masters of Qigong advise that one needs to spend most of one's practice in releasing tension down to earth and connecting with the nurturing solidity of the earth before one is able to receive the spaciousness and love from heaven. An analogy may be of trying to shine a beam of light through the top of a bottle which is full of mud. The light beam would not penetrate very far. However, if the mud was first of all washed through the bottle and out into the earth through holes in the base of the bottle then, and only then, would the light be able to shine through the bottle and down into the earth.

Thus, in order for us to benefit from the light from heaven we have to first of all clear out the mud. Many of the practices of Qigong are dedicated to this aim – clearing out the mud from the system. This may involve movements such as swinging the arms or bouncing movements, shaking movements or directed breathing. To clear out the mud one also has to train one's awareness, to allow the feet to open up and melt into to the ground, so the mud from the body can be released into the ground. This process may take many years.

When one has released sufficient 'mud' (or stagnant Qi) for the light to shine through and when one's awareness can be kept in the present moment so that one can give permission for the light to shine through, then one can be ready to receive 'heaven'.

Again it is important to point out that this process does not involve a forcing or a 'pulling in' of heaven but rather adopting an attitude with which one can allow oneself to *receive* the Qi of Heaven, which is always there, if only we can find the way to allow it to enter us. This attitude necessarily involves the development of compassion for oneself and others. If the compassion isn't there, the opening will not occur. There are no shortcuts to heaven.

For people with mental health problems, most authorities in Qigong would not recommend opening up to the Qi of Heaven without first having spent considerable time, creating a clear enough vessel into which that form of spiritual support can enter. For people going through an experience of psychosis, the main benefit of Qigong is in helping to create a sense of being 'centred and grounded' from which they can develop their confidence in being able to survive the psychotic phenomena (Mills and Whiting 1997; Mills 2001b, 2002).

I have used Qigong to help people of different religious faiths to work in this way (Mills 2000a). I have found that one does not have to use the language of Qigong, but can adapt that language to the faith of the client concerned. For example, if I am working with a Christian client I may say:

> If you were to allow yourself to receive the love of God, which part of your body do you feel that love would enter through? If that love of God was to be represented by a coloured light, then what colour would it be for you? So if you were to allow that possibility just now of allowing that particular colour light to enter into that part of the body and allowing it to circulate through your body, how would you have to change your posture, to change your way of being, to change your attitude towards yourself and others, so as to allow that light to come right into your very being? (Mills and Whiting 1997; Mills 2000a)

Who may benefit?

Just about anyone who wants to! As with any therapy, the recipient has to perceive some credibility in the approach and also the recipient has to want to help themselves through this modality. Someone who is convinced that the answer to their problems lies in developing a verbal understanding of their situation would be better off taking that route. Someone who wants to feel energetically and physically more 'solid' without having a desire, or perhaps an ability, to analyse verbally where their fragility came from, is a more likely candidate. The 'modality' with which we interact with our world, is, to my mind, crucial in determining the form of therapy with which we are most likely to benefit.

I am therefore not advocating that Qigong should be routinely given out to all people with mental health problems. It is my experience however that for those people who wish to work with their kinaesthetic/energetic experience in a direct way, then significant gains can be made.

In one-to-one therapy I have found that people can use Qigong to help discharge the 'bound energy' of post-traumatic stress disorder and of panic attacks. In group settings I have used aspects of Qigong with people with a diagnosis of psychosis. By developing a sense of 'centre' it becomes easier to cope with the 'fragmentation' of psychosis (Mills and Whiting 1997; Mills 2001b). Probably one of the most rewarding settings, where I have used 'therapeutic Qigong' is that of the acute inpatient ward. Readers familiar with these will be aware of the typical lack of any therapeutic input beyond medication. This is largely due to the rapid turnover of residents and staff, and so traditional verbal psychotherapies are not appropriate, due to the complete lack of consistency. Using Qigong, however, each session stands alone and it is my experience that Service Users in a state of 'fragmentation' often benefit enormously from a non-verbal opportunity to 'gather themselves together', to become more centred and grounded and to receive a 'nurturing beyond words'.

Finally it is my experience that health professionals also have a strong need to centre themselves while they are facing the turmoil of the emotions of others. If one can find a way to centre and replenish one's own energy, then one is more likely to be able to pass on that ability to others. I would therefore strongly recommend the practice of Qigong for any health professionals who would like to improve their ability to cope with the distress of others (Mills 2000b).

Research questions

It is my opinion that we have lost a great opportunity, in the development of therapies, by going down the 'one size fits all' route and investing millions of pounds of research money in trying to find out which therapy is 'the best'. A far more useful question, to my mind, is 'how can we ascertain which individual is most likely to benefit from which approach'. We acknowledge that some people are very sporty whereas others prefer poetry, others again prefer art whereas others prefer dancing. Yet for some reason we do not acknowledge that these individual differences are likely to affect what sort of therapeutic approach people are likely to engage in. Instead we assume that people's way of interacting with their world is irrelevant and what is important is the 'therapy' itself.

If there is ever any 'scientific' research into Qigong for mental health problems I think it needs to address this question: 'What sort of *person* (not what sort of diagnosis) is more likely to benefit from a kinaesthetic/energetic therapeutic approach as opposed to a verbal therapeutic approach.'

Useful websites

www.nigelmillstherapies.co.uk
Describes the background and current clinical work of the author.

www.energyarts.com
Gives details of training in Qigong in the USA and Europe and self-help audio and video material from the Qigong teacher Bruce Frantzis.

www.Qigong-southwest.co.uk
Gives details of training in Qigong available in the South West of England.

www.dao-hua-qigong.com
Gives details of training in Qigong in London and some self-help audio and video material from the Qigong teacher Zhixing Wang.

References

Frantzis, B. (1993) *Opening the Energy Gates of the Body*. Berkeley, CA: North Atlantic Books.

Frantzis, B. (1999) *The Great Stillness*. Fairfax, CA: Clarity Press.

Jahnke, R. (2002) *The Healing Promise of Qi. Creating Extraordinary Wellness through Qigong and Tai Chi*. New York: McGraw-Hill, Contemporary Books.

Levine, P. (1997) *Waking the Tiger: Healing Trauma*. Berkeley, CA: North Atlantic Books.

Mills, N. (2000a) 'Working with the client's sense of spiritual nourishment.' *Transpersonal Psychology Review 4*, 2, 23–25.

Mills, N. (2000b) 'Therapist burn-out or therapist glow? Some light from the East.' *Clinical Psychology Forum 146*, 30–33.

Mills, N. (2001a) 'Working with the body in cognitive therapy.' *Clinical Psychology 4*, 25–8.

Mills, N. (2001b) 'The Experience of Fragmentation in Psychosis. Can Mindfulness Help?' In I. Clarke (ed.) *Psychosis and Spirituality*. London: Whurr.

Mills, N. (2002) 'The Experience of the Fragmented Body in Psychosis. Can Mindfulness Help?' *Journal of Critical Psychology, Counselling and Psychotherapy*, winter edition, 220–226.

Mills, N and Allen, J. (2000) 'Mindfulness of movement as a coping strategy in multiple sclerosis. A pilot study.' *General Hospital Psychiatry 22*, 425–31.

Mills, N., Allen, J. and Carey-Morgan, S. (2000) 'Does Tai Chi/Qi Gong help patients with multiple sclerosis?' *Journal of Bodywork and Movement Therapy 4*, 1, 39–48.

Mills, N. and Whiting, S. (1997) 'Being centred and being scattered: a kinaesthetic strategy for people who experience psychotic symptoms.' *Clinical Psychology Forum 103*, 27–31.

Segal, Z., Williams, M. and Teasdale, J. (2002) *Mindfulness Based Cognitive Therapy for Depression*. New York: Guilford Press.

Weiner, D. (1999) *Beyond Talk Therapy: Using Movement and Expressive Techniques in Clinical Practice*. Washington: American Psychological Association.

Holy Love

He writes poetry
Thinking he is a poet
Writes about hardship
And despair
About being lost
And insane
About hopelessness
And pain
And rejection

Until he finds faith

Then he writes about
Beautiful things
That comes with it
Like love
A holy love
With Heaven in mind!

Khazim Reshat

CHAPTER 15

SPIRITUAL PRACTICE DAY BY DAY – CONVERSATIONS WITH THOSE WHO KNOW

Mary Ellen Coyte

Spiritual practice. So many different things. Shaped by many different things. Geography, history, science, beliefs, motivation, experience, feelings…life.

Discovering and fostering my own spiritual practice has been driven by my attempts to escape the clutches of chronic depression and suicidal thinking. Although 'driven' implies a sense of purpose and energy, quite unlike anything I felt in the worst decades of wading and drowning in the thickest of darknesses, with hindsight I think there was something of that nature within me, however hidden, faded and feeble. A puttering motor at the bottom of a deep, murky pond.

Eventually, during moments of spiritual practice, this motor was fired into a more lively, and life-giving state, giving me hope that things could change. Things *have* changed and continue to change, for the better, and, for me, it is my spiritual practice that is now the cornerstone of my well-being.

But my story is just one of zillions. In an attempt to capture something of the nature of spiritual practice, this piece also draws on other people's experience. It includes things I have read but it is a chance for you, the reader, to eavesdrop on conversations I have had with survivors of mental distress and those who work in mental health services. What is spiritual about what they do, and how does it help them?

Each of these people is very clear about what a spiritual practice is for them. Rather than define what it is, I hope their words speak for themselves.

I would have loved someone to have invited me to explore this realm many years ago, giving it authority and credence, yet being my companion on the journey, alongside me in my explorations. So, as well as giving a glimpse into other people's lives, this is a greeting to those on similar journeys and a warm invitation to the curious. An invitation to wonder, explore, consider and even reconsider.

Doing and being

There seems to be both a doing and a being about spiritual practice and these can be both separate and closely connected. For some people an essential part of their spiritual practice and mental health involves taking action to make the world a better place:

> Getting eco-conscious and campaigning made my spirit feel good.

On the other hand one can engage with an activity, a doing, which allows one to be still and 'be'. The stillness may be a stillness of movement, or an inner stillness, or both. These kinds of 'doing' might include meditation, being in nature, writing a poem, painting or listening to music.

For one person I spoke to, spiritual practice is more about a state of being:

> For me it's about awareness which can apply to everything. It's not about a mental thing, it's a heart and body thing. A sensory awareness and an emotional awareness of my own feelings, it's about opening up to the moment through body and feelings.

My conversations revealed that those who experience mental distress, and those who work with them in psychiatric care, use a great variety of spiritual practices.

Three stories from real life

The very personal stories from the following three people give a taste of the diversity of spiritual practice and how it can relate directly to specific mental states and well-being.

SHAMANIC JOURNEYING

> One approach I take to dealing with my psychosis, for want of a better word, is to use shamanic journeying. This involves travelling to realms outside day-to-day reality with a clear intention of why I

am doing it…in some ways being in a journey is similar to delusional states that I have been in. The main differences are that journeys typically last 30 minutes rather than a couple of months, there is a supportive environment and also set techniques for leaving ordinary reality and, most importantly, coming back.

I had always been a wilderness kind of person, but, having been in West Africa during my gap year, there was a definite increase of attraction towards earth-based spirituality. When I first became 'psychotic' I was very preoccupied with the phase of the moon and things culminated with a trip up Glastonbury tor in the middle of a very wild December night…in some ways earth spirituality was pretty much hard-wired into my perspective of being 'mad' and has continued to be a major driver. I first started reading seriously about shamanism about 18 months later when I was in day hospital. I was drawn very strongly to it as it seemed to offer some very applicable techniques to negotiate the changing realities of being psychotic.

MEDITATION

I have tried all kinds of meditation. Years ago I couldn't do it at all as my negative thoughts took over. However, through psychotherapy and other things, I moved on. So I took a few tentative steps, learning mainly from books, and was able to get into it more easily and trust it held some value for me. It was while I was meditating once that I became aware that a small flame had appeared inside me. And then I knew that there *had* been something missing all these years and that feeling something was missing had been a key cause of my anxiety and contributed to my depression… I had been right to keep searching. It had been awful sensing something was missing and not being sure exactly what it was, how to find it or how to put it in place. I always floated above the earth, never able to fully engage with this world. Now I felt I had an identity. Something had come home to me and I had come home to myself.

DANCING

I have realized as an adult that my need to dance helped me to survive and recover from my earlier years when I was emotionally and mentally abused. The sensation of being able to move my body and express things and emotions I could not put into words gave me the security I needed to grow up and has helped me learn about myself and the world around me when no one else was willing to do so. Dance has become a spiritual outlet for the rest of my life, improving and enlightening me every step of the way.

These experiences show how spiritual practice can have a direct bearing on mental well-being and clinically diagnosed mental distress. A purely clinical approach to mental distress, and a general ignorance of spirituality (including in some faith communities), can define and foster many so called mental health problems. These stories demonstrate the concept of breakdown-to-breakthrough which allows us to see mental distress as a difficult but ultimately positive experience if we can move through it in an appropriate way, not necessarily looking for cure but to find some kind of healing.

If spirituality or religion is included in this concept breakdown can also be seen as an opportunity or invitation, in some views an invitation by God, to develop our spiritual selves, bring it into balance and increase our spiritual understanding.

As far as I know the three people who told me these stories had no knowledge of the concept of breakdown-to-breakthrough, but that is the way their paths led. By instinct, by listening to their bodies and their deeper selves, they found their way to a spiritual practice which supports their mental health. This was not an overnight discovery, but something that evolved. Other people living with mental distress, who are less autonomous, might welcome support to find out what would help them to 'break through'.

Through my conversations I learned that some spiritual practices are common to many people who experience mental distress.

Other spiritual practices
PRAYER, AFFIRMATIONS AND SCRIPTURE
Prayer, affirmations and scripture can help on a day-to-day basis as a general practice and also in coping with the small and large crises of life.

For many people prayer is the mainstay of their spiritual well-being. In religious terms this includes talking to God about everything and God listening to, and answering, prayers.

In times of crisis several people I spoke to would manage to pray:

Help me! Help me!

which they did, indeed, find helpful.

The use of extemporary prayer can sometimes be too taxing especially during trauma and at these times saying well-known prayers, or anchor prayers, is a great comfort, perhaps using a string of beads such as the Christian rosary, Hindu mala, or the tasbih of Islam. People also find it helpful to repeat a comforting phrase from religious scripture or repeat an affirmation.

Religious affirmations usually involve extolling the virtues of God, rather than the self as in: 'Oh God you are so magnificent'. Much of the unhelpful impact of religion on mental distress is due to concentration on negative messages of sin and shame and an image of God as vengeful and retributive. Religious affirmations can change the focus of attention away from this to the positive attributes of God. Secular affirmations such as 'I love and approve of myself' focus the attention on the self and can have a powerful impact, especially when they are part of a belief system that encourages one to embrace the idea of a higher power, or the Universe, as a positive force and resource.

Holy Scripture can also be a strong source of support:

> Although I left the church, one thing that has helped is the promise that Jesus came to give life in all its fullness [The Bible, John 10:10]. It gives me hope – I want *that* kind of life. It helps me get angry with God and make demands, not put up with my depression – God promised a better life. It can help me not kill myself – what would I be like as *that* person, can I wait to find out?

ANGELS

Personally I have found the concept of angels very helpful. I decided to try communicating with them as they seemed to having nothing but positive attributes of kindness and gentleness, colour and light. In my harsh world of that time I saw them as a way of communicating with a welcoming spiritual realm when my God was a merciless, male being.

Since then I have noticed that people of all faiths and none have a special affection for angels. Nearly everyone I have spoken to, sometimes complete strangers, whether or not they have mental distress, likes the idea of them and believes in them.

> I believe people are angels. We are all angels.

> I call on the angels for help. It always works.

> When I feel helpless I ask them to help others and that makes me feel better.

FORGIVENESS, BLESSING AND THANKS

Those with mental distress have usually had very difficult circumstances to contend with either resulting in mental distress or due to it. The practices of forgiveness, blessing and thanks, secular or religious, are very healing:

> I pray for forgiveness for others. It helps heal the past and can help one to cope better with the present: When I have difficult feelings

about someone such as anger, fear or envy I bless them, imagine them feeling loved.

Others found it useful to say thank you for a difficult situation, for the opportunity to find out what it could teach them. They might be open to their sense of God or The Universe to help them deal with anger or other difficult feelings.

RITUAL

Three benefits of ritual, when your life has been turned upside down through mental distress, are its supportive structure, its familiarity, and its reference to a time when life was more under control. Rituals associated with religion carry their own spiritual meaning and value which can be very personal.

Where there are ritual requirements of faith which cannot be carried out because, for example, the hospital cannot provide the means, this can induce guilt on top of other mental health difficulties.

For others the discipline of ritual is a blessing and a curse especially when it is linked to feeling one has to follow rules.

> I'm not very good at routine. I don't know if that is a reaction to having tried to follow rules in the past which were not helpful to my mental health. I do do rituals, but not on a regular basis. I have ceremonies, sometimes based on Wiccan rituals, and I enjoy the creativity of that very spiritual experience – choosing what items to use and words to express something, choosing gemstones and flowers.

CONNECTION

> What worked for me in terms of spiritual care at the [National Health Service Day Centre] was pure respect and affection, human warmth and connectedness. That was the healing thing. So different from the negative authority voice. It was life-affirming. It has that mystery too, the mystery of what happens between people – a quality of respect in the widest, deepest sense of the word.

Feeling we belong is very important for most people. Mental distress can make us feel we don't belong anywhere because we are different and other. We can feel that we don't even belong to ourselves. Membership of groups, such as a running club, campaigning organization or, indeed a mental health service, as in the quote above, can provide spiritual support of a secular nature.

Because of fear and stigma, faith communities sometimes cease to be a source of comfort to those with mental distress who may feel they don't belong there any more. Where faith communities work well, providing loving acceptance, then belonging to one can be a vital source of support.

> I happened to meet the chaplain when I was out shopping and she asked me if I wanted her to come to my home to give me Communion. That really touched me, not just that I could have Communion, but that she had offered without being asked.

But, for some, there are other kinds of connection which are a necessary part of spiritual awareness in dealing with mental distress. These involve feeling connected to something, perhaps beyond ourselves, which may be a Deity or sentient Higher Power or a sense of connection with nature or creativity:

> When I am depressed connecting to nature, that spiritual place, is one of the only things that will get me moving and when I am manic it will calm me down.

or to other non-sentient realms as understood in physics:

> I am taken with those ideas from Buddhism and quantum physics that all things are connected. I find that inspirational, the implications are massive and it fires my imagination. It puts value on the choices I make. It is very easy to feel powerless in the world especially regarding poverty and the arms trade and the environment BUT the idea that what I do can influence... I choose to believe that it is meaningful for me to act as if that is the case. In depression, how dead and unconnected one feels, but this is a very different experience – the alive-ness of being part of a trembling system.

Practitioner experience

I spoke with practitioners about their experience of integrating a spiritual approach to care. There was a theme of dislocation and subterfuge – the isolation of working with others, particularly managers, who did not have the same vision, and finding ways to implement spiritual care which was not generally agreed upon.

An occupational therapist, who had a comprehensive vision of spiritual care, said:

> We have staff who think we only do OT to distract people from their mental health problems, whereas I think OT is a way for service users

to connect with their own spiritual centre. Imagine the difference in these perceptions for the kind of care a service user will get.

A student nurse who had found Buddhism gave him tools for managing his own mental distress also found it valuable in his nursing practice:

> It helps me to be more patient and I am less distressed by others getting angry. I am stronger and can be more assertive, not putting up with the shortcomings of other staff – for their benefit and the patients...the important thing is to do everything with love. I think, even with restraint, the patient will feel a difference if you do it with love.

Practitioners and spiritual 'being'

When a service user is seen to be at risk of self-harm or suicide, but their preference is to stay at home rather than go into care, it must be difficult for their practitioner to adopt a sense of 'being', allowing the service user to have their wish rather than give themselves a sense of safety.

There is a powerful example of active being by the psychiatric nurse Peter Wilkin in Barker and Buchanan-Barker (2004). He is with Aaron who has decided to kill himself and wants to stay at home:

> I knew that it was vital that I did nothing – nothing other than being... I wanted to relinquish all responsibility and hand it over to [the ward]. But...I took hold of his intentions with the whole of my being...I could think of nothing better to say than 'I will be here for you at exactly the same time again next week'. (Barker and Buchanan-Barker 2004, p.161)

Over the next three days Peter thinks of Aaron often and then gets a phone message from him saying 'see you as arranged'. At their meeting he hears that Aaron did indeed go out to kill himself. Aaron's recall of what happened next is hazy, although it included seeing 'an angel's face'. Wilkin felt that:

> we had entered the same story; become the characters ... The bloodless shadow that had blacked out Aaron's soul had lifted. A soft light waxed, now–deeply down–he was different...we never questioned 'why?' (Barker and Buchanan-Barker 2004, p.162)

Exorcism and spirit release

Many service users have been told by their faith community that they have the devil in them and have been unhelpfully subjected to exorcisms. There is evidence that, in a minority of cases of mental disturbance, people have become inhabited by unhelpful spirits. There are well-developed techniques for communicating with such spirits in a loving way and helping them to move on. The Spirit Release Foundation works with such cases and some psychiatrists include it in their practice.

As one psychiatrist, a Hindu, told me:

> When I was a Senior House Officer, so didn't have much authority, a 14-year-old girl came in who was growling, speaking in an unrecognizable language and voice and had lost control of her body, she almost looked like she was having a seizure. However, she was conscious. All sorts of tests were done and high doses of diazepam used with no result, but I think everyone knew this was different. I voiced it saying 'Perhaps she's been taken over by a spirit?' which we all passed off as a joke but I think others thought the same.
>
> I happened to be on call that night and she had been in this state for 24 hours. Since I was alone I had the opportunity to take the action I thought was appropriate without fear of censure. I spoke the names of God to her for 20 minutes. I stopped when I saw a difference in the girl and decided to go and get some sleep.
>
> After I woke up the nurses reported that soon after I left, the girl sat up, a completely different person, saying 'Where am I?' The girl later reported that 'All I remember about the last two days is you, it was like you were calling me out.'

Context for spiritual practice

For the people I spoke to there was a context for their spiritual practice.

This might have started from belief in a religion or theory or the theory was found through experience.

> I wasn't really trying to make sense of anything anymore, just sensing what I responded well to. I'd done some meditation on the chakras[1] and found it helpful. Then I read this book that linked the

---

1   Chakras are points on energy pathways in the human body and act as step-down transformers affecting the flow of energy. They relate to emotional development and this is one of the things that affects how open or closed the chakras are and, therefore, the energy flow. Some would say that the energy comes from a spiritual ground which surrounds us.

chakra system to mental health diagnoses and spiritual awareness [Corry and Tubridy 2001]...this made sense of a lot of things both in me and in the spiritual realm beyond me. So I hadn't been looking for something to make sense of it all but then I realized that I had actually found something that did.

The context might be a formal religion or philosophical tradition; a belief in a sentient divine being or higher power not allied to any religious tradition; a thorough knowledge of, and belief in astrology, a belief in one's dreams as messages from the soul or psyche; a commitment to 'sort oneself out' perhaps by finding out how to be happy and at peace with self-respect and love for oneself and others. It might also be a belief in the powers of nature either within the context of creation spirituality or paganism or with no such wider beliefs. It might be an understanding of the interconnectedness of all things, maybe with a belief and wonder at the findings in quantum physics, or a belief in energies such as auras, and the meridians, chakras and kundalini.[2] It could be a belief in past lives and soul journeys. It could be a combination of several of these. These were all mentioned to me in my conversations. And it could equally be a belief in things I have not named. In essence, the contexts for spiritual practice are as many and varied as spiritual practice itself.

I have focused on spiritual practices which people are drawn to because they ease their own emotional and spiritual pain or confusion, or the pain of those they work with. I have not looked at aspects of spirituality which people have found unhelpful.

Some people are confused by, or critical of, those who seem to cherry pick from different spiritual traditions. The conversations I had show that those who strive to relieve and make sense of their situation, by exploring a variety of spiritual practices, are not without moral compass, and, far from being frivolous, are usually grappling with some of the deepest issues of being human as well as their own mental distress. They might also find that adherence to a strict regime has aggravated their madness or dis-ease.

And of those who remain in a faith community because they value it some, Christians in this case, felt that it was expedient to keep silent about some of their own beliefs because of the experiences which underpinned them.

I do have to negotiate the church's beliefs versus my own, for example regarding a deeper psychology or seeing visions.

---

2   Kundalini is a Sanskrit word defined in Western terms as a psycho-spiritual energy thought to reside in the sacrum. It is aroused either spontaneously, or through spiritual discipline, to bring new states of consciousness.

> [Through psychosis] I do have intense experiences of God, a power-
> ful personal relationship. I have felt like God. I wouldn't tell them in
> church. They would be shocked and say it was madness.

Those who move away from their faith community often do so because they
cannot cope with this kind of subterfuge or lack of congruence. They need
to find a faith community in which they can feel more fully accepted, or a
belief system which accommodates the whole of them.

What does all this mean?

What is this pot pourri of fragments? What does it mean in practice for those
in mental distress and those who work with them?

To me they are a hymn to the variety of experience and practice. They
are a tale of exploration and trial and error, a response to the unfolding of
experience and an interest in making sense of the world. They are also
about journey and change, allowing the soul or psyche to unfold, evolve,
giving it the space and opportunity to grow. They are not about instant
answers or quick fix solutions. They are not necessarily about answers and
solutions at all.

By and large the approaches of psychiatry and the dominant religions of
the 20th century have not reflected the groundswell in diversity of search for
meaning.

We who experience mental distress are given models of belief by psychiatry and religion which often do not encompass our experience. We struggle
at the edge trying to make sense of our situation. Where we have the ability
and courage to frame our experience in our own spiritual terms we can find a
way to a meaningful centre. There are practitioners in both religion and psychiatry who are able to embrace our experience and support us but they may
find themselves at odds with their colleagues.

Our stories are a wealth of information for fostering good mental health
for those in distress and a resource for developing scientific and spiritual
thinking for those who are prepared to listen.

Acknowledgements

I would very much like to thank the many contributors to this chapter: Abina
Parshad-Griffin, Jim Clark, Alan Sanderson, Alice Hicks, Brian McDonald,
Chas de Swiet, Chetna Kang, Chris Melville, Francis Chantree, Geoff
Ravalier, Julie Weston, Natalie Watts, Noel Took, Pippa Woods, Sarah-Jane
Wren and all those who remain anonymous.

Useful websites

www.shamanism.co.uk
Eagle's Wing Centre for Contemporary Shamanism.

www.spiritrelease.com
The Spirit Release Foundation promotes the understanding of spirit attachment and the practice of spirit release through Spirit Release Therapy.

www.quietgarden.co.uk
The Quiet Garden Trust encourages the provision of a variety of local venues where there is an opportunity to set aside time to rest and pray. These may be in private homes and gardens, retreat centres or churches, inner city areas.

References and resources

Barker, P. and Buchanan-Barker, P. (2004) *Spirituality and Mental Health: Breakthrough.* London: Whurr.

Breggin, P. (1993) *Toxic Psychiatry.* London: HarperCollins.

Chopra, D. (1989) *Quantum Healing: Exploring the Frontiers of Mind/Body Medicine.* London, New York, Toronto: Bantam Books.

Corry, M. and Tubridy, A. (2001) *Going Mad: Understanding Mental Illness.* Dublin: Newleaf.

Coelho, P. (1998) *Veronika Decides to Die.* London: HarperCollins.

Eastcott, M.J. (1979) *'I' The Story of Self.* London: Rider and Company.

Hay, L.L. (1996) *You Can Heal Your Life.* Middlesex, UK: Eden Grove Editions.

Minns, S. (2002) *Be Your Own Soul Doctor.* London: Cico Books.

Kabat-Zinn, J. (2005) *Full Catastrophe Living.* London: Piatkus.

Nelson, J.E. (1994) *Healing the Split: Integrating Spirit into our Understanding of the Mentally Ill.* New York: State University of New York Press.

Nicholls, V. (1999) *The Courage to Bare our Souls.* London: The Mental Health Foundation.

Nicholls, V. (2002) *Taken Seriously: The Somerset Spirituality Project.* London: The Mental Health Foundation.

Pattison, S. (2000) *Shame: Theory, Therapy, Theology.* Cambridge: Cambridge University Press.

Scott, M. (1983) *Kundalini in the Physical World.* London: Arkana.

Vickers, S. (2000) *Miss Garnet's Angel.* London: HarperCollins.

We Without Purpose

We stand in line,
We without purpose
And watch
Mother Theresa
Jesus Christ
and Ghandi
Perform their miracles.

The poverty of we without purpose
is more acute than the pennies in our pockets which won't
become pounds.

Guilt not gilt

We reap the condemnation of not having saved the world
For us it is a struggle to find our own soul let alone save it
To find our own house let alone build one for others
Find our own water let alone slake another's thirst.

'I am the living water'.

We see it when it rolls and thunders through Mary Seacole,
Galileo and Theresa of Avila
And we watch
And wonder.

We did our bible study. We sought the light. We tried to save the
world.
But our souls were buried. Our purpose has been as
archaeologists,
Excavating the titanium gauze that was our birthright obliterated
with the plaques of other people's lives.

For this we have been no burden on the state.

And now it is done we flower and flourish and fly.
And so our time has come later.

We have had no visible purpose
We have suffered and we have found treasure
If our breath lasts we will have the outward signs of purpose
accomplished
And if not
we will
nonetheless
have fulfilled our purpose.

Mary Ellen Coyte

CHAPTER 16

HOW DIFFERENT RELIGIOUS ORGANIZATIONS CAN WORK CONSTRUCTIVELY TOGETHER

Azim Kidwai and Ali Jan Haider

> And vie with one another to attain to your sustainers forgiveness and
> to a paradise as vast as the heavens and the earth, which awaits the
> God conscious, who spend for charity in times of ease and in times of
> hardship, and restrain their anger, and pardon their fellow men, for
> God loves those who do good. (The Qur'an 3: 133–4)

In the Qur'an, God the Almighty highlights the blueprint for inter-personal
relations, with the fundamental principle being righteousness. The Prophet
Muhammad further reinforced this in his famous last sermon, when he made
clear that God has said: 'We have made you into families and tribes that you
may recognize one another. Verily, the most honorable in the sight of God is
he who is most righteous amongst you.'

Righteousness and pursuit of this is inherent in most faiths, and consequently in the religious organizations which represent them. Ergo, this is a
value common to those religious organizations which have a will to work
together.

Through the course of this chapter, three core concepts will be explored,
which represent the terms upon which religious organizations can constructively work together. These concepts are as follows:

- *Shared principle methodology:* This is essentially the identification and
  utilization of shared concerns between different religious
  organizations for the mutual benefit of their communities.

- *Quality management:* Religious organizations can seek to operate like corporate entities and use quality management methodologies as the basis of their engagement.

- *Organizational competence:* The final element of this discussion will look at what organizations have to do internally before they can engage with other religious entities. This essentially means, considering 'How', in terms of the structures and competence required by each.

In order to provide clarification of these concepts, each will be explored individually, as follows.

Shared principle methodology

> Good people do not need laws to tell them to act responsibly, while bad people will find a way round the laws. (Plato)

Regardless of their religious denomination, organizations seeking to work constructively together essentially do so for the good of their congregations and communities at large. A key to constructive working relationships is fostering that 'good will' for the benefit of developing and sustaining inter-faith relationships. As Thomas Paine famously said, 'Greatness of a nation is provided on principles of humanity' and clearly the principle is shared between nations and religious organizations.

Organizations can work creatively together through identification of shared principles and values. This, essentially, means using commonality as the basis for maturing their relationships. This principle is a recognized way of working together, and is the backbone of the inter-faith movement. Initiatives throughout the world involving different religious bodies have been established on this very principle.

This can be appreciated through the Jewish/Muslim project in Wisconsin, which is one of the largest inter-faith projects in the USA, involving two major student religious groupings. Its value is expressed in the founder's words surrounding the endeavour:

> Our Jewish Muslim connections first began when I sent an email to the Muslim Student Association member list at the University of Wisconsin, Madison, asking if anyone was interested in working together to create a Jewish Muslim student organization that would aspire to celebrate both religions and cultures on campus. I already knew two Jews, Alan and Michal, who were passionate and willing

to give their time and effort to create this group. I had met Alan, an orthodox Jew, in my Arabic class while Michal, a conservative Jew, was referred to me from many sources who told me of her similar aspirations. Both individuals were very passionate about creating a perennial group that integrates Muslims and Jews into one cohesive community. A group rising from a shared human struggle under oppression of political forces and media propaganda, bound together by humanity. After my mass email, I received a response from a Muslim student, Maryam.

On that particular day she had actually visited my Arabic class and it was immediately after clearing out her email mailbox when she came across my email and read it for the first time. She went back to my Arabic class to see if my class was still there, but due to an untimely fire drill, class had already been dismissed. Her response to my email was optimistic and clearly displayed her excitement to be part of such a group. She ended that first email with the words, 'Thanks so much for showing so much interest in doing something like this; I think it's really honorable'. I knew she was the person I was looking for... (Luxenberg 2005)

This shared concern to learn about another people is clearly able to bear fruit. However, the merit of such a shared principle approach goes further. Its greatest effect is through an identification and utilization of shared values from the religions themselves, using them as a basis for development.

Despite the media's creation of a clash of civilization concept among different religions, one finds that most faiths and, consequently, their representative organizations, will share certain core principles. For example, Islam, Judaism and Christianity agree on the basic 10 commandments as laid out in Exodus 20:17 (The Bible, King James Version) as core rules for civilization. Henceforth, projects working on the two commandments, 'Thou Shalt Not Kill' and 'Thou Shalt Not Steal', through public order programmes, easily win support and participation from different religious institutions.

For example, in Bradford, West Yorkshire, police are seeking to work with both the Diocese of Bradford and IslamBradford (an Islamic Educational Trust), to combat gun crime and gangster culture. Interest by both organizations has been recognized and a process has been established for all three organizations to work together. Henceforth, the shared principle of honouring human life and property is being used as the basis for constructive working together.

The concept of shared principle working goes beyond those issues which benefit society as a whole, as effective relationships can and do emerge, even in situations which are only of benefit to specific religious organizations and their congregations. This can be illustrated by some interesting work concerning possession and exorcism under way in the city of Bradford.

In Mental Health services the phenomenon of 'possession' is increasingly becoming recognized as a state of mental distress. The phenomenon is defined by the Crystal Reference Encyclopedia as, 'The control of a living person by an entity lacking a physical body'.

In order to deal with this in Bradford, the Mental Health services provider, Bradford District Care Trust (a NIMHE Pilot Site for Spirituality), is hosting a pilot scheme seeking to manage states of possession. The project is being led by an Islamic organization, the Spiritual Care Foundation (SCF). SCF provides an Islamic talking therapy for Muslim service users complaining of possession.

The therapy essentially involves dialogue between the 'possessed' and a Muslim cleric. The cleric talks through the situation with the person complaining of possession and recites to them chapters of the Qur'an to support them and take them on a path to recovery. A far cry from the Hollywood interpretation of exorcism, the therapy is founded on supporting an individual to take control of their life.

Through recognition that Roman Catholic service users have also seen such a therapy as of potential benefit, SCF are now establishing a relationship with the Catholic Church and their designated exorcist. This co-operation between the two different faiths has been founded on two sets of principles; those relating to the religion and to its followers:

- Religion:
    - recognition of possession as an actual state
    - recognition of a religious based intervention
    - the recognition of a social responsibility by the individual's affiliated religious organization/institution.

- Followers of religion:
    - the need for inclusion
    - the need for support at a time of distress
    - recognition of a consequential diminished responsibility
    - the desire to have their concerns taken seriously.

The reason this relationship is made possible is recognition of shared principles; both those of creed and those of religious practice. An example such as this should indicate that religious organizations of all sizes can work

Box 16.1 The National Spirituality and Mental Health Forum: A summary background and purpose of the Forum

The concept of the Forum was initially discussed in the first half of the 1990s. The idea grew out of an old HEA (Health Education Authority) publication committee, which produced the book *Promoting Mental Health – The Role of Faith Communities Jewish and Christian Perspectives*. This was the first time that a government agency had worked together with religious organizations and funded a publication concerned with mental health. The book was published on World Mental Health Day, October 1999.

From the following year, 2000, meetings of the original committee continued to take place at Mentality, the mental health promotion charity (based at the Sainsbury Centre for Mental Health). The title given to the group was the Spirituality and Mental Health Forum, as it was increasingly concerned with the holistic and spiritual dimension to mental well-being.

A series of reports had proved the lack of understanding of mental illness, let alone the importance of spirituality as an important component part in a person's recovery programme. Cultural misunderstandings between patients, their families, the clergy, chaplains and the clinicians, were causing and continue to cause frustration in the provision of the caring services. One of the questions debated was, how could the Forum and its concerned members successfully challenge the existing restrictive and restricting models of mental illness; assist in satisfactorily influencing NHS mental health service providers; and bring about positive change? There was a great need to develop mental health services that understood and respected spiritual, religious and cultural differences.

By December 2003, the membership of the Forum had grown to some 50 participants. The secretariat was then taken over by the Jewish Mental Health Alliance. Thereafter, members/participants in the Forum grew to over a thousand, which brought about the need for incorporation and its independent charitable status.

Meetings have since taken place every two to three months and are held at different secular, religious/faiths premises. Presentations are made by users of services/survivors, providers and carers. The meetings allow exchanges between representatives of the various faiths and beliefs, and those of no particular religious affiliation: mental health professionals, service users, carers, chaplains, educators and others who attend from all parts of the country.

The need to improve understanding and harmony between the different faith communities and those of no faith was well recognized and this was considered an important part of the Forum's remit. The Forum facilitates the necessary inter-action to take place, while at the same time providing material from presentations and debate for the further study of spirituality in medical schools, universities and other educational and training establishments.

To some extent spirituality shortens the distance between ourselves and whomsoever or whatsoever created us; it is a form of telecommunication between our minds, bodies and 'God' or that 'Life Force'. Whatever interpretation one may place on it, spirituality is the breath of life within us, life's energy which enables us to see and enjoy things, and gives us the strength to overcome life's difficulties.

The main purpose of the Spirituality Forum is to benefit service users of the mental health services in the UK and to promote a more holistic approach to recovery. Coupled with this prime motive, to support carers and all engaged in the provision of mental health services.

All faith communities have their own specific needs, and there is a very important role that their chaplains and lay chaplains have to play, in supporting people through their periods of mental distress. The Forum provides a centre for debate and the essential exchange of views. The Mental Health Chaplains Group affords chaplains with further understanding of spirituality and support.

Since the Department of Health closed down the HEA and created NIMHE, the Forum has become a good sounding board and support to the NIMHE Spirituality and Mental Health National Project (directed by Professor Peter Gilbert). As the National Project has developed dialogue for the implementation of spirituality in mental health services, so too has liaison and interest increased with the Forum.

In November 2006, the Forum joined NIMHE and the host University of Staffordshire, in jointly convening the first-ever comprehensive Symposium on Spirituality in mental healthcare. The

Symposium involved all nine of the religions liaised with by the Department of Health, the Humanists and a powerful group of user voices.

The Forum provokes much food for thought, and is a paradigm for the future development and recognition of spirituality as an essential part in recovery from physical, as well as mental illness. The monitoring of the National Project is now a joint responsibility of the Forum with NIMHE (part of the Care Services Improvement Partnership).

Finally, at a time of communal unrest between certain faiths and beliefs, the Forum considers it even more important to prove, by its actions, how well communities from different cultural and religions backgrounds can work together; recognizing and respecting their differences, while forming bonds of friendship and co-operation between us for the common good.

Martin Aaron
Chair, The National Spirituality and Mental Health Forum

together on even very specific issues, by putting their followers at the heart of their activity.

Therefore, this discussion of shared principle methodology should illustrate, that, if the terms of engagement (between different religious organizations) are mutually beneficial, then constructive working relationships can emerge. The key to success is working on principles which are genuinely shared and respected, rather than anything which maybe politically appropriate.

Quality Management

Quality management methodologies and models have played an instrumental role in the development of organizations and corporations since the 1960s. With the example of corporate working there are many lessons which can and have been learnt by religious organizations.

In order to appreciate this, two management models will be explored here, with examples of how they have essentially been applied to yield very positive results, effectively illustrating how different religious organizations can work constructively together, using modern management methodology.

VALUE DISCIPLINE METHODOLOGY

The Value Disciplines model of Michael Treacy and Fred Wiersema (1997), describes three generic value disciplines. Any organization must choose one of the following value disciplines and act upon it consistently and vigorously:

Operational excellence

Superb operations and execution, often by providing reasonable quality at very low cost. The focus is on efficiency, streamlining operations, supply chain management, 'no frills' and volume counts. Most large international organizations are following this discipline.

Product leadership

Very strong in innovation and brand marketing, operating in dynamic markets. The focus is on development, innovation, design, time to market and high margins in a short timeframe.

Customer intimacy

Excel in customer attention and customer service. Organizations tailor their products and services to individual or almost-individual customers. The focus is on relationship management; delivery of products and services on time and above 'customer' expectations, lifetime values, reliability, and being close to the customer are key.

Treacy and Wiersema argue that any organization must choose to excel in one value discipline, where it aims to be the best. This does not mean the other two dimensions should be neglected, but rather that the organization should aim to be at least satisfactory in the other two.

Using this model and focusing on customer intimacy provides religious organizations with a major opportunity to work with one another. As the focus of attention becomes the individual, all available resources can be directed towards delivering on their expectations and requirements.

If we take this model to the healthcare setting, we can see how it can be used to organize activity and deliver for patients through the chaplaincy function.

The East London City Mental Health Trust has a department of Spiritual Religious and Cultural Care (see also Chapter 9). They seek essentially to provide spiritual, religious and cultural components to the care of service users with a view of tailoring their care pathway to their individual profile. The department has representatives from religious organizations, such as Jewish Care and the Church of England, and also successfully pools resources which are non-specific. Knowledge of the health and social care system is shared by team members, and administrative and managerial resources are pooled across the department (and economies of scale achieved), while the different religious organizations involved deliver to the needs of their own people.

This can be appreciated by a case study from the Trust which shows a very positive outcome for a service user through different organizations. This essentially means building their relationship upon the value discipline model.

Case Study: James (From the East London and City Mental Health Trust, Department of Spiritual, Religious and Cultural Care, Homerton Hospital Mental Health Unit)

Name: James (not his real name)

Age: 63 years

Faith: Jewish

Marital status: Divorced

Diagnosis: Schizoaffective disorder

Background:

James was brought up in East London. His parents were Jewish and both he and his brother were brought up in a traditional Jewish home in which all the festivals were celebrated and a kosher home was maintained. His father died when he was young.

James has a chronic psychiatric history dating back to 1961. He married in his late twenties but, due to his mental illness, separated from his wife, who together with their son went to live in Canada.

Since his first breakdown, James has been admitted to a number of NHS mental health hospitals, staying for different lengths of time depending on his mental state. James's last admission to hospital was over three years ago and when we, representatives of the Jewish faith, met him from Jewish Care.

The Department of Spiritual, Religious and Cultural Care is a group of people coming from three main religions: Christianity, Islam and Judaism. While patients are being looked upon from a clinical perspective, our department is advocating considering their spiritual, religious and cultural needs.

This, we believe, will deliver a more comprehensive and holistic support towards achieving a sense of well-being. This is done at present by visiting the various wards, talking to the patients (those who wish to talk to us), advocating for them if requested, talking to the professionals involved in their care, providing seminars and training to staff on related issues and, last but not least, making links with the respective family and community.

With this in mind, we met James on a weekly basis. James not only was able to tell us about his mental health problems and its effects upon him, but also about his Jewish upbringing and the mark it left on his life.

While everything else in a person's life may be shattered and disintegrated, one aspect of their life that they may hold very dearly, is that sense of identity and belonging that makes them feel real people.

For James, the interaction we offered enabled him to be acknowledged and be respected as a person, and not just someone with a mental illness. We were able to support James so that his spiritual, religious and culture care was acknowledged as part of his needs for long-term support. This was achieved by working in partnership with the various professionals involved in his care and utilizing team resources and knowledge.

He is now living in the rehab ward attached to the hospital with the prospect of moving in the near future to Jewish accommodation.

Susan Garcia and Moshe Teller
Co-ordinators for the Jewish Faith

From the case study, one should be able to see that by making the needs of the customer, i.e. service user, the core value and term of engagement, constructive partnerships can be achieved, which enable representatives of different religious entities to genuinely aid people of their faith and support their recovery.

RESULT ORIENTATED MANAGEMENT

The result orientated management (ROM) methodology aims to achieve maximum results based on clear and measurable agreements made upfront. ROM is primarily a management style based on the thought that people work with more enthusiasm if:

- they clearly know what is expected of them
- they are involved in establishing these expectations

- they are allowed to determine themselves how they are going to meet these expectations, and

- they obtain feedback about their performance.

Such an approach enables religious organizations to work with others who share a common goal. Despite there being many issues which divide religious organizations, there are also many which can unite them; and if organizations use the appropriate principles as shared objectives, they can move forward constructively and work together to achieve positive results.

A fine example of such working can be seen in the movement which is currently under way, to use magnetic resonance imaging (MRI) to establish cause of death. Necropsy is not allowed by many religions, particularly Islam and Judaism, and this can be the cause of major emotional distress for families of the dead facing the procedure. In recent years a range of both Jewish and Muslim organizations have sought to support the effort to allow MRI to be used as an alternative to necropsy for determining cause of death. Despite major differences in the two religions, and a weakened relationship in recent years, both have stood united on this issue.

The result they are focusing on is to have MRI as the coroner's first option for establishing cause of non-suspicious deaths and deaths suspected to be from small vessel coronary artery disease.

Therefore using result-orientated management can enable religious organizations to work constructively together and make substantial achievements.

VALUE-BASED MANAGEMENT

> Surely my prayer and my sacrifice and my life and my death are for God, the Lord of the worlds. (The Qur'an 6:162)

Positive values are vital and can be used to bring diverse organizations together through an organized focus. The value-based management model is based on establishing a specific mission, working through a strategy to achieve it, and ensuring it is appropriate to the cultures of the relevant organizations; the glue for the mission, strategy and culture being shared values.

As religious organizations often share a mission, they also often share some core values, which can be used as the basis of engagement with other religious organizations. A valuable case study to illustrate this, relates to Oxleas NHS Trust in London, which has essentially achieved a multi-faith infrastructure. The Trust has a platform for different religious organizations to work together successfully, and is based on a clear mission, strategy and culture, underpinned by values which a number of religious organizations can relate to. An understanding of how they have been able to successfully co-ordinate input from churches, mosques and synagogues, can be appreciated through simply considering their mission, strategy and culture:

- *Mission:* To deliver a spiritual and cultural care service, focusing on bringing peace and inspiration to an individual and supporting them to arrive at a solution to their problems, or an answer which helps them.

- *Strategy:* We work in line with the Trust's Equality and Diversity Strategy and the Trust-wide approach to delivering a person-centred service; that is, all staff, service users and visitors will feel welcomed and respected and, in particular, have their spiritual and cultural care needs acknowledged. The service will implement an evidence-based approach while continually exploring new ways of working.

- *Culture:* We all share a common humanity that needs to be acknowledged and respected. The service provides a space for individuals and groups to explore their spiritual and cultural needs. Being free of direct responsibility for treatment, the basis of our work is the establishment of voluntary, interpersonal relationships.

However, before different religious organizations can work together, they typically require some internal development. Consequently, the final concept for discussion in this chapter looks at what must be present or developed inside organizations to work with other religious organizations.

Organizational competence

Edgar Schein (2004), Professor of Management at Massachusetts Institute of Technology (MIT) argues that the key to successful organizational development is harnessing the appropriate culture for a successful market delivery, as 'to understand the culture is to understand your organization'.

With this in mind, if religious organizations can harness a culture whereby dialogue and genuine working is seen as positive, and inter-faith relationships are underwritten by respect, then different groups could work together quite easily. 'Culture surrounds us all, and we need to understand how this is created, manipulated, managed and changed' (Schein 2004).

Schein provides a framework for doing this through identifying three levels of culture, starting with 'Underlying Assumptions', going up to

'Espoused Values', to finally the 'Artefacts' which together mould the organizational culture.

Religious organizations can use such methodology to understand their emotional intelligence and then use this as a basis for identifying what needs to change or be done, to ensure they can work together harmoniously.

Such an approach can seem to be very corporate; however, it has real usability for organizations of all sizes. A sound example of this is a social project, which is the product of such an approach, in Bradford, between two major religious organizations, the Salvation Army and the Jamiat Ahl-Hadith, a Muslim organization representing 15 per cent of Bradford's Muslims. The Jamiat Ahl-Hadith wanted to work with the Salvation Army on a project with the homeless, to provide hot meals once a week, and an opportunity to talk through any issues they might have with ministers of religion from both organizations.

After an internal assessment by the Jamiat Ahl-Hadith, it was identified that the internal cultures were generally appropriate to build a positive relationship. However, there might be issues surrounding the 'artefacts', as they wanted to run the project from the mosque. Consequently, they renovated one floor of the mosque and established it as a community centre and invited the Salvation Army at that point. The project has now been established for five years and representatives of both organizations work closely together to provide the service. Therefore, the relationship yields hot meals and counselling opportunities for homeless people and genuinely seeks to make attendees feel valued. The relationship seeks to promote good mental well-being among attendees and an opportunity for engaging with people who they generally wouldn't otherwise.

Such projects are increasing in number, due to the rise of organizational psychology and development theories in society in general, so we find religious institutions increasingly recognizing the importance of generating organizational inter-faith competence.

The three broad concepts explored here should give an insight into just how religious organizations can constructively work together. The core message which emerges from the discussion, is clarity in the terms of engagement. All case studies that have been documented here have a common thread and that is:

- clarity in purpose
- clarity in position
- clarity on the terms of engagement.

Unquestionably, religious organizations have a similar purpose, in that they seek to provide support and guidance to their congregations and be a source of solace for the community at large. Therefore, if they establish sincerity and clarity in their purpose, they can unquestionably work together.

The concepts discussed in this chapter simply seek to shed light upon some of the ways in which different religious organizations can work constructively together. There will be others but if, in the current climate, just one of these were used, major social enlightenment could be achieved. It would appear that the key is to export core principles of inter-personal relations to inter-organizational relations.

It seems appropriate to close with the famous words of Galileo, which essentially point to the direction we need to take, which is that pertaining to natural behaviour: 'I do not feel obliged to believe that the same God who has endowed us with sense, reason and intellect has intended us to forego their use' (Galileo Galilei).

Bibliography

Cole, G.A. (2003) *Management Theory and Practice.* Andover: Thomson Learning.

Luxenberg, H. (2005) *The Jewish Muslim Project (JMP).* Available at www.mideastweb.org/jewishmuslimdialog.htm (accessed 20 September 2007).

Martin, J.D. and Petty, W. (2000) *Value Based Management: The Corporate Response to the Shareholder Revolution.* Oxford: Oxford University Press.

Paine, T. (2000, first published 1792) *The Rights of Man.* London: Dover Publications.

Plato (360 BCE 1956) *Crito* (2nd revised edn). Essex: Prentice Hall.

Schein, E. (2004) *Organizational Culture and Leadership* (3rd edn). New York: Wiley.

Treacy, M. and Wiersema, F. (1997) *The Discipline of Market Leaders: Choose Your Customers, Narrow Your Focus, Dominate Your Market.* London: Perseus Books.

Reflection: The Muslim Community and Mental Health Care
Luthfa Meah

This reflection explores a number of personal worldviews and issues that are unique to Muslim clients concerning mental health and distress. It highlights particular issues that mental health professionals need to take into account in the care process.[1]

Mental distress is increasing among ethnic minorities. Research has found that black ethnic populations are more likely to be hospitalized under the compulsory sections of the Mental Health Act 1983, than the ethnic majority (Hussain 2001, pp.6–9). However it is also the case that minority ethnic populations are reluctant to use Mental Health services, both at the primary and secondary care stage. The Government is aware of the need to improve the mental health of minority ethnic populations, as well as the need to provide culturally appropriate and competent services (Bahl 1999, pp.13–14). Overcoming communication barriers between mental health professionals and the community is seen as the key to service improvement. As an aspect of the same, it is important to examine the issues involved when dealing with Muslim clients in mental healthcare.

One of the main reasons that Muslim clients are reluctant to utilize mental health services is because there is often a sense of mistrust towards the medical treatment provided. Patients and families give explanatory reasons for mental and emotional disturbances that are culture bound and often not so well understood by healthcare professionals.

The two most common explanatory causes are *Jinn* (Spirit) possession and black magic (*jhado*). Muslims believe that there is another creation besides humankind – that is the *Jinn* (Spirits). Regarding creation the Quran (the Holy Book for Muslims) states: 'I only created the *Jinn* and men to worship Me.'[2] The *Jinn* is believed to be a creation invisible to the human eye, but the *Jinn* share their dwelling on earth and are found mostly in 'deserts, ruins, and places of impurity like dunghills, bathrooms, and graveyards' (Ashour 1989, p.25). Among the *Jinn*, some are thought to be believers following the guidance of the Quran, and some are non-believers who transgress and interfere with humankind. Possession could happen for various

1   I am indebted to Imam Shafiqur Rahman and Imam Abdur Raqib (Chaplains in mental health) and to Aliya Parvin (a Muslim clinical psychologist at St Clements Hospital) for their assistance in field-work related to this study.
2   Quran, 51: 56, Trans. Ali, A.Y., IPCI, South Africa, 1934.

reasons such as envy or jealousy of the *Jinn* or the *Jinn* being intruded upon in its private sphere where it takes revenge on the person.

There is belief also in evil forces, which are thought to derive from the *Shaytan* (Devil), from which the phenomenon of black magic is thought to exist. *Shaytan* is the name given to the Jinn that is 'malicious and has become wicked' (Ashour 1989, p.8). The belief is that envious people engage in black magic in order to bring about harm upon someone to whom they are hostile. This is achieved by befriending the *Shaytan*, doing what is pleasing to it and in return the *Shaytan* would assist with its powers. Muslims are taught in the Quran to take refuge in God from all types of evils. The two most often recited prayers by Muslims, are as follows:

> I seek refuge with the Lord of the Dawn, from the mischief of created things; from the mischief of Darkness as it overspreads; from the mischief of those who practise secret Arts; and from the mischief of the envious one as he practises envy.[3]

And:

> I seek refuge with the Lord and Cherisher of Mankind, the King of Mankind, the God of Mankind, from the mischief of the Whisperer of evil, who withdraws after his whisper, the same who whispers into the hearts of Mankind, among Jinns and among Men.[4]

Muslims believe that both *Jinn* possession and black magic are the cause of mental disturbance that might otherwise be diagnosed as schizophrenia, anxiety and phobic states, depression, obsessive compulsion disorder, hysteria and loss of memory, and so on. Muslims traditionally go to the Mosque for treatment and ask the Imam for protection prayers, exorcism from any *Jinn* possession and amulets to wear in order to ward off any black magic. Holy water (*pani pora*) can also be given to drink for further protection. It is often because of such popular beliefs in *Jinn* possession and black magic, and the religiously designated treatment that is usually sought first that mainstream medical treatment is viewed as secondary and culturally inappropriate.

Another reason why Muslim clients are reluctant to utilize mental health services is the institutionalization of mental healthcare itself. In Muslim communities, the traditional approach would be to care for those who are mentally disturbed within the family network. In these communities it is not

---

3   Quran, 113.
4   Quran, 114.

the norm for elderly people and those who are mentally disturbed to be put into 'Care Homes'. Such practices would be viewed as ethically wrong, as it is always the family duty to take care of the elderly and the sick, with much religious piety attached to it. Hence the institutionalization of mental healthcare is somewhat new within the Muslim community.

The Mosque, as an institution, plays an additional pivotal role in providing mental healthcare to the Muslim community. The Mosque in Islam is not just a religious institution but also a social and a political one. The Friday congregational prayer is compulsory for Muslims to attend. It is like a community gathering where people embrace each other after the prayer and express their concern for each other. In this sense it is a community centre. The Mosque could be viewed as a medical centre also (traditionally in Muslim countries it has been so), in the sense that spiritual prescriptions are sought from the Imam.

Further, the prayer acts as a spiritual therapy for both physical illness and mental disturbance. The Mosque has useful healing resources and potential within itself to help the promotion of mental health. The Muslim community in the UK needs to ensure it mobilizes and utilizes the resources that are at its disposal as effectively as possible so that it can be at the forefront of 'future planning and programming in the mental health field' (Baasher 1984, pp.588–93).

Muslim women compose a significant number of users of mental health services. Thus, when providing mental healthcare, service providers need to take into consideration the specific needs of Muslim women, who can be seen as a 'minority within a minority'. First, the aspect of segregation of men and women is a very important part of Muslim public life. Men and women are instructed to dress modestly when outside in public, in order to curtail immorality and promote decency in society. Segregation is meant to help sustain the moral fibre of society (Henley and Schott 1999, p.513). When interacting in society, Muslim women prefer to go to women only services where available. For example, Muslim women would prefer to visit a General Practitioner that is female rather than one that is male. Consciousness for segregation is most often at the back of a Muslim woman's mind. One mental health facility I visited provides female only dormitories in all wards, a user-friendly service which is highly appreciated by the Muslim women clients. The need for female only doctors for treatment is not seen as a matter of great urgency from Muslim women patients, as the nature of treatment in the mental health field is not so much physical as psychological and communicative. However, it is known that Muslim women clients are much more at ease when communicating with female staff. It is important to be informed about the cultural and religious etiquette of clients. This both helps to avoid any embarrassment, and does not add to any distress already being experienced.

Second, with the growth of the number of Muslim clients in mental healthcare in recent years comes growing recognition of the need to provide Muslim chaplains for these clients. As a result there are now Muslim chaplains in hospitals providing spiritual care, but these are mostly men. It can be argued that the provision of more female Muslim chaplains for Muslim women clients would increase the benefits women clients receive from spiritual care services.

It is important that mental health services and professionals are aware of daily Muslim rituals and that they make provision for clients who want to perform them. For Muslims, it is a religious obligation to pray five times a day – 'at dawn, just after mid-day, in the mid-afternoon, immediately after sunset, and at night before going to bed' (Henley and Schott 1999, p.513). As prayer is proven to be a useful aid for psychological healing, it is even more important that prayer facilities be provided, although it is recognized that prayer can become a source of obsession for some people. Not all mental health institutions provide separate prayer facilities for Muslim clients. Due to the nature of Muslim prayer, shared prayer space with other faith communities is not always appropriate. However, one must acknowledge that the lack of this type of prayer facility is mainly due to shortages in funding and space.

Muslims have specific dietary needs. Certain food and drink are prohibited for Muslims to eat and drink, like pork and alcohol. The meat has to be killed in a special way in order to for it to be *halal* (permitted) to eat. If Muslims do not receive strictly guaranteed *halal* food, then they would eat strict vegetarian food instead. The NHS has been aware of Muslim dietary needs and has provided *halal* food for some years now. However, extra care needs to be taken with food arrangements during the month of Ramadan. The month of Ramadan is when Muslims fast from sunrise to sunset. Just before sunrise, Muslims have a substantial meal or breakfast. Just after sunset, when they can eat, they need a substantial meal. Fasting is not a religious obligation on people with mental disturbance, as the Islamic law exempts them. However, many clients choose to fast perhaps because they do not consider themselves to be ill, or they may also fast to gain control and become free from distress.

A final consideration is the relationship between Islam and mental health. Muslim professionals working within the mental health field argue that Islam provides a holistic approach to mental health and well-being. The suggestion is that: 'Islam gives great care to prevention. The Islamic daily programme is rich with many pieces of advice provided to lay the foundation of a programme which protects Muslims from disease whether physical, psychological or social' (Azayem 1984, pp.562–77).

Furthermore, the belief aspect of the religion can be seen to promote mental heath. There are seven articles of faith – (1) Oneness of God; (2) God's Angel; (3) God's Books; (4) God's Messengers; (5) The Day of Judgement; (6) Destiny or fate; (7) Life after death – all of which one must believe in order to be a Muslim (Abdulati 1997, p.27). The last two articles are the most influential for one's psychological, emotional and spiritual disposition and perception. Religion is central to the life of the majority of Muslims. When afflicted by any illness, the Muslim has a strong conviction in God's Will and the good in it and hence comes to terms with it. The Muslim looks upon the after-life with a great deal of optimism. Ahmed contends that the believer 'remains undaunted in the face of the greatest calamity and never leaves command over his patience. He takes the view that whatever has occurred was decreed by God and no command of God is devoid of wisdom or purpose' (Ahmed 1984, pp.579–83). Thus, faith can provide inner strength and be a great resource in terms of one's emotional stability. This being so, it is important for mental health professionals to be open to and develop an understanding of the cultural framework that Muslim clients come from, and to display a readiness to incorporate the Muslim paradigm as much as possible within the care programme. This will help Muslim clients be more comfortable with the statutory mental healthcare provision, and could encourage more willingness from the Muslim community to utilize the services provided.

In conclusion, good practice in mental healthcare must incorporate the worldviews, issues and religious and spiritual needs specific to the Muslim community, some of which have been outlined above. Muslim clients are deeply embedded in their alternative explanatory models on mental illness/disturbance. Perhaps it will never be possible to fully remove the gap in understanding concerning the nature, causes and treatment of mental disturbances between every Muslim client and every mental health professional, as each one views these matters from his or her respective framework. However, it is important that Muslim clients are encouraged to maintain their cultural and religious values. Indeed, it can even be 'unreasonable and unrealistic to expect them to abandon their culture and religion… Indeed for their own emotional stability and mental health, it is important that they do not' (Henley and Schott 1999, p.74).

References

Abdulati, H. (1997) *Islam in Focus.* Egypt: El-Falah Foundation.

Ahmed, B. (1984) 'Depression – psycho-socio-biological factors: role of Muslim physician.' *Proceedings of the Third International Conference on Islamic Medicine 3*, 579–83. Jeddah, Saudi Arabia.

Ashour, M. (1989) *The Jinn in the Quran and Sunna.* Trans. Bewley, A., Dar Al Taqwa. London.

Azayem, G. (1984) 'The Islamic model in the field of mental health.' *Proceedings of the Third International Conference on Islamic Medicine 3*, 562–77. Jeddah, Saudi Arabia.

Baasher, T. (1984) 'Islam and mental health.' *Proceedings of The Third International Conference on Islamic Medicine 3*, 588–93. Jeddah, Saudi Arabia.

Bahl, V. (1999) 'Mental illness: a national perspective.' In D. Bhugra and V. Bahl (eds) *Ethnicity: An Agenda for Mental Health.* London: Gaskell.

Henley, A. and Schott, J. (1999) *Culture, Religion and Patient Care in a Multi-Ethnic Society: A Handbook for Professionals.* London: Age Concern.

Hussain, A. (2001) 'Islamic beliefs and mental health.' *Mental Health Nursing 21*, 6–9.

CHAPTER 17

ORGANIZATIONAL HEALTH: ENGAGING THE HEART OF THE ORGANIZATION

Sarajane Aris and Peter Gilbert

I am human, you are human

In July 2006, the National Patient Safety Agency (NPSA 2006) published statistics on the incidence of rape and sexual assault in NHS Mental Health services. The results were shocking and disturbing (see also Jackson 2006). In their investigative report July 2006, the Healthcare Commission highlighted an oppressive, institutional regime, within the Mental Health Service, serving people with learning disabilities in Cornwall (Healthcare Commission 2006). People were shocked, but not, perhaps surprised, that the institutional culture of oppression, which had been so prevalent within the old long-stay hospitals, had resurrected itself in a different environment.

June 2005 saw a BBC1 *Panorama* programme run a story of institutional abuse in wards caring for elderly, frail people in a Brighton general hospital, through the lens of an undercover nurse (Undercover Nurse, *Panorama* BBC1 July 2005). Because of the stark nature of the visual images coming through on the television screen, there was a profound sense of revulsion and dismay in those watching it. This was not some remote corner of a developing world starved of resources; it was not in a country devastated by earthquake or tsunami; it was a general hospital in the prosperous south-east of the UK in the 21st century!

The images of very elderly, frail, helpless people being bullied and starved, even of water, made many viewers sad and angry. What made people angrier, however, was the bland response from senior management. There was the usual tired litany of excuses, coupled with the mantra of complaints procedures, due process, action plans, etc; in effect, a reliance on systems, but apparently nothing which told us that senior managers had enough of a concept of leadership to get out of the penthouse suite and down on to the ward front line to see for themselves what was happening and put things right! (see Gilbert 2006a).

To counter these events, we recently heard a story, told by two night staff in a hospice: a man lay dying, with medication blunting the physical pain, but in emotional turmoil. At 2 o'clock in the morning, he told the night staff that he felt that his hour of passing was near and he needed to unburden himself to someone who would listen. Although not a man with a formal faith, he requested to speak to the Chaplain. The night staff rang the Chaplain at home, who promised to come as soon as possible, but his house was over an hour away, down country lanes. When the Chaplain eventually arrived, he found the patient peacefully asleep and snoring quietly! The two night staff were white-faced and in tears. They had listened very carefully to the man unburdening himself of a fearful trauma and the heavy weight of guilt that he bore. In many ways, that load had been transferred to their backs and they were carrying it, so that the teller of the story could rest easy through the night.

The Chaplain sat them down, made them a cup of hot chocolate and listened to them as they passed the burden to him, so that he could both understand where the man was coming from when he met him in the morning, and also support the staff who had carried that weight. Examples of good practice such as Imran Soobratty and his staff's use of 'protected time' in the Camden and Islington Health and Social Care Trust abound (see Case Study).

Case study: Patient Protected
Therapeutic Engagement Time (PPT)

'I come to hospital because I have a story to tell you and you are here because you wish to hear my story. Yet I leave hospital without having told my story and you not having heard it.' The above statement by a service user who was on Topaz Ward (Highgate Mental Health Centre) in 2005 was echoed by other users: 'If the staff could only spend more time with us instead of being in the office,' and the staff stating: 'And I thought that we were here to look after patients instead of being in the office answering the telephone and doing paper work.' These remarks and the Acute Care collaborative logo: 'Try out small changes to make a difference in the clinical setting', gave birth to the idea that we could somehow set aside uninterrupted time to devote to patients; it would bring happiness and satisfaction to both patients and staff. Hence Topaz Ward introduced the concept of Protected Therapeutic Engagement Time (PPT) as part of a project sponsored by the Acute Care Collaborative in June 2005.

PPT meant that staff would close the ward office for three hours (Protected Time) in the morning and devote it to direct patient care, (Therapeutic Engagement), only. Very often patients come to hospital because ill-health has caused disruption to their activities of daily living, to such an extent that they find great difficulty in doing the simple things that we often take for granted, like talking about their problems and finding solutions, building and maintaining relationships, maintaining their safety and the safety of others, eating and drinking, maintaining balance between rest and work and other activities that promote good mental health. PPT creates the opportunity for patients admitted to hospital to tell their story and for the staff to contribute to a happy ending. In the words of the patient who returned nine months later for a visit: 'You've got it. You have created an environment that is conducive to recovery. I can now tell my story to somebody who is there to listen.'

This project was presented at the King's Fund and has since been adopted by many hospitals across the country. At the Highgate Unit it has led to a significant reduction in incidents/violence and increase in positive contact between ward staff and patients.

Imran Soobratty
Ward Nurse Manager

What is it, then, which makes some front line staff react with humanity when facing the kind of situations which none of us relish, and what is it that makes others react either with an oppressive abuse of power, or simply with indifference? This is a pertinent question at any stage in history, but it is particularly acute now, when there is both huge attention on the NHS and Social Care organizations in this country, but also research which shows that recovery from severe mental illness may have a better chance of success in so-called developing countries, than those which devote significant resources to statutory Mental Health services (see Harrison, Hopper, Craig *et al.* 2001). Our firm belief is that, especially in human services, it is only by engaging the heart that really effective organizations will be created and maintained. A failure to do so leads to organizations which are essentially vacuous and hollow.

Staff at many different levels within services in the UK, express concern both about a lack of leadership and 'old paradigm' models of leadership in operation (see Alimo-Metcalfe 2005 and Gilbert 2005) and a culture (see Mannion, Davies and Marshall 2005) which does not focus on making life better for those who use services and their carers.

Ken Jarrold, one of the doyens of NHS management, in his valedictory speech to the Institute of Health Management (Jarrold 2005) stated that the NHS needed to create 'the right relationship with staff, which, in turn, will deliver the right relationship with patients'. He continued by saying that: 'values are worthless unless they are lived' (see Chapter 2 in this book) and that 'everyone, at all levels, needs to behave towards others as they would wish others to behave towards them' (Jarrold 2005, p.12).

Beverly Alimo-Metcalfe (2005), in her recent research on NHS management, talks about the need for 'transformational leadership'; a leadership approach that talks about 'sculpting a shared vision; a shared meaning of the purpose and the process of the work-role activities of a group of individuals who come together to achieve a common aim' (Alimo-Metcalfe 2005, p.69).

Community or confinement – a brief historical perspective

In their *History of Care in the Community from 1715 to 2000*, Peter Barlett and David Wright, from a legal and history of medicine perspective, respectively, comment that '"care in the community" holds the dubious distinction of being universally supported in principle, and universally condemned in practice' (Barlett and Wright 1999, p.16); how we got to what Peter calls a state of 'care in collision' (see Gilbert 2003, ch. 2) is a long and complex story. At its heart it involves humankind's innate need to differentiate for purposes of evolutionary security (see Haidt 2006); and in the UK a concern, not always well achieved, to balance the liberty of the citizen against the safety of that individual citizen and society as a whole (the tension over a replacement for the 1983 Mental Health Act for England and Wales is an illustration of this).

Less explicit is a desire to limit public expenditure, perhaps not unreasonable in itself, but hypocritical and dangerous when cost cutting is dressed up as a beneficent attempt to provide people with more independence. From the 1970s onwards, therefore, some hospitals for people with mental illness (and also those for people with learning disabilities) were closed and re-provided for on an ethical basis, with the care of the present and future user population in mind. Unfortunately, many others were based on a desire to offload vulnerable people from the NHS on to the burgeoning social security budget and the private sector market in the early years of the Thatcher government (Gilbert and Scragg 1992, ch. 1).

With stigma still a problem in many countries, it is instructive to look at the ancient world and see that the manifestations of mental distress were usually tolerated and often honoured. Despite the fact that Ancient Greek society placed such an accent on rationality, Plato, in his *Phaedrus* quotes Socrates as preaching that: 'the greatest blessings come by way of madness, indeed, of madness that is heaven sent' (quoted in Gilbert and Scragg 1992, p.27). Jewish society also accorded respect, even reverence, to those who were deemed to be uttering what might be prophecies, and Mosaic Law recognized the appointment of guardians for those who were not in full possession of their faculties.

St Paul, in his first letter to the Corinthians (1:25) points out to his audience that: 'God's foolishness is wiser than human wisdom and God's weakness is stronger than human strength' and Christian monasteries gave succour to people with mental health needs and learning disabilities. The Qur'an urges Muslims to clothe and speak kindly to those made vulnerable by mental distress. Islamic communities set up some of the first centres devoted to the humane care of people with mental illness (*maristan*) and also in the tabulation of medical ethics, reminded 'physicians that they were charged with maintaining both body and soul' (Sheikh and Gatrad 2000, p.35).

Although it would be naïve to glorify the pre-industrial period as a golden age, it does appear that the enclosure of common lands from the 17th century onwards, and the advent of the Industrial Revolution, fractured many social and economic ties and exposed those who were functioning at some level in a traditional society, to the icy glare of modern production. Professor Andrew Scull contends that 'many of the transformations underlying the move towards institutionalization can be more plausibly tied to the growth of the capitalist market system and to its impact on economic and social relationships' (Scull 1984, p.24).

With a second industrial revolution in train at the moment (see Sennett 2006) we need to keep a wary eye on historical precedent. Bauman talks about today's 'strangers' being perceived as a 'problem' because of 'their tendency to befog and eclipse boundary lines that ought to be clearly seen' and living 'perpetually with the "identity problem" unsolved' (Bauman 1997, pp.25–26).

Historians of the progressive liberal school, such as Kathleen Jones (e.g. Jones 1972) saw a steady march of progress in Mental Health Services. Michel Foucault, Andrew Scull and others would see the growth of the system as primarily self-serving, and increasing identification of difference, categorization and deviance. It was Foucault who talked of 'the great confinement', and who remarked on the irony that 'the Classical Age was to reduce to silence the madness whose voices the Renaissance had just liberated, but whose violence it had already tamed' (Foucault 1961/2001, p.35).

Coming up to the present day, Clare Allan, in her searing novel *Poppy Shakespeare* (Allan 2006a) quotes Anton Chekhov: 'since prisons and madhouses exist, why, somebody is bound to sit in them'. In her article accompanying the launch of the novel, Allan demonstrates how the human need to categorize can raise the spectre of the institution at all times and in all settings.

Allan describes how passing a door into an institution meant entering 'a different world' (Allan 2006b). She speaks of her diagnosis as being 'validating', proving that her problems were not just imaginary, but also 'limiting, desperately so' (p.7). She also recalls how other people craved to know her diagnosis, for, as the sociology of deviance tells us, we so often need to define the other to define ourselves.

Although the walls in services are never completely impervious to movement between community and institution, there is always a tendency for even progressive services to ossify and stagnate; for our human need to differentiate to confine the 'stranger' or 'other'; or, indeed, we may confine ourselves.

The nature of organizations

At Staffordshire University, on the Social Work Degree course, there is a module on organizations, because it is increasingly important for students to consider the fact that they will be working in and for and into organizations for much of their professional life. How that organization is set up and functions will profoundly affect those who use services, informal carers and the staff working for and with it. We ask students not only to look at their placements in terms of shared values, strategy, structure, style of leadership, skills, staff and systems (see Gilbert 2005, ch. 2), but also to visit and consider a range of other organizations: supermarkets, leisure facilities, restaurants, GP surgeries, schools, informal clubs, etc. to ascertain if they do, in the words of the advert: 'what it says on the tin?'!

Organizations often vaunt their mission statements and list of values; but are these so much candyfloss, or are they lived and breathed? Gareth Morgan, in his seminal work: *Images of Organization* (Morgan 1997) provides us with a number of metaphors for the way that organizations are configured. Tellingly, however, he starts with the metaphor of 'organizations as machines' and quotes the 4th-century Chinese sage Chuang-Tzu. The latter refers to an old man working in his fields as saying:

> He who does his work like a machine grows a heart like a machine, and he who carries the heart of a machine in his breast loses his simplicity. He who has lost his simplicity becomes unsure in the strivings of his soul. (Morgan 1997, p.12)

The etymology of 'organization' comes from the Greek *organon*, meaning a tool or an instrument; and the Romans carried this into the Latin as *organun*, meaning an implement. Although many modern corporate bodies would prefer to use another metaphor of Morgan's: 'organizations as organisms', there is a tendency for organizations to revert to an institutional model, as we noted with the brief historical overview above. Just as Richard Dawkins talks about 'the selfish gene' (Dawkins 1976) for the human species as a whole, one might well talk about the 'selfish organization', because organizations tend to revert to the self-seeking of organizational ends, and it is imperative that we are not naïve about this (see also, Barratt 2006; Covey 1992; Linstead, Fulop and Lilley 2004; Mullins 2002; Rooke and Torbert 2005).

What makes a spiritually healthy organization?

Organizations need to fulfil their aims and these may involve numerous stakeholders; for instance, shareholders, suppliers, customers, staff and other partners in a retail industry. In a commercial enterprise it would be naïve to think that profit is not a major driver. But when Marks and Spencer, the giant of the High Street clothes retailers, came under sustained pressure a few years ago and a new CEO, Stuart Rose, was called in to restore its fortunes and to repel a takeover, it was no surprise to most women shoppers, who had been saying for years that M&S lines were dowdy and the service was poor. In the commercial world, you cannot make a profit without pleasing customers and motivating staff. Uninspired staff is the surest way to send profits plunging! In reporting the continuing distress caused by mixed-sex wards in the NHS, a national newspaper spoke of: 'the distressingly casual attitude towards the provision of small comforts' (*The Independent*, 24 November 2006, p.40).

In Health and Social Care one would think that this would be taken as read; but, in fact, Ken Jarrold has spoken of 'bullying and harassment at all levels' (Jarrold 2005), and the Secretary of State for Health in her address to the NHS Confederation (16 June 2006) warned that she would 'stamp out' (an interesting use of language!) '"macho" bullying' in the NHS.

In an era when demographics are working against us and we need young people to enter caring professions, we have to create organizational environments which people actually want to join.

Sociologists and commentators (e.g. Bauman 2000; Bunting 2005; Handy 2002; Schwarz 2005; Sennett 2006) have commented that work subsumes an increasing amount of our time and, therefore, we not only need to think through our work/life balance, but also how our working environment can connect to our deeper purposes around meaning and identity – how it can touch our essence (see Merchant and Gilbert 2006).

In America, in the mid-1990s, influential thinkers and research institutes predicted that 'the issue of meaning' would 'become more and more important in companies' (see Biberman and Whitty 2000, p.67). In the UK, Roffey Park Institute's annual survey began to pick up the concept of 'meaning' in the workplace becoming more significant for an increasing number of employees as the 1990s moved into the new century. In their 2004 publication, Linda Holbeche and Nigel Springett outlined the possible reasons for this upsurge:

- People generally spend longer at work than on other parts of their lives.

- Change and the 'dog-eat-dog' ethic in many workplaces are making relationships more transactional and mistrustful.

- Reported higher levels of employee cynicism over a range of issues, including 'hollow' ethical policies…which cause people to doubt the purpose of their organization and the integrity of leaders.

- Community as a whole has undergone a moral/values transformation in recent decades, to a more commercial, secular society.

- The plethora of 'alternative' therapies…suggests that many people are experiencing the lack of community spirituality – they want to fill a 'God-shaped hole'.

- Society in general, and employees in particular, are becoming increasingly mistrustful of people in authority, especially leaders.

(Holbeche and Springett 2004, pp.3–4)

Charles Handy, in his book *The Hungry Spirit* (Handy 2002) says that the argument of his book 'is that, in our hearts, we would like to find a purpose bigger than ourselves because that will raise us to heights that we had not dreamt of' (p.9).

Progressing from her original research, Holbeche, in *The High Performing Organization* (2005) points out, that even in the private sector, with its greater resources for change management processes, 75 per cent of all transformation efforts are thought to fail, and that what is needed is achieving the paradox of dynamic stability: organizations which can innovate and respond to customer need, while staying true both to core values and the key aims of the organization. A sure recipe for disaster, however, is frenetic, frequent and ill thought through initiatives, which are launched and de-bunked in a flash! Both public and private sectors in the UK are notoriously short-term in their thinking, while research from North America (see Collins 2001; Collins and Porras 2000; Gilbert 2005; Holbeche 2005) is indicating that organizations that are healthy and well functioning at their heart show the following transformational qualities (Barratt 2006):

- Leadership, at all levels, which is focused on essential purpose and integrity.
- Leaders who are authentic and demonstrate the values they espouse.
- Values which inspire and are deeply rooted at all levels.
- The creation of a culture which encourages both innovation and long-term purpose – 'dynamically stable' (Abrahamson 2000).
- Establishing 'a human community of successive generations of people' (Holbeche 2005, p.20), through a developmental culture.
- Engaging all those who have a stake in the organization.
- An 'ethos of compassion and trust' (Tehan 2007).

Perceptive observers of organizations like John Whitmore (1997) speak of the importance of understanding and working with the levels of organizational consciousness and culture to create a spiritually healthy organization. Figure 17.1 shows how all elements have to cohere together so as to create the essential relationship at the front line, which we are all meant to be striving for. Richard Barratt (2006) refers to 'values based leadership', and the need to encompass four key dimensions: physical, emotional, mental and spiritual to achieve a positive cultural transformation (see also Goleman 2006).

This sense of integrity and authenticity running through the organization, is not only a moral imperative, but a pragmatic one as well. In such a fluid environment, as that in which we now operate, we never know when we may be professional one day and user the next; someone's manager on Friday and their employee on Monday! The old adage: 'Never step on someone's face on the way up the ladder, because they may pass you on your way down again' is never truer than it is today!

The NIMHE Spirituality Project and Organizational Health

In the context of the NIMHE Project on Spirituality, there are a number of instances when organizational health is key. This is demonstrated by both the Pilot Sites (see www.nimhe.org.uk) and the Mental Health Foundation's research into organizations providing spiritual care (see Gilbert and Watts 2006).

The Pilot Sites are, in some ways, an anomaly in today's public services. They have a framework in which a number of elements can be considered (see Box 17.1), but there are no performance indicators or targets. The aim is to build on the good work already being done by the organizations themselves and their communities; through engagement, sharing good practice (see Sewell and Gilbert 2006), research and regional events (see also Gilbert and Nicholls 2003).

When the Pilot Sites had an England-wide symposium in May 2006 at Lincoln University, it was very evident that the Trusts who were most committed to a spiritual approach were the most dynamic and value-driven organizations. An example would be the Sussex Mental Health Partnership Trust, which, despite being in the process of a major merger across the county, of 2 1/2 Trusts in the spring and summer of 2006, managed to put on an inclusive conference, where it launched a comprehensive Spiritual Care Strategy (Sussex Partnership Trust May 2006). It was noticeable that the Board, chief executive and senior managers were very much in evidence during the day, with a high level of interaction and integration with users, carers and faith communities.

Leadership at all levels

Leadership is key to organizational health, but there is considerable discussion about what kind of leadership is most effective in large, modern organizations, often with a global reach, and increasingly driven by information technology. Jim Collins, in perhaps the most thorough study of leaders of successful businesses, believes that in the long term, the most successful are those leaders who have 'a paradoxical blend of personal humility and professional will. They are more like Lincoln and Socrates than Patten or Caesar' (Collins 2001, pp.12–13). That has a lot of truth in it; but most people we

Box 17.1: Areas which pilot sites are invited to focus on, as set out in the NIMHE Framework Document

- The values and mission of the organization.
- How humane and spiritual approaches are recognized, supported and celebrated.
- The assessment of spiritual and religious needs, and care practice in a broad sense.
- Recognizing and responding to an individual's spiritual needs.
- Recognizing and responding to an individual's religious needs.
- Chaplaincy services (multi-faith).
- Partnership approaches to faith communities.
- Partnership approaches to community groups with a spiritual dimension.
- Education and training programmes for staff.
- Recognizing the spiritual and religious needs of staff.
- Assisting faith communities in their understanding of mental health and how they can work appropriately with services.
- Published materials.
- Issues such as diet, space interpreters, etc.
- Sacred space.
- Links between the Spirituality Agenda and other relevant agendas, e.g. Social Inclusion, Values, Recovery, Workforce, etc.

speak to also say that they wish to know that, in human services, their leaders are somehow alongside them. This authenticity, visibility and journeying with and together, has to run through the organization like lettering through a stick of rock (Table 17.1).

Table 17.1 Levels of organizational health

Governance	Board setting strategic direction and ensuring the organization sticks to its core values and tasks.
Strategic leadership	Chief executive and executive Board being both transformational and transactional (Peck, Dickinson and Smith 2006).
	'Walking the talk' – visibility.
	Organizational transformation requires the presence of leaders who are Strategists and Magicians (Rooke and Torbert 2005).
Operational leadership	Enabling not blocking.
	Setting the tone.
Front line leadership	Facilitating, developing and supporting good practice.
Practitioner leadership	Walking with people in discovery and recovery.
	Taking the risk of empowerment. Innovating from the front line up.

Working with Social Work students in a variety of practice placements, it is very clear that leadership is the key to creating the difference between inspiring and dispiriting services. Front line managers who really focus on the interlocking circles of mission, team and the individual (Adair 2002) create teams which provide the services that people require. Senior managers create a culture, which enables rather than disables (Schein 2004 and Gilbert 2005, ch. 6). In fact, Schein is fond of saying that, the most important thing that leaders do, is create the right culture.

Conclusion

As we saw in Chapter 1 of this book, the Jewish faith has a concept of *ru'ach*; a Hebrew word meaning both breath and spirit, and giving the concept of *invigorated life*. This is what we desire from the organizations we work for. We do not wish to work for organizations which demean, devalue and depress. Instead, we want to work for organizations which both espouse and live values which are *heart-based*, with that essential empowering dialogue, which is imperative in human services: 'You are human – I am human.' Too often the scandals in human services demonstrate that the dialogue is: 'I am human, but you are different and less than human.' Figure 17.1 shows how this elemental relationship needs to be supported by inspiration and real learning (Senge 1998) running right through the whole system. If I am acting as a psychiatrist, social worker, nurse, etc. one day am I a highly-competent

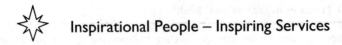

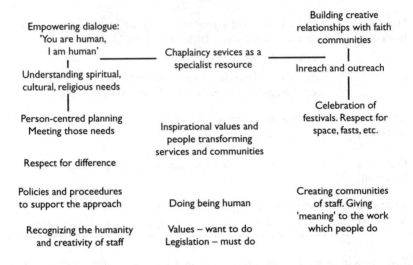

Figure 17.1 Inspirational People – Inspiring Services (Gilbert 2006b)

professional? If then I am taken ill the next day and taken into a hospital to address my physical or mental health needs, am I somehow less than human, somebody passive to be done unto, rather than to be worked with?

This I:thou dialogue will not be sustained in the large and complex organizations today, unless there is support for that right across the board, in terms of its values, strategy, policies, supervision, systems, structures, partnerships, relationships and community support. Many commentators feel that the Postmodern era has seen a breakdown of communities and, if this is so, then perhaps organizations need to provide and create communities of meaning, because if we don't do 'being human', what do we do? It is by engaging the heart of the organization that we will create organizational health.

Bibliography

Abrahamson, E. (2000) 'Change without paying.' *Harvard Business Review* July–August 2000, 75–9.

Adair, J. (2002) *Inspiring Leadership.* London: Thorogood.

Alimo-Metcalfe, B. (2005) 'Leadership; Time for a new direction?' *Leadership 1*, 1, 50–71.

Allan, C. (2006a) *Poppy Shakespeare.* London: Bloomsbury.

Allan, C. (2006b) 'Defining moment.' *The Guardian*, 19 April 2006.

Barlett, P. and Wright, D. (1999) *Outside the Walls of the Asylum: The History of Care in the Community 1750–2000*. London: Athlone.

Barratt, R. (2006) *Building a Values Driven Organization; A Whole Systems Approach to Cultural Transformation*. London: Butterworth-Heineman.

Bauman, Z. (1997) *Post Modernity and its Discontents*. Cambridge: Polity Press.

Bauman, Z. (2000) *Liquid Modernity*. Cambridge: Polity Press.

BBC1 (2005) 'Undercover nurse.' *Panorama*, July 2005.

Biberman, J. and Whitty, M. (eds) (2000) *Work and Spirit: A Reader of New Spiritual Paradigms for Organizations*. Scranton: University of Scranton Press.

Bunting, M. (2005) *Willing Slaves: How the Overwork Culture is Ruling Our Lives*. London: Harper Perennial.

Collins, J. (2001) *Good to Great*. London: Random House.

Collins, J. and Porras, G. (2000) *Built to Last* (3rd edn). London: Random House.

Covey, S. (1992) *Principle Centred Leadership*. London: Simon and Schuster.

Dawkins, R. (1976) *The Selfish Gene*. Oxford: Oxford University Press.

Foucault, M. (1961, this edition published 2001) *Madness and Civilisation*. London: Routledge Classics.

Gilbert, P. (2003) *The Value of Everything: Social Work and its Importance in the Field of Mental Health*. Lyme Regis: Russell House.

Gilbert, P. (2005) *Leadership: Being Effective and Remaining Human*. Lyme Regis: Russell House.

Gilbert, P. (2006a) 'We need leaders at all levels with heart and guts.' *Open Mind 138*, March/April 2006.

Gilbert, P. (2006b) 'Flying High: presentation to the NIMHE Pilot Sites.' 3 May 2006.

Gilbert, P. and Nicholls, V. (2003) *Inspiring Hope*. Leeds: NIMHE.

Gilbert, P. and Scragg, T. (1992) *Managing to Care*. Sutton: Community Care/BPI.

Gilbert, P. and Watts, N. (2006) 'Don't mention God.' *A Life in the Day 10*, 3, August 2006.

Goleman, D. (2006) *Social Intelligence: The New Science of Human Relationships*. London: Hutchinson.

Haidt, J. (2006) *The Happiness Hypothesis: Putting Ancient Wisdom and Philosophy to the Test of Modern Science*. London: William Heinemann.

Handy, C. (2002) *The Hungry Spirit: New Thinking for a New World*. London: Arrow Books.

Harrison, G., Hopper, K., Craig, T. *et al.* (2001) 'Recovery from Psychotic Illness: a 15- and 25-year international follow-up survey.' *British Journal of Psychiatry 178*, 506–517.

Healthcare Commission (2006) *Investigation into Services for People with Learning Disabilities at Cornwall Partnership NHS Trust*, HCC, 5 July 2006.

Holbeche, L. (2005) *The High Performance Organization*. London: Butterworth-Heinemann.

Holbeche, L. and Springett, N. (2004) *In Search of Meaning in the Workplace*. Horsham: Roffey Park Institute.

Jackson, C. (2006) 'Out of sight.' *Mental Health Today* September 2006.

Jarrold, K. (2005) 'The NHS – Past, Present and Future.' Speech to the Institute of Health Management 23 November 2005. Available at http://society.guardian.co.uk/health/story/0,7890,1648297,00.html (accessed 17 October 2007).

Jones, K. (1972) *A History of the Mental Health Service*. London: Routledge and Kegan Paul.

Linstead, S., Fulop, L. and Lilley, S. (2004) *Management and Organization. A Critical Text*. Basingstoke: Palgrave Macmillan.

Mannion, R., Davies, H. and Marshall, M. (2005) *Cultures for Performance in Health Care*. McGraw-Hill/Open University Press.

Merchant, R. and Gilbert, P. (2006) 'The Modern Workplace: Surfing the Wave or Surviving the Straightjacket?!' *Crucible*, Autumn 2006.

Morgan, G. (1997) *Images of Organization.* London: Sage.

Mullins, L.J. (2002) *Management and Organizational Behaviour* (6th edn). Harlowe: Pearson Education.

National Patient Safety Agency (2006) *Safety in Mind.* London: NPSA.

Peck, E., Dickinson, H. and Smith, J. (2006) 'Transforming or transacting? The role of leaders in organizational transition.' *British Journal of Leadership in Public Services 2,* 3, September 2006.

Rooke, D. and Torbert, W. (2005) *Seven Transformations of Leadership.* Harvard: Harvard Business Review.

Schein, E.H. (2004) *Organizational Culture and Leadership* (3rd edn). San Francisco: Jossey-Bass.

Schwarz, B. (2005) *The Paradox of Choice: Why More is Less.* London: Harper Perennial.

Scull, A. (1984) *Decarceration: Community Treatment and the Deviant – A Radical View* (2nd edn). Cambridge: Polity Press.

Senge, P. (1998) *The Fifth Discipline: The Art and Science of the Learning Organization.* New York: Doubleday.

Sennett, R. (2006) *The Culture of the New Capitalism.* Yale: Yale University Press.

Sewell, H. and Gilbert, P. (2006) 'Leading and learning.' *British Journal of Leadership in Public Services 2,* 1, March 2006.

Sheikh, A. and Gatrad, A.R. (eds) (2000) *Caring for Muslim Patients.* Oxford: Radcliffe Medical Press.

Sussex Partnership Trust (2006) *Spiritual and Religious Care Strategy: A Working Document.* Brighton and Hove: Sussex Partnership Trust.

Tehan, M. (2007) 'The compassionate workplace: leading with the heart.' *Journal of Illness, Crisis and Loss 15,* 3, 205–218.

Whitmore, J. (1997) *Need, Greed or Freedom; Business Change and Personal Choices.* London: Element.

SIMBA's Black Diversity

Here I sit and think of SIMBA
A tiger born in Camberwell, South London
But with his roots firmly embedded
In the Black nations of the world – Africa, Asia, the Caribbean
In countries like Antigua, Egypt, Ghana, India, Jamaica, Nigeria,
All bathed in sun and heat
Vibrant energy rising up through the roots
Uplifting and enriching the tiger's soul.

Here I sit and witness SIMBA
Diversity personified, marked differences
In skin colour, hair texture, facial features
Beauty in all its forms. Voices, dialects, accents
All differences openly acknowledged, accepted and respected
Each providing a new and distinctive facet to the whole
Forming a precious jewel, sparkling in its glory
Proclaiming to the world the unique multiplicity of SIMBA's
being.

Here I sit and consider SIMBA
Black people openly acknowledging the importance of the spirit
Intangible, indefinable, a powerful force that is always present.
For some, in the form of their own Gods
Be they Rasta, Christian, Muslim, Hindu or Jewish
While others have spiritual beliefs of their own making
Drawn from the sacred core that exists in us all
To make us human, humble, capable of love and compassion.

Here I sit and reflect on SIMBA
And see some clear in their faith, drawing strength
As they cope with the struggle of their fractured lives
And use their prayers and rituals to heal and revive the soul.
But for others confusion reigns, and their gods move further
away
And prayers are not enough to stop the pain or devastating guilt
And accepting blame seems to be the only way, maybe through
that confession
Making way for redemption, and hope for faith once more.

Here I sit and pray with SIMBA
That each of us may find some peace within ourselves
And come to understand our place and purpose in the world.
That the spiritual bonds we form one with another
And the common experiences we share
Will help us to understand, respect and support each others
struggles
And celebrate our joys as we use our united strength to triumph
over adversity
And show the world how, in spite of everything,
Our spirituality survives and the soul remains intact.

Premila Trivedi, October 2000

MATTERS

SECTION D
Education and Training

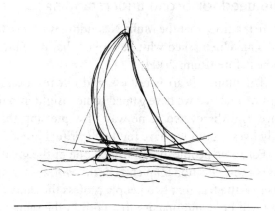

CHAPTER 18

A PLEA FOR BROAD UNDERSTANDING: WHY MENTAL HEALTH PRACTITIONERS NEED TO UNDERSTAND SPIRITUAL MATTERS

Christopher MacKenna

The need for broad understanding

There is a story that the Mulla Nasruddin was once found walking aimlessly at 4 a.m. When asked why, he replied that if he knew, he would have been home before (Rumi 2004).

The human heart is restless, and our restlessness will not be assuaged until we feel that we have gained some insight into the meaning of our existence, and discovered some way of expressing this understanding in our daily lives – until we have found a spiritual home.

For some people, home will be one of the great world faiths, but – and this is a complication for mental health workers trying to make sense of spirituality – the fact that two people profess the same faith does not mean that they will hold and practise that faith in the same way. Besides, these days, many people develop their own spiritual insights and intuitions which draw on diverse sources – ecology, reincarnation, and Goddess worship, among many others. Yet other people, who eschew the 'spiritual', still find spiritual meaning in the arts, or politics, or science, or other aspects of everyday life.

This huge diversity of spiritual interest and allegiance is fully represented among users of mental health services, but here we have an added complication. Not infrequently, in the mental health field, we find people expressing beliefs which may strike even sympathetic health professionals as symptomatic of illness, and nothing more.

Faced with this bewildering variety of spiritual interest and activity, how can we make sense of this intimate and many-layered dimension of the lives of those for whom we care?

A broad understanding in practice

The thoughts which I want to put forward in this chapter are driven by a cluster of convictions.

First, some form of spiritual outlook or religious practice is vital for human well-being; but religion and spirituality need to be understood in broad terms. From the mental health point of view the key question is, what sustains this person's spirit? That is, what gives them the courage, hope, vision and interest to go on living? A vital spirituality may not always appear to be very 'spiritual'. In a recent interview, Nick Cohen said, 'My family's religion is really Socialism' (Jones and Spanner 2006, p.16); and Simon Jenkins said, 'If I have got any religion…it is the religion of history, and local history being real for people' (ibid., p.21).

One way of getting beyond the multiplicity of spiritual and religious expression is to begin by asking ourselves, What sustains this person's spirit? What has power, or energy to *animate* them?

Second, given human diversity, it is inevitable that there will be many religious and spiritual traditions. In this field, there cannot be a 'one size fits all' approach. Even within the traditional religions we find an extraordinary diversity of culture, language, belief and practice; and in the Western world, at least, the rapidity of social change, and the speed of technological and scientific innovation and discovery are ensuring that new possibilities are constantly appearing which challenge and inspire the human spirit. Spirituality is always in process of evolution.

Third, religious and spiritual beliefs and practices exist in more benign and in more pathological forms: it is as dangerous to idealize spirituality as it is to dismiss it. Inevitably, our mental states influence our spiritual outlook, and sometimes this outlook will be coloured by mental disturbance. It is, however, a mistake to imagine that apparently 'psychotic' forms of spiritual thinking are 'nothing but' the workings of the illness. However chaotic or apparently disturbed, they deserve respectful attention because they are both an accurate expression of what the sufferer believes s/he is experiencing, and also a vital framework within which – perhaps alone – some vestiges of meaning can be preserved.

We need to look for the 'gold' in even the most garbled or unpromising spiritual expressions.

Fourth, however difficult it may be, mental health professionals need to cultivate humane and generous attitudes in this area because, even if they see themselves as unspiritual or non-religious they will, inevitably, encounter deeply held beliefs among those for whom they care; and, if they are spiritual/religious people, they will still have to relate sympathetically and intelligently to people whose beliefs will sometimes conflict directly with their own. Such encounters can be disturbing and challenging to the health professional's own sense of identity, and will often make us uncomfortably aware of our ignorance and lack of existential understanding. These can be frightening, but also, potentially, growth-full experiences; and it may well be that our understanding of professional supervision should be expanded to include the spiritual/existential questions which arise for those working in the mental health field.

Spirituality confronts us with ultimate questions. In this area, mental health professionals are quite as exposed and vulnerable as those for whom we care. Like Nasruddin, we are all in search of a spiritual home, whether we know it or not.

These are sweeping statements. To earth them, I want to present three 'cameos' which give some idea of the bewildering range of spiritual expression which we regularly encounter in the mental health field, and through which we can tease out some of its underlying common features.

Three spiritual witnesses

The first extract is taken from a medico-legal report, prepared in the case of a patient who was mounting a legal challenge to his compulsory hospitalization for paranoid schizophrenia:

> The culminating point of the patient's delusional system is his belief that he has a mission to redeem the world, and to restore mankind to their lost state of bliss. He was called to this task, so he asserts, by direct inspiration from God, just as we are taught that the Prophets were. Nerves in a condition of great excitement, as his were for a long time, have precisely the property of exerting an attraction upon God. He maintains this is touching on matters which human speech is scarcely, if at all, capable of expressing, since they lie entirely outside the scope of human experience and, indeed, have been revealed to him alone. The most essential part of his mission of redemption is that it must be preceded by his *transformation into a woman*. (Freud 1911, pp.16–17, text slightly edited)

The second extract is from a publisher's memories of one of his most cele-brated authors:

> I once asked Muriel Spark why she had become a Catholic. Her answer fascinated me. She said: 'Because it is the only thing that has stopped me going mad.' Many might question whether it had entirely done the trick, but the fact that she was aware of the turmoil within was certainly a source of enormous creativity. Indeed it gave her the spark of genius. Her conversion to the Catholic Church gave her the capacity to cope with her contradictions and this is what made her a great novelist. [However] The irony with Muriel Spark was that the inner turmoil could transform itself into a kind of venom or hatred that seemed entirely irrational. (Baird-Smith 2006, p.23)

The third extract is from the Epilogue to one of Carl Jung's monumental studies of Alchemy:

> Alchemy, with its wealth of symbols, gives us an insight into an endeavour of the human mind which could be compared with a reli-gious rite... The difference between them is that the alchemical opus was not a collective activity rigorously defined as to its form and content, but rather, despite the similarity of their fundamental prin-ciples, an individual undertaking on which the adept staked his whole soul for the transcendental purpose of producing a *unity*... Alchemy...has performed for me the great and invaluable service of providing material in which my experience could find sufficient room... (Jung 1970, paragraphs 790 and 792)

Three very different people; three very different worlds of experience and belief; three very different forms of spiritual expression; what they have in common, though, is the relief which all three people found in a narrative, a vision, a story, a practice, which gave expression to the most vital aspects of their experience, and also provided a container for them.

JUDGE SCHREBER

Judge Schreber, whose religious beliefs were outlined in the first cameo, mounted a successful legal challenge to his hospitalization, and was appar-ently able to live at least an outwardly normal life for another five years – until his condition deteriorated following his wife's stroke. Believing in their universal importance, he published his own account of his religious beliefs in the year following his release from hospital.

We can imagine that the belief that God wished to redeem the world through transforming him into a woman endowed the Judge with enormous dignity, and perhaps enabled him to survive an experience which might otherwise have destroyed him. From a psychiatric point of view, of course, the grandiose and apparently bizarre nature of this conviction suggests a psychotic state of mind. However, if we resist the urge simply to dismiss it with this label, we may be able to see that Judge Schreber's belief is also a very concrete expression of ideas found in many religious traditions: the soul is feminine in relation to God. In the Christian tradition, for example, Mary symbolizes those who create a 'virginal' (i.e., open, uncluttered, receptive) state of mind which is favourable for 'impregnation' by the Holy Spirit. Schreber's belief that he was the chosen instrument of God's universal saving purposes can be interpreted in a similar way: religious believers often believe that they are children of God, but in a way which allows for symbolic understanding. In psychotic states of mind, when the ego is possessed by the force of a powerful idea, there is no room for symbolic understanding and the result is a concrete equation: 'I am the unique Son/Daughter/Spouse of God.'

Instead of dismissing Judge Schreber's beliefs as if they were merely a by-product of his psychosis, we should ponder them. What is happening when the symbolic becomes concrete? Is concretization simply the effect of the illness? Or, could it be one way in which the mind responds to unbearable stress? We need to keep this question open.

MURIEL SPARK

Despite occasional violent antipathies, which sometimes reached delusional intensity, Muriel Spark was a successful novelist who delighted in Luther's saying that ridicule is our most effective weapon against the devil. Her conversion to the Roman Catholic Church enabled her to live with her contradictions: Catholicism provided the stories, rites and symbols which grounded, contained and, to her satisfaction, explained her otherwise unbearably conflicting impulses; not least, her sense of the reality and power of evil (Baird-Smith 2006, p.23).

Spark was not alone in having to live with an almost overwhelming – and therefore utterly terrifying – sense of the reality of evil. In schizoid states of mind, people not infrequently find themselves tormented by diabolical laughter, or they may hear mocking voices ridiculing them and taunting them with horrible accusations. Often it is difficult for the bystander to understand what is going on. Are these voices the distorted – or, perhaps, not so distorted – memories of cruel, bitter words which lacerated the child when he, or she, was too young to do other than believe them? Or, are they a partial personification of the sufferer's own vitriolic self-hatred which has had to be split off from their ego consciousness in a desperate attempt to protect the ego from their poisonous effects? Or, again, might it be that the fragile ego of the sufferer is somehow picking up from the collective psyche some aspects of the vast cruelty of the human race, and taking it too much to heart – as if they were personally responsible for all the evil in the world?

These are huge questions, but they deserve our thoughtful attention. Those whose lives are untroubled in these ways can have no understanding of the terror and despair, but also of the metaphysical hunger which may be generated in the hearts of those who experience such taunts. Martin Luther knew these things (Bainton 1994, pp.362–4), so did Muriel Spark; and both of them were comforted by the discovery that the mocker could be mocked. How so? Because their faith taught them that, no matter how awesome the power of evil, and no matter how debased their own lives might be, the power of God's love is always greater. In this way, their religious beliefs took their terror seriously while, at the same time, containing it within an ultimately benign frame of experience and belief.

CARL JUNG

Jung's mental state is a matter for discussion. Donald Winnicott, the eminent paediatrician and psychoanalyst, once suggested that Jung had suffered from childhood schizophrenia, but had had the strength to heal himself (Winnicott 1989, p.483; MacKenna 2000). If this is true, then his achievement of a measure of sanity was due, in no small measure, to the years he spent exploring the psychological and spiritual implications of alchemy. As he says:

> Alchemy…has performed for me the great and invaluable service of providing material in which my experience could find sufficient room. (Jung 1970, paragraph 792)

Looked at from outside, alchemy might seem to typify the mad, esoteric systems which sometimes gain such a tenacious hold over disturbed minds. It belongs to the pre-scientific age when enthusiasts were apparently obsessed by the idea of turning base matter into gold. Alchemical texts are replete with weird diagrams and strange personifications of chemical elements. Yet it was this antique world, with its grotesque, erotic, violent and sometimes beautiful imagery which finally provided Carl Jung with an adequate symbolic universe into which he could project his turbulent inner world.

From an early age – as Jung explains in the autobiographical chapters of *Memories, Dreams, Reflections* (Jung 1995) – he had lived with a terrible secret: he *knew* God. And what he 'knew' was that God was not like the Christian God of his father's preaching. For Jung, God is light and God is darkness. God is good and God is evil. The wonder and the terror of this knowledge threatened to tear Jung apart so, all through his life, he was in search of some means of holding the opposites – even if he was crucified by them – but in such a way that, ultimately, God himself might be redeemed, as God sought salvation through unfolding his conflicted unconscious life into human consciousness.

In his memoirs, Jung paints a poignant picture of his childhood self, haunted by this wonderful but terrible secret which could not be shared with another living soul. The world of alchemy – when he found it – not only provided him with a map of the path which, unconsciously, he had been walking, but also furnished him with a community. Not an ordered community, like the church, but a disparate group of pioneering alchemists who, over the centuries, had staked their souls (and sometimes their lives, given the explosive nature of their experiments) on a quest which – Jung believed – was not so much about transmuting base physical matter into real gold but, rather, the quest for psychological integration and transformation.

Some practical implications

From a psychological point of view, it may be significant that Muriel Spark found a container for her disturbance within an existing religious community – though her relationship with the church remained characteristically acerbic and embattled; Carl Jung had partly to discover, and partly to create a community of his own (which he did, quite successfully); but Judge Schreber – despite the publication of his religious beliefs, which he believed to be of universal import – remained in a community of one.

Donald Winnicott once wrote:

> Should an adult make claims on us for our acceptance of the objectivity of his subjective phenomena we discern or diagnose madness. If, however, the adult can manage to enjoy the personal intermediate area without making claims, then we can acknowledge our own corresponding intermediate areas, and are pleased to find a degree of overlapping, that is to say common experience between members of a group in art or religion or philosophy. (Winnicott 1980, p.16)

Judge Schreber made claims for the objectivity of his subjective phenomena and was judged to be in a psychotic state of mind.

However, as we have seen, even manifestly disturbed spiritual visions can be understood, if interpreted as concretized forms of widely shared spiritual motifs and beliefs. This demands an imaginative and sympathetic response, as well as a very delicate and tactful process of discernment on the part of mental health professionals – especially if we are concerned that the beliefs being expressed may have dangerous implications for their possessor, or for other people. In these circumstances, our response will largely be determined by our role in relation to the person concerned, and the quality of our relationship with them.

As a religious person, I have no difficulty in engaging seriously with what may sometimes strike me as gross spiritual delusions because – if pressed to accept them at face value – I can always say (quite truthfully) 'I will need to pray about this, because God hasn't shown this to me yet'. Then, if at all possible, I will see whether I can make any connections between the spiritual vision, or experience, being presented, and more balanced religious perceptions – as I have attempted to do in my reflections on Schreber, Spark, and Jung. In doing this I am hoping to establish some rapport with, and to reinforce, more balanced parts of the other person's mind – which I believe continue to exist, even in grossly disturbed conditions.

Non-religious health professionals will need to find ways of responding which respect their own integrity. One approach might be to accept what the patient says, apparently at face value, and then to respond with the feelings which that experience would evoke – if it happened literally – to us. For example, 'That sounds terrifying/really exciting/terribly upsetting' – or whatever. Another way forward might be to respond straightforwardly, in terms of what the patient has said. For example, a parish priest once reported feeling totally stumped by a patient who confided, 'I am a tree.' The priest might have found a way forward, though, had he simply said, 'I wonder what sort of tree you are?' Or, 'What season of the year is your tree in?' Questions which might have elicited precious information about the patient's emotional and spiritual state. What we need to avoid, if we can, is either just ignoring the patient's spiritual communications, or, ponderously rephrasing them in our own psychological or psychiatric language; reactions which may well be experienced as rejection, or as desecration.

The 'man in the street' equates madness with what he takes to be nonsense. Sometimes he is right, but sometimes he is wrong – and we can be wrong too. Festus thought that Saint Paul's great learning had driven him mad (The Holy Bible, Acts of the Apostles 26:24); and, on the day of Pentecost, a whole section of the crowd thought that the disciples were drunk because they were speaking in tongues (The Holy Bible, Acts of the Apostles 2:13). Paul might have been mad, and the disciples might have been drunk, but many of the people who listened to them found that their teaching chimed with their own spiritual intuitions, and so the Christian church was born. Hopefully, a broad understanding and appreciation of spiritual matters will guard us against making the automatic assumption that, because we are mental health professionals, our preconceptions must be right, and those of our patients wrong. Indeed, in this area – perhaps above all others – they may prove to be our teachers.

The importance of community

Mental health professionals who have no involvement in organized spirituality, or religion, may be unaware of the enormous benefits which many people find through participating in a community of faith. Equally, health professionals who adhere to one religious persuasion may find it difficult to be supportive of other faith groups – as may religious leaders involved in the mental health field. Both reactions are understandable, but we must resist the temptation to exercise control over other people's lives and learn to trust their ability to discern their own needs. As I suggested earlier, the key question is, what sustains this person's spirit? What has the power, or energy genuinely to animate *them*?

Faith communities vary enormously, but most provide certain key ingredients which can be profoundly reassuring. For example, they:

1. Offer a story about the meaning of life within which we can locate our own experience.

2. Confer a sense of identity: e.g. child of God.

3. Hold us in time while opening a door on eternity.

4. Provide a moral compass, with an opportunity to acknowledge guilt and to receive the assurance of forgiveness.

5. Assure us of the ultimate justice of life.

6. Offer a pathway to healing, even if full healing is assumed to occur beyond the confines of this life.

7. Have rituals which cover the developmental crises of life: birth, puberty, marriage, death; as well as a perspective on what comes after death.

8. Draw people together in community.

9. Negotiate the tension between our longing for an ideal and the necessity of having to cope with reality.

10. In prayer, meditation and worship provide an outlet for our frustrations, anxieties, and longings; as well as a container for conscious and unconscious processes and for transcendent experience.

Many people will not wish to associate with others on their spiritual quest; but some will, and some may need support in venturing out beyond faith communities which have failed to nurture them. As mental health workers, the more broadly informed we are about spiritual and religious issues the more likely we are to be able to assist others on their quest. For the journey is long and many, like Nasruddin, are wandering in the night.

References

Bainton, R. (1994) *Here I Stand: Martin Luther.* Oxford: Lion Publishing.

Baird-Smith, R. (2006) 'Keeping the Devil at bay with laughter.' *The Tablet,* 22 April 2006.

Freud, S. (1911) 'Psycho-Analytic Notes on an Autobiographical Account of a Case of Para-noia (Dementia Paranoides).' In J. Strachey (ed.) *The Standard Edition of the Complete Psycho-logical Works of Sigmund Freud, Volume XII.* London: The Hogarth Press.

Jones, S. and Spanner, H. (2006) 'Of English and Welsh descent.' *Third Way 29,* 3, 16–21.

Jung, C.G. (1970) *Mysterium Coniunctionis: An Inquiry into the Separation and Synthesis of Psychic Opposites in Alchemy.* London: Routledge and Kegan Paul.

Jung, C.G. (1995) *Memories, Dreams, Reflections.* London: Fontana Books.

MacKenna, C. (2000) 'Jung and Christianity: Wrestling with God.' In E. Christopher and H. McFarland Solomon (eds) *Jungian Thought in the Modern World.* London: Free Association Books.

Rumi (2004) *Selected Poems,* tr. C. Banks. London: Penguin Books.

Winnicott, D.W. (1980) *Playing and Reality.* London: Penguin Education.

Winnicott, D.W. (1989) 'Review of Memories, Dreams, Reflections.' In C. Winnicott, R. Shep-herd and M. Davis (eds) *Psycho-Analytic Explorations: D.W. Winnicott.* London: Karnac Books.

Reflection: Church on Sunday Morning
Peter Bates

> Like a collage of photo fragments, the following story is fiction built
> from the truth spoken by my friends and by my own heart.

Sunday morning and prescribed lethargy pins me down under the duvet.
Perhaps I'll feel livelier when I get to the service, although Jane, my psychiatric nurse, looked worried when I mentioned church the other day.

Nowadays I walk to church. Before Sunday shopping I could get my
favourite seat on the bus so that I could watch without being watched and
get out without speaking. Jane says brisk walking will help my mood, but
sometimes it expands my thought balloon until it presses against my skull. At
those times, I find the church building comforting in its ancient solidity. I
picture myself as part of a long line of humanity in which each tiny marcher
brings their fears and their laughter, their babies and their dead through this
old red door.

Richard is on door duty. He knows to say hello and let me pass. Others
he shakes warmly by the hand or even hugs, but that sort of thing is not for
me. I go and sit with Sue and Dave, who nod to me and then resume their
companionable silence. We are in the same group that meets every Wednesday evening, and though I don't say much, it means more than I can say to
have some people who have known me half my life. Last Wednesday I
clawed uselessly against a quicksand of despair as other people talked and
said their prayers aloud, but afterwards Dave offered me another cup of tea
and we talked a bit. It was kind, but I am *so* tired of relationships in which I
view myself or am viewed by others as the needy one, and I am poor
company when I need company too much.

Back here in church the music group are finishing their sound check.
Thankfully it is not too loud, but last week it made my ears buzz and I have
enough weird acoustics in my head already. Who's that playing a flute?

Doug is leading the service. He knows I use mental health services so I
don't need to hide it from him, and often asks me how I'm getting on.
Having a few friends outside the system who know but don't mind counter-
balances the fear I expect from others. His version of pastoral care is to sit
down beside you, chat, say a prayer and then offer to help decorate your
lounge. I never accept, but he means it.

The service has started and the church is filling up now – most of the
families with young children seem to arrive five or ten minutes late, which
always strikes me as odd, given how serious most of them are about their
faith. Sometimes the music group start with children's songs and invite

everyone to join in with the actions, but I'm safe enough sitting next to Dave as he never moves a muscle. A few people seem to love the naïve words and clap along with the song or raise their hands in the air, but I just find this part of the service irritating.

After the songs, Doug introduces the prayers of confession. Church leaders who treat their people like naughty children just make me angry and I'm not one of those horror-movie junkies who feasts on bad feelings, but the words of confession can still sear me with self-loathing. Today Doug briskly moves us on from confession to forgiveness. The sharp pain of confessing and the rush of forgiveness feels a bit like cutting did when I was first ill. I remember a recent lecture on recovery where we were told that forgiveness is a vital step on the way to acceptance and escaping the trap of the past.

Then the children go out to their Sunday School groups and the notices are given, followed by a teenager called Alice who comes to the front to explain that she is off to Africa for a month to work in schools. She explains how she felt that God led her to go and how sponsors miraculously appeared to help fund the trip. Her gauche exuberance has the congregation smiling and nodding, but it's a world away from my mundane half-life where things are endured rather than fixed.

The prayer time provides a space for me to recalibrate my inner yard-stick, think of God and others, and connect with longings. The absurd requests for peace in the world reach beyond the dull injunctions of common sense and help us lift our eyes to the horizon, clarify our goals and set to work.

Next we settle down for the Bible reading and sermon. Today it's Janet's turn to preach. She was off work for a few months last year with depression and seems to understand what people's lives are actually like. The sermon explores how hope and thanksgiving are central to the Christian faith. That recovery lecturer said it is hope that sustains us on the journey. Perhaps my Christian hope in God's goodness will help me find a recovery path. And thanksgiving helps to form a positive mental discipline that appreciates kindness in others and abandons the role of gloomy victim.

The sermon is personal, vulnerable and devotional. Janet explains that, on the positive side, Alice and others have spiritual experiences in which they believe that God meets them, motivates them, helps and heals them. But there is also a negative side, where suffering is not relieved. Sue and Dave's daughter is back from a death dance with anorexia, but Colin's young wife is dead. God sometimes intervenes with help and healing, and sometimes doesn't. No one knows why. To view God as disengaged would resolve the conflict, but be a hopeless retreat, no more true to our experience than the opposite escape into naïve optimism where every sorrow is mended through faith. Janet ends by saying that, like a child reaching out her hands for a butterfly, our church seeks healing through prayer, but we know it doesn't always land on us.

I love that image of the butterfly. I know that my mind has a habit of latching on to an idea and going over it again and again, so I try to get it on to gentle images. This is harder than people tell you it is. As soon as I realize that I am ruminating on something pleasant, then it's as if another part of my mind hunts out the unpleasant alternative topics to think on – like trying to think of holidays while in the dentist's chair. But perhaps I can be still for a while and give the butterfly a chance to settle.

After the sermon we sit together in silence for a time and then quietly sing '*When the darkness closes in, still I will say, blessed be the name of the Lord*'. Both modern song lyrics and the ancient psalms occasionally validate my experience and point me forward. Nobody seems to have noticed the tear on my cheek as a tsunami of feelings rushes in from nowhere. Rather than drown I go to the kitchen for a drink of water.

When I get back to my seat, the service has moved on to Communion. The familiar words and shared ritual helps me feel connected when I don't know who I am, when I have nothing to say, when the quicksand has swallowed me whole. There's a blend here of childlike trust in the mystery and grown-up responsibility as I choose to stand, walk forward and kneel at the rail.

Just before the last hymn, a woman comes forward to describe a vivid mental picture she has had that might contain a message from God for someone. I don't know her name. Is it a psychotic moment, a spiritual experience or an over-active imagination? The kindly invitation is a far cry from the sarcastic accusations I sometimes hear before sleep.

Doug follows up by explaining that members of the prayer team will be available at the end of the service. He says that team members work hard to avoid putting pressure on people. You don't have to tell them anything or explain yourself before they pray for you. They also resist giving advice in their conversation or disguising it in their prayers. One day I might overcome my feelings of self-consciousness, shame and unimportance and ask, but not today. Perhaps Dave would agree to come along and support me.

The final hymn and blessing sends us out from the building and from a preoccupation with ourselves to enrich the lives of other people. Tomorrow I'm going to the Volunteer Bureau with Jane. For now, though, I make a swift exit as the service ends, rather than stay for coffee and small talk.

CHAPTER 19

PROMOTING SPIRITUAL WELL-BEING IN THE WORKPLACE – TRAINING AND SUPPORT FOR STAFF

Frances Basset and Thurstine Basset

Introduction

In this chapter, we reflect upon some of our experiences from a combined time of 62 years working in the health and social care sector. We reflect on our involvement as both practitioners and teachers. We also explore both useful theory and practical examples of addressing spirituality in our work as teachers.

Experience in the workplace

Throughout our years of working in health and social care our general experience is that spirituality is not acknowledged and even sometimes suppressed – partly this has been due, during the latter part of the 20th century, to suspicion of and alienation from established religion within an increasingly secular society.

We both come from families that would state their religion as 'Church of England', but have long since ceased to attend church services or to read the Bible. Prayer is something to be used only in very difficult times, almost as a last resort in a crisis. In seeking a deeper meaning to life, we have come to very personal understandings of spirituality through reading, studying, working, communicating and just living in the modern world.

Looking back in time we remember that health and social care staff who were practising Christians, were often viewed with suspicion in the second half of the 20th century. There seemed to be a fear that they would somehow force their religious views onto their clients, rather than just use their religion as a philosophy to underpin a career in the caring professions. In the circumstances many staff just kept their religious views to themselves. We were recently reminded of this climate of suspicion when we told a mutual work friend about a colleague who had just retired from work. 'Oh yes – I remember him, he was a nice chap but he was a Christian', was the response.

While the concept of holistic care has been advocated by a variety of theorists and educationalists for many years, the integration of a person's 'spiritual needs' during ill health have been markedly absent. The space on the patient assessment form under 'spiritual needs' is often marked with 'C of E' or is simply bypassed with 'not applicable'. Where academics have attempted to integrate the spiritual side into nurse education (Watson 1999) many front line nurses have struggled to translate this into a workable format. As modern healthcare becomes increasingly reductionist the need to bring in meaning and human values becomes ever more urgent. Concerns with new pharmaceuticals, new techniques and disease management create an ongoing challenge to holistic care.

The time is certainly right for a re-birth of spirituality. We work in a system that is perfectly at ease with itself in referring to older people who have nowhere to go and remain in hospital as 'bed-blockers' and a bad day at Accident and Emergency is sometimes described as 'we had a lot of rubbish to deal with today'. A young acquaintance of ours took a job in a day unit at a local hospital and was surprised that the announcement that one of their long-term patients had died took the form of a post-it on the staff notice board with just their name and the time of their funeral on it.

Sometimes the way the NHS is described through television and other media makes it sound more like a war zone than a place of care and compassion.

The 21st century has thankfully seen a revitalizing of the importance of more 'artistic' approaches in health and social care, with the acknowledgement that the 'scientific' approach of the previous century hasn't come up with all the answers. There is also an awareness that the UK has become a multi-faith society, and one of the major plusses of our more multi-cultural society is that it has opened the eyes of many of us to the diversity of faiths throughout the world. Recent generations of people who grew up without a spiritual tradition are also beginning to look for some deeper meaning to life.

'Holism' is now part and parcel of health and social care policy and hopefully practice too, yet it is hard to apply holistic Eastern principles within a Western medical classification system that so clearly separates the 'physical' from the 'mental'. This is clearly represented on Denmark Hill in South London. On one side of the road in Kings College Hospital, which deals with physical illness and on the other is the Maudsley Mental Hospital. The road, Denmark Hill, runs through the middle of these two renowned hospitals in a visual representation of the truly non-holistic system that exists and that we must somehow all work within.

We will revisit the East/West debate later in this chapter, but it is clear that what is needed is some kind of fusion of the two approaches, building on their strengths and minimizing their weaknesses.

Teaching and learning about spirituality – theory

It is important at the outset of any discussion about teaching and learning in the field of spirituality that we define our terms. In our teaching and training, we use the term 'spirituality' within its broadest sense as opposed to the term religion. Ken Wilber's (2001) concept of 'deep spirituality' is useful. Wilber (2001, p.76) suggests that spirituality 'involves in part a broad science of the higher levels of human development'. Wilber claims we have available to us different levels of conscious awareness; not just matter, body and mind, but also soul and spirit. Whereas religion may be taught and followed (translative), spirituality is to be experienced from within (transformative).

In 1979 Sir Alistair Hardy carried out a survey in the UK asking: 'Have you ever been aware of or influenced by a presence or power, whether you call it God or not, which is different from your everyday self?' Hardy (1979) published his results after receiving 3000 responses and later these were presented by Hay (1990) in a simplified form which captured the essence of those experiences:

- a patterning of events in a person's life that convinced them that they were meant to happen

- a sense that all things are 'One'

- an awareness of a sacred presence of nature or God

- an awareness of being looked after in some way.

Greely and McCready (1973, cited in Firman and Vargiu 1980) carried out a national opinion survey in the USA asking: 'Have you ever felt as though you were close to a powerful spiritual force that seemed to lift you out of yourself?' When the results were published in the 1970s responses were drawn from as many as 70 million people who were willing to admit that they had experienced this sense of higher consciousness frequently (Hay 1990). An awareness of this feeling of connectedness, or higher sense awareness is what we refer to as spirituality.

We believe that profound experiences such as these can give value and meaning to our lives as they provide a sense that our inner worlds are not so separate from the world outside of ourselves. It can be assumed from studies of this nature that these types of experience are actually very common despite often being taboo and rarely talked about.

At a personal and one-to-one level we, as teachers and trainers, aspire to teaching with a level of self-awareness and openness that acknowledges that these experiences are real for many people.

There is a growing body of psychotherapeutic, educational and managerial literature seeking to combine East/West approaches to spirituality health, and healing. We now explore some of the writers that we have found useful when working with this approach.

Roberto Assagioli founded a particular form of counselling and therapy in 1910. He named this psychosynthesis (as opposed to psychoanalysis). Assagioli suggested that in addition to Freud's emphasis on analysis and the subconscious (instinctive, repressed material, etc) the human psyche also consisted of a super-conscious (creative, inspiring) layer. His egg model of the human psyche offers one way to understand this.

Assagioli stressed that it was from the higher unconscious that we receive intuitions and inspirations. These may be artistic, philosophical or

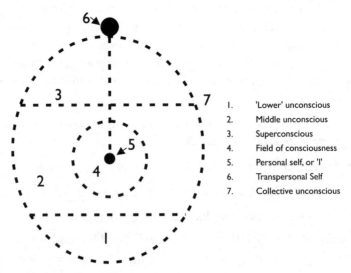

1.	'Lower' unconscious
2.	Middle unconscious
3.	Superconscious
4.	Field of consciousness
5.	Personal self, or 'I'
6.	Transpersonal Self
7.	Collective unconscious

Figure 19.1: Our Psyche (Assagioli 1965)

scientific, ethical imperatives and urges to humanitarian and heroic action. In this realm Assagioli suggested, are the latent spiritual energies (Assagioli 1965). It is important to note that the distinction between the 'lower' and 'higher' unconscious or superconscious, is developmental, not moralistic. The lower unconscious merely represents the most primitive part of ourselves which is not bad, just earlier.

Assagioli saw the superconscious as all that we still can reach in the course of our evolution. Connection with the Transpersonal Self is a rare occurrence which may result from the culmination of years of discipline; although for others, it may be a spontaneous extraordinary experience. This Transpersonal Self lives at the level of universality, of the wider vision of the whole (Ferrucci 2004). It is our belief that this Transpersonal Self is not only accessible thorough our superconscious but can be equally experienced from lower unconscious material whereby the notion of, 'breaking down to break through' suggests that in times of utmost despair people may have flashes of great joy and feelings of connectedness to something greater. In this sense the Transpersonal Self might realistically be drawn at both ends of the egg.

'Well-being' from a psychosynthesis stance suggests a reconnection from parts split off (repressed) through the life course. Assagioli talks about the need to re-connect the I–Self pathway, whereby the 'I' is viewed as a paler reflection of the Transpersonal Self. Through empathetic failures and other painful experiences we repress both our subconscious and superconscious energies. Assagioli saw this reconnection to our sense of I and ultimately between I–Self as a form of homecoming where healing could take place. It is important to note that while Assagioli was interested in the world religions of Buddhism, Hinduism, Christianity and Judaism, he did not believe psychosynthesis should be used in this way. Assagioli, whose primary identity was that of a psychotherapist (not a minister) claimed that psychosynthesis 'took people to the door, but stopped there'.

Following in the footsteps of Assagioli, contemporary writers such as Kornfield (1994), Wilber (2000), Welwood (2000) and Tolle (2005) have all made legitimate links between Western models of psychology and Eastern concepts of spirituality and thus the growing body of knowledge known as integrative spirituality has flourished. As Welwood points out (Welwood 2000, p.xi), 'While the traditional spiritual cultures of the East have specialized in illuminating the timeless, supra-personal ground of being – the "heaven" side of human nature – Western psychology has focused on the earthly half – the personal and interpersonal.' Essentially we believe that this is about combining the best of our Western scientific/psychological understandings with the Eastern concept of mindfulness. Kornfield (1994) for example, advocates the benefit of engaging in psychotherapy combined with a contemplative, meditative practice.

It is not just in the field of psychotherapeutic literature that this paradigm has been espoused. Over the last ten years the field of integral spirituality has been linked into the world of corporate management and organizational behaviour. Writers such as Zohar (1997) stress how Western organizations would do well to take these ideas on board. Zohar suggests that if organizations are to develop and bring about transformational change they too, need to be cognisant with their deeper spiritual values and meanings. This means re-thinking traditional organizational structures to go beyond the purely 'mental level' of managing change to incorporate what Zohar refers to as the 'New Science'. As she points out, Western organizations continue to model themselves on a 'Newtonian' paradigm:

> The billiard ball was Newton's metaphor for the atom, the smallest bit of matter. As described in his mechanistic physics, each atom (billiard ball) was isolated in space and time from every other. The atoms bounced about in a void, connected to each other by forces of action and reaction, their movements determined by iron laws of motion that assured universal order and predictability. Each atom was circumscribed by a hard and impenetrable boundary. None could get inside the other. When they met, they experienced collision and one or both was knocked off its course. The billiard ball and game has become a familiar metaphor for the Western organization. (Zohar 1997, pp.100–101)

Rather than managing and leading our organizations from this separated, reductionist model, the new science incorporates an integrated East/West, or as Zohar refers to, a 'quantum' approach to structure and change. Zohar sees 'quantum' organizations as having flexible boundaries – these flexible boundaries being a synthesis between the rigid boundaries of the West and the ambiguous boundaries of the East. Similarly 'quantum' organizations use dialogue, combining conflict and control from the West and cooperation from the East.

Zohars' quantum model combines East/West approaches and recognizes that organizations need to integrate their approaches if they are to truly transform themselves.

Practical examples from teaching and learning

Having explored some of the theory that we find useful in raising and exploring the topic of spirituality with learners, here are two examples of successful approaches and useful resources from our wider links and our practice as teachers/facilitators:

CLIENTS AND PROFESSIONALS IN TRAINING AND LEARNING

CAPITAL (Clients and Professionals in Training and Learning) is an organization from West Sussex made up of people who have been or currently are users of mental health services. This organization acknowledges the importance of spiritual beliefs. One member, Laura Lea writes:

> For many people mental illness may be experienced as a process of fragmentation and disintegration. Recovery and well-being should therefore be focused on restoring a sense of wholeness. We are body, mind, spirit and soul. Holistic care needs therefore to include care for any spiritual needs. (Lea 2004)

Lea suggests that people are searching to gain some meaning and explanation from their experience of mental distress and that this search is at root a spiritual task. This should be at the heart of mental healthcare.

> The often religious nature of symptoms and the existential crisis experienced by people going through mental health problems are surely clues that there is something going on beyond the here and now that might be of significance or value to them. (Lea 2004)

Lea makes a plea for workers to be at least interested enough to ask about spiritual matters.

CAPITAL members regularly return to the theme of spirituality and this mirrors the great importance attached to spirituality by many service users who have consistently championed spirituality in a climate which has not only been unresponsive but also has often pathologized spiritual experience as a symptom of mental illness. Indeed it is service users rather than mental health workers whom we can thank for putting spirituality back on the agenda for mental health services.

We would encourage all mental health trainers and educators to be involved in some way with an active service user group.

THE JANKI FOUNDATION FOR GLOBAL HEALTH CARE

The Janki Foundation for Global Health Care is a healthcare charity dedicated to positive human development, and to working to research and promote a spiritual model of modern healthcare. We have found their training package 'Values in Healthcare – a spiritual approach' to be an excellent programme for exploring spirituality. The seven modules (each module is one day in length) in the programme are:

1. *Values* – inner values and values at work.

2. *Peace* – being peaceful and peace at work.

3. *Positivity* – being positive and positive interaction at work.

4. *Compassion* – finding compassion and compassion in practice.

5. *Co-operation* – understanding co-operation and working in teams.

6. *Valuing yourself* – self-care and support at work.

7. *Spirituality in healthcare* – exploring spirituality and healing and spiritual care in practice.

One problem with these materials however is getting to a situation where staff can give seven days to this training.

One of the authors was, however, involved in a one-off day conference organized by a Sussex-based Doctor/Healer network in conjunction the British Holistic Medical Association. The conference explored Spirituality in Healthcare and the approach was based on the training materials produced by the Janki foundation.

This day really broke the mould of the traditional 'medical/nursing' conference as the facilitators shared details of their own spiritual journeys and how this had motivated and enriched both their lives and their professional work. Healers, doctors, lay people and nurses all sharing their thoughts and feelings with great honesty created a much needed non-hierarchical space. Being able to speak about these issues from the heart (as well as from the head) enabled others to contribute in a more accessible way. The subject matter became grounded in a personal everyday non-academic way and was really brought to life. This 'levelling' environment enabled the sharing of similarities of experience, which is such a rare thing given the hierarchical nature of healthcare professions and institutions.

Systems for promoting spiritual well-being in the workplace

There is a danger here that interesting and useful educational and developmental initiatives will simply fizzle out and die when transplanted to a workplace where there is no support and no fertile ground for a more spiritual approach to working with people in mental distress.

There are some obvious ways for allowing this approach to flourish. Our experience has been that the following work practices are very variable, with some excellent examples mixed with their complete absence in some services:

- Workplaces need to have good support and supervision policies which work in practice.

- Supervision needs to address staff members' needs for support and development as well as the need for their work to be managed within the policies and procedures of the organization.

- There need to be avenues for both formal and informal individual support in the workplace.

- Support groups for staff can be an excellent way to build morale and avoid burn-out.

- There may be some scope for spiritual advisors/mentors in the workplace.

- Action learning sets. We have had some success with running these; an example is included below.

The action learning set was made up of five senior nurses with a facilitator and took place within an NHS trust. The set met monthly and was facilitated with group agreements and regular process reviews. The set evolved and while the main purpose was to provide managerial and professional development support, set members reported a much deeper sense of connection and support from both the facilitator and each other. This was a level of support which they had never experienced before despite many years of working in the NHS. One member also felt able to make positive changes of a much more personal nature, which in turn, energized and strengthened her role as a leader. The set stayed together for five years and members remained in contact well beyond its closure.

It was unfortunate that this model was not adopted more widely across the NHS trust as members often expressed how, 'it kept them in the job' and how the set enabled them to see beyond major difficulties of a professional or personal nature.

The challenge is inevitably how to get the acknowledgement and discussion of spirituality more into the mainstream, but the dawn of a new century (indeed a new millennium) is showing positive signs.

'Matters Spiritual' are very much more on the agenda. If you doubt us on that, these are the words of a former captain of the English Rugby team, Lawrence Dallaglio, when speaking about a 'totally cathartic experience' which led to a reconciliation with his family following an injury which 'allowed us to get back together and move on to a different chapter in our lives. It might have seemed like a rugby disaster to some but I felt almost spiritual about it. I was clearly meant to be back home sorting out things with my family'. (*The Guardian*, 17 January 2006). If rugby players can talk about spiritual matters, then surely health and social care workers can also take the plunge.

References

Assagioli, R. (1965) *Psychosynthesis – The Definitive Guide to the Principles and Techniques of Psychosynthesis*. London: Thorsons.

Ferrucci, P. (2004) *What We May Be – Techniques for Psychological and Spiritual Growth through Psychosynthesis*. New York: Tarcher Penguin.

Firman, J. and Vargiu, J. (1980) 'Personal and Transpersonal Growth.' In S. Boorstein (ed.) *Transpersonal Psychotherapy*. Palo Alto: Science and Behaviour Books.

Hardy, A. (1979) *The Spiritual Nature of Man*. Oxford: Clarendon Press.

Hay, D. (1990) *Religious Experience Today*. London: Mowbray.

Janki Foundation for Global Health Care (2004) *Values in Healthcare: A Spiritual Approach*. London: The Janki Foundation for Global Health Care.

Kornfield, J. (1994) *A Path with Heart – A Guide through the Perils and Promises of Spiritual Life*. New York: Bantam.

Lea, L. (2004) 'Body, mind and soul.' *Mental Health Today*, September 2004, 35–7.

Tolle, E. (2005) *A New Earth – Awakening to Your Life's Purpose*. London: Penguin, Michael Joseph.

Watson, J. (1999) *Postmodern Nursing and Beyond*. Edinburgh: Churchill Livingstone.

Welwood, J. (2000) *Toward a Psychology of Awakening – Buddhism, Psychotherapy, and the path of Personal and Spiritual Transformation*. Boston: Shambhala.

Wilber, K. (2000) *One Taste – Daily Reflections on Integral Spirituality*. Boston: Shambhala.

Wilber, K. (2001) *A Theory of Everything – An Integral Vision for Business, Politics, Science and Spirituality*. Dublin: Gateway.

Zohar, D. (1997) *Re-Wiring the Corporate Brain – Using the New Science to Rethink How We Structure and Lead Organizations*. San Francisco: Berrett-Koehler.

Yours

I write to tell you of my
experience of illness and life.

I was born premature
And was not meant to be

So, from birth I made sure
the world knew me.

I ranted and raved as a child.
Tried to take my own life as an
adolescent

But, learnt as an adult that
Life and death are not within
my control

Life took my arrogance and
Indestructibility of youth, and made
me humble and destructable with age
The glow of having and the shiver
of not having

The pure pain of suffering and the joyous vibrancy of life

The rays of the beating glistening sun, and the icy stillness of the
turning clear ocean

Pours onto my body.
While the vastness of the universe
Swallows me up

Some say I am ill for my sins
Others say God loves me, so he tests me
I say he blesses me, for I have my own

I do not judge, nor expect to be judged
For I know I was meant to be.

Fatima Kassam

CHAPTER 20

AWAKENING THE HEART AND SOUL: REFLECTIONS FROM THERAPY

Brian Thorne

I am delighted to have the opportunity to share with you some of my reflections as I try to make sense of my experience as a therapist over the years. I do this within the context of my Christian faith and its practice since boyhood and of my struggle – often rather unsuccessful – to be properly human.

The starting point for me is the trustworthiness of the client and of his or her experience. As a person-centred practitioner, I operate from the basic assumption that my client knows where it hurts and is the best possible guide to finding the way through to healing and wholeness. My task is to be along-side, to honour and respect my client's inner world and to help him or her discover meaning and direction by tapping into the wisdom and resources which he or she inherently possesses but has lost sight of in the passage through life. I discover that this trusting of the client is not fashionable in the context of the 21st century insistence on quick results and cost-effective therapeutic methodologies. Diagnosis, goal setting, cognitive-behavioural programmes seem to be the order of the day with the client placed in the role of willing or unwilling learner of how to live his or her life. True, efforts are made to understand the client's experience but such efforts are often directed principally towards establishing a diagnosis and working out a treatment plan which the client may feel able or unable to own and about which he or she is unlikely to have been consulted in any depth. My desire to trust my clients, let alone be guided by them, can in such a culture, be perceived as naïve, foolhardy or even irresponsible. And yet most therapeutic and medical practitioners seem to expect their clients to trust *them*. It is strange that a reciprocity of trust is not as a matter of course either expected or considered appropriate.

Trusting a person, of course, confers value upon them – even if, in reality, they are not on the evidence trustworthy or certainly do not consider themselves to be so. To be perceived as a person of value, however, is for many in our culture a rare experience and this is particularly true, I believe, of those who find themselves hitting the buffers, suffering breakdowns or falling prey to distress and disintegration which can lead to hospitalization.

Wordsworth in his 'Intimations of Immortality' refers to the newborn child as 'trailing clouds of glory'. The infant, he tells us, 'comes from God who is our home'. Why is it, then, that so many of us apparently have no sense of that glory, no concept of ourselves as wondrous beings bearing the marks of divinity? The answer to that question is almost certainly complex and its fullness unknowable. Two factors, however, seem fairly clear.

In the first place we live nowadays in a culture which seems increasingly to assume that we are anything but glorious. On the contrary, the unwritten message seems to be that we are probably at heart lazy, incompetent and dishonest and therefore need to be constantly observed, appraised and chivvied. I do not recall a time in my life when there has been so much built-in surveillance in almost all walks of life. The obsession with raising standards and being cost-effective and efficient coupled with the advent of the litigation-conscious mentality means that almost everyone is looking over his or her shoulder to see who's watching. A perfectly proper concern for justice, fairness and protection of the vulnerable has led, I would suggest, to a culture of blame and contempt where it is difficult for anyone to feel good about themselves let alone that they have within them the seeds of divinity.

And then second, there is the common failure to welcome newcomers into the world. The newborn need mirrors to be held up to them – loving, tender, empathic mirrors – if they are to have a sense of their own natures and to perceive their own value. Instead, it seems, the fate of so many people is to have distorting mirrors held up to them or in some cases no mirrors at all. Instead of empathic understanding they receive constant criticism, denigration and, in the worst cases, abandonment or abuse. Worst of all, perhaps, is to experience no response at all but simply neglect and indifference. So many studies of those who as adults experience the shipwreck of mental breakdowns or disturbance reveal the lack of empathic responsiveness which they received as infants and children. They have not known what it is to be prized and understood or to have reflected back to them the image of their own intrinsic worth and loveliness. They cannot recognize their true selves because nobody has held up the mirror to them so that they can see their own quality and beauty. On the contrary the distortions that they do receive often convince them that they are useless, stupid and even evil.

Sadly this lack of what we might call 'empathic mirroring' is sometimes exacerbated by early experiences of particular forms of dogmatic or bigoted religion. I still remember, with much anguish of spirit, an occasion in Paris more than 20 years ago when at a conference for psychotherapists I convened an impromptu seminar for those interested in the relationship between psychological and spiritual growth. Within half an hour of the start, almost the whole group was in tears as one member after another talked about their experiences at the hands of the churches – both Catholic and Protestant. I still remember some of their stories.

There was the man brought up in Catholic boarding school where the staff – mostly priests – inflicted a vicious round of humiliating punishments for the smallest misdemeanours and seemed to derive sadistic satisfaction from dealing out frequent corporate punishment to lonely and frightened young adolescents. There was the woman who had had her mouth washed out with soap by a nun for saying 'shit' and then been made to stand barefoot in the chapel for an hour without moving. There was the account of a Calvinist minister who had told a 15-year-old that she was possessed by the devil and should on no account enter a chapel building.

The stories were not only of priests, nuns and ministers, but also of parents whose religious beliefs and practices seemed to make it impossible for them to relate to their children without at the same time judging or condemning them and making them feel so burdened with guilt that life was almost intolerable.

For me that impromptu seminar was saved from turning into a complete nightmare by the contribution of a Swiss woman who told how as an adolescent she, too, had felt utterly guilty, unable to find any virtue in herself and totally despairing. In her distress she had rung the bell of a house of the Jesuit fathers and had collapsed sobbing into the arms of the priest who opened the door to her. Strangely enough he did not welcome her in but instead himself left the house and taking her arm walked for two hours with her in a nearby park. At the end of that time, she said, her despair had lifted and for the first time for years she felt that she had value. It was only some years later that she discovered that the priest who had walked in the park with her was Fr Pierre Teilhard de Chardin.

For the moment I need to pause and to reflect with great sadness on those countless individuals over the years who have come to seek my help because they were so loaded with guilt life had become well nigh impossible. None of these people as I recall had done anything particularly appalling – there were no murderers or rapists, arsonists or swindlers. They were afflicted, however, by a guilt which was elusive but all-pervading, a sense of being in the wrong, of never being able to please those whose love they craved, of being eternally without value. They might as well have stepped out of the pages of a novel written by Franz Kafka.

Against such a depressing background it is, to my mind, little short of miraculous that in the lives of so many people, the heart and soul are awakened by what appears to be the direct intervention of spiritual reality. The difficulty, of course, is to recognize such an intervention when it comes and to be able to hold on to its authenticity in the face of the scepticism or outright ridicule of others. Most difficult of all, perhaps, is to hold on to it when others deem it to be madness or the unmistakable evidence of psychosis.

Of course, discriminating between the false and the authentic is not always easy. Some so-called spiritual visitations are clearly, under another guise, the sinister internalizations of judgements passed by all-too-human agents in the past. When the apparent intervention reinforces a sense of guilt, unworthiness and hopelessness it needs to be rejected as false – the treacherous reinforcement of the distorting mirror which has so harmed the individual in the past. Authentic spiritual breakthroughs, I would suggest, bring in their wake an altogether different message. It is as if against all the previous evidence the person is left with a sense of well-being, of being acceptable, loveable, of worth.

Sometimes, too, the world which was previously hostile and threatening reveals a new beauty. I remember a client of mine whose life history was appalling: rejection, abuse both sexual and physical, expelled from school, a failed and violent marriage – and yet this person in all her very real misery and distress brought into the room a sense of there being a still centre. It was almost uncanny – how could she with such a history of suffering, injustice and brutality communicate a kind of peacefulness in the storm? One day she explained the mystery. As a young child – after a beating from her mother – she had fled from home, rushed down the street and in through the open door of the village church. And there, through her tears and terror, she had looked at a statue of Christ with a child in his arms and had heard him say: 'Don't be afraid. I will love you always even when you forget me.' As a child there was nothing to block the entry of that experience – no questioning scepticism, no distrust of subjective knowledge, no scientific method. What is more nothing in her past experience would seem to have prepared her for such a startling revelation of the loving heart of the universe. And that one experience – a matter of a few minutes only – has sustained her over the decades. In the midst of a life of often unspeakable abuse and deprivation her heart and soul have remained awake because as a child she had met with the living God.

For most of us, perhaps, such apparently direct intervention of spiritual reality into our lives is unlikely to occur – and yet recent research suggests that as many as two in five of us do undergo positive mystical experiences which we are then reluctant to take on board or even to discuss with others. It is as if we cannot believe that we are by nature desirable or desired and dismiss such experiences as wishful thinking or just plain mad. Be that as it may, for most of us intimations of spiritual reality will come to us through our relationships with others. And that is why it is so important – to return to where we started – that those who strive to help those who are in mental disarray never lose sight of the inherent beauty and wisdom of the one who suffers and never forget that they themselves are of infinite worth and beloved to all eternity. It is through such relationships that not only can suffering be alleviated but the heart and soul awakened to new life and new hope.

Acknowledgement

This chapter was adapted from a presentation given at a Mental Health Foundation conference in 2000 entitled 'Awakening the Heart and Soul'.

Restless Sea

I'm always on the move,
Restlessly active, that's me.
Surging and ebbing,
Like the tide-torn sea.

I sense God spoke to me once,
At least it seemed so.
I wasn't meant to be where I was,
Somewhere else it seemed!
I wasn't told where to go,
The light faded too soon:
Not the full Damascus!
Not the completed picture,
Just a trailer,
Jigsaw pieces for me to play with.
Dom helped –
I find God without a human face difficult
To envisage.

Years later…
When the tomb door was shut on me,
So sand silted up my ears,
My eyes, my brain, and heart.
The crypt sealed with a metal trapdoor –
Tight! Bolted down.
Then, it was human hands
Reached down to me
And pulled me up.

Because I couldn't hear,
Couldn't bear,
The music,
I sought the comfort
Of my faith family
And listened to the rhythm
The measure of the psalms
The rhyme and rhythm bore me up,
Like the waves…beating, carrying.

The listeners delved,
And dug out the silted, cloying sand.,
With their ears and hands,
Listening with the ear of the heart.
They digested the grit for me.
So, another conversion
In conversation,
Communion
In communication

Flow and ebb, blue on blue,
The restless sea,
The restless heart,
But there is a me, and there is a you.

Peter Gilbert, December 2006

CHAPTER 21

MENTAL HEALTH CARE: THE ULTIMATE CONTEXT FOR SPIRITUAL AND PASTORAL FORMATION

Julia Head and Mark Sutherland

Where are we coming from?

In the late 1970s, the Chaplaincies of the Bethlem and Maudsley Special Health Authority under John Foskett and St George's Hospital under Ian Ainsworth-Smith, pioneered the introduction of non-accredited Pastoral Care Courses modelled on the method of Clinical Pastoral Education (CPE). For a number of years these chaplaincies ran a joint programme divided between acute and mental health settings. Eventually the programmes separated, and in the 1980s St George's chaplaincy stopped running a separate programme. The Bethlem and Maudsley programme continued into the mid-1990s, at which point it stopped. One reason for the cessation was that the staff did not want to take the route of seeking accreditation for the programme. Consequently, student numbers began to dwindle with the movement in higher education towards accredited courses.

In 2000 the Maudsley re-introduced a small CPE style course for four students. The programme combined the previous Maudsley Pastoral Care Courses and more specific CPE elements. In the following year, a second course for eight students was run on similar lines. The moderate success of these courses exposed also an area of difficulty. Although senior chaplains within the Maudsley team oversaw both courses, they had been run by supervisors who, while bringing CPE-based experience, were not working chaplains and were unfamiliar with the healthcare context in which the course took place. Reviewing this approach led to the conclusion that we needed to embed the CPE model more firmly into the healthcare context in which the students were placed, and which provided the raw material for their learning. Two direct changes have resulted from this review process:

- The working chaplains have taken back direct input into and management of the programme – an arrangement more typical of CPE programmes and introducing little change to the traditional model.

- There has been significant modification of the traditional model concerning seminar work.

Where do we find ourselves?

CPE is a pedagogical model focusing exclusively on the learning experience and on personal and professional development processes. There is little focus on the dissemination of content, making it essentially *content lite*. Within the UK context, the numbers of pastoral practitioners who have experienced the CPE process are few, but those who have feel deeply indebted to this experience. CPE changes lives, and among its adherents this is regarded as a strength, which it undoubtedly is. However, there is a downside to a situation where, among a larger ministerial community, only very few have had this particular life-changing experience. It leads to an excess of evangelical zeal among the 'converted' which expresses itself in the all too familiar cry 'this is the only way'. This naturally puts off the majority who are made to feel that they have to convert, or be damned. This tendency towards exclusivism is built into much CPE culture and in our view results from three factors:

- the dynamic within all religious communities towards the assertion of exclusivity, which is compounded when the holders of the 'truth' perceive themselves to be a misunderstood minority

- the general ignorance among CPE's exponents of its connections to the wider educational culture of experiential and developmental pedagogy

- the general perception of CPE as a North American import.

CPE is not an exclusive model. It is but one example of a wider approach seen in other areas of education. Most particularly CPE shares an approach taken within the traditional[1] psychotherapy and counselling trainings and in the educational discourse of *learning from experience* advocated by Freire (1972, 1974, 1985) and Knowles (1977, 1984). A wider recognition of CPE's broader pedagogical connections could go some way to modifying its rejection within mainstream British theological education. In this way CPE could inform, and be informed by the larger body of experiential learning.

How has our experience shaped our current response?

These insights, together with our now substantial experience of running CPE programmes, have led us to critique the essentially North American imported model of CPE. One of the historic weaknesses of much pastoral care, and CPE in particular, has been its aversion to theory. Thus, even when pastoral practitioners operate well in one-to-one interaction they are unable often to articulate a coherent understanding of the *how* and *why* of what it is they do. This has led us towards the inclusion of more content-based material into our programme in an attempt to counter two areas of weakness in contemporary experientially-focused spiritual and pastoral education, namely:

- lack of knowledge concerning viable theoretical models of human spiritual and emotional development and relationship dynamics

- lack of expertise in building living theology from actual, rather than abstract, human experience.

In our education programme, we have retained the key process elements of supervision, clinical placement, and experiential group. However, the traditional seminars in pastoral theology and pastoral skills have been strengthened by a content-focused infusion of ideas introducing wider reading and discussion in the areas of religion and mental health, and pastoral psychology.[2] The experiential focus on personal and professional self-development as the primary tool for spiritual and pastoral care remains our paramount consideration. Students are encouraged to explore their personal experience in tension with the process and content of a programme operating within specific clinical and social contexts (hospital and community). They are further encouraged to discern within their own experience, past and present, the construction of their personal and pastoral identities under the

---

1   We are referring to the vocational, personal process focused trainings rather than the purely academic, increasingly university-based models of psychotherapy and counselling training.

2   Our content concerns mental health and emotional development. Importation of our model to other pastoral care settings might require theoretical content that draws on other areas of health care theory more relevant to the setting.

influences of the social and political discourses of power, class, ethnicity, gender and sexual identity.

The setting for the programme is mental health care. However, the purpose of this is not to create pastoral workers who will operate predominantly within mental health settings. Nor is it simply to acquaint pastoral workers with issues affecting people who have mental health needs. Mental health dynamics offer the greatest challenge to negotiating personal, emotional and spiritual lives. They offer also the richest rewards in developing and deepening personal capacities for self-understanding as a basis for standing alongside others. Together with this, the addition of the seminar content has provided a wider and deeper background of theoretical knowledge against which the developmental process of the student's learning takes place.

Emerging from our engagement with, and resulting critique of, the imported model of CPE we have begun to forge what we regard as a contextualized working philosophy shaped by two key influences:

- our debt to the philosophical legacy of the CPE Movement, which has given us our primary psycho-spiritual focus on the personal-professional interface of the student's development

- the influence of the multi-faith context within a *modernizing*[3] health service and the development of a psycho-spiritual approach.

Currently there are different approaches to embracing multi-faith inclusion in the development of healthcare chaplaincy. One such view privileges religious difference through the creation of a series of vertical silos each representing a different, historically conditioned, faith tradition serving the needs of an individual faith constituency. Our approach has been to develop what we call a psycho-spiritual focus on the deeper commonalities between all faith traditions.

Within all religions there exists a deeper strand reflecting the universal elements within spiritual experience. These deeper strands, while not homogenous, are to a very great extent mutually comprehensible and facilitate considerable cross-boundary communication and pastoral working. This is because psycho-spiritual experience emerges out of the direct encounter between the human and the Divine or Cosmic Ground permeated

---

3   Modernizing here refers to the revolution in culture shift within the NHS known as the
     Modernization Agenda. This is an attempt to move health service organization away from its
     historic hierarchical, bureaucratic, top–down control and command culture with its privileging of
     professional interests towards hierarchically flatter, networking, learning organizations able to
     place the needs of the patient at the heart of the design for service delivery.

through the dynamics of human consciousness. That is, beneath their historical, cultural and philosophical differences, all religious traditions speak with noticeable similarity about human encounter with the Divine/Cosmos.

These universal aspects of spiritual experience are highly significant at points of life crisis such as illness and distress. Understood against this background the developmental, self-reflective model of spiritual and pastoral care at the heart of CPE offers an approach capable of presenting reassuring familiarity which is attuned to meeting individual spiritual needs at points of crisis. Such an approach requires a certain kind of formation in training and it is to this that our attention has been focused in our programme.

Our programme has developed within a Spiritual and Pastoral Care Service operating within a secular mental healthcare context. We articulate universal principles through our core value statement:

> Chaplains will not discriminate between persons on the basis of faith community, gender, ethnicity, class, or sexual orientation.

Our approach emerges from our core belief that the chaplain's role is to *follow the other's articulation of need*. To do otherwise is to impose upon the other our definition of usefulness, which in turn shapes our perception of their need. For many people in mental distress labels pale into insignificance beside a more urgent need for someone able to listen to, and accompany them, amid frightening and disintegrating experiences.

We are in the fortunate position of having financial support from our Board of Trustees for the programme. This allows us to take this inclusive working philosophy into the multi-faith arena through the offering of bursary places for students from minority faith communities. Within the designation minority faith communities we include Black-led Pentecostal Christianity. Students from faiths other than Christianity have the opportunity to take their places in a multi-faith learning situation. Within this situation each student is encouraged to make the necessary connections between practising a psychologically informed pastoral care, as it has developed in our secular institutions of healthcare, and their own particular theological tradition of personhood and care.

Aspects of our programme now carry full accreditation from the Chaplaincy Academic and Accreditation Board, the advisory body to the three professional chaplaincy organizations in the UK. For those students who are interested in pursuing development as healthcare chaplains, these points count towards being eligible to apply for, and maintain professional accreditation on the Chaplaincy Register. Although not in force at present, within the foreseeable future only persons eligible for registration will be able to apply for Chaplaincy posts.

What have we learned from the changes we have made?
STUDENTS
The programme has been developed in response to various factors, including:

- the urgent need for suitably trained chaplains in all healthcare sectors
- the need to extend pastoral care training to faith communities other than Christianity
- the better targeting of chaplaincy input in clinical settings
- the need to respond to new priorities in mental health service provision.

Our programme is suitable for all faith community leaders, teachers, pastors, pastoral carers, counsellors, chaplains, theology students, and others wishing to develop their self-understanding as the foundation for spiritual and pastoral care practice. The programme is directed towards the health of the community (public health) in that we aspire to accept those students who we consider will return as a resource to their local contexts.

We have experienced difficulty on occasion in recruiting individuals from minority faith communities for a variety of reasons. This difficulty is not so much concerned with differing theologies, but more with the fact that individuals may come from non-conventional educational backgrounds, and educational competence can fall below the standard required for the type of course we offer.

We have noted also that minority faith communities can be largely internally self-referencing with limited participation in wider culture, including religious culture. This can lead to views of spiritual and pastoral care that are highly authoritarian, which can be compounded when individuals struggle with low levels of psychological insight and capacity for self-reflection. This latter aspect is the main difficulty encountered within the educational programme with students from a whole variety of traditions and backgrounds. With any individual it shows itself in adherence to rigidly held beliefs and ways of being in relationship and in ministry that can tend to objectify and patronize the person being 'cared for'. This requires fairly high levels of input throughout the programme regarding personal and professional development.

We anticipate always that the programme experience will highlight clashes of personal and religious culture. However, we do hope to provide students with a well-supported space in which to explore and negotiate these challenges to self and an individual's deeply held values and to interpersonal relationships.

EDUCATIONAL EXPERIENCE

The programme includes what is often a difficult mix of the experiential and the theoretical, which makes this an intensive experience for the students.

The experiential elements comprise mainly the placements, supervision and the professional development group (experiential group).

Placements

Role negotiation in placement takes a long time and can be discerned through the many questions that students bring to supervision. Negotiation of 'What am I here for?' and 'What do the staff and patients think I'm here for?' are just two of the frequently asked questions highlighting the dilemma between 'doing' something to feel useful and just 'being' in the tension very often of not knowing what to do to make things better. This place of chaos is about the students surviving the experience for themselves.

Students on placement are designated as Chaplaincy Assistants, working within the operational and philosophical policies of the Spiritual and Pastoral Care Service. In their placements, students are directed to exercise spiritual and pastoral care for Service Users, their significant others, and staff, respecting confidentiality at all times. They are to learn from the experience of working with others under stress and how religious and spiritual resources can be utilized in an appropriate and helpful way. In addition, they are to integrate into the work patterns of the setting by attending nursing handovers, management and case discussions, community meetings and so on.

Supervision

Supervision attends to the students' current personal and professional development through asking the question, 'how does this material relate to, or arise from the present context of the student's experience?' However, the line dividing supervision from counselling is a fine one. The work may trigger off personal issues, taking the students beyond their immediate task of relating their personal development to their professional development on the course. Where this is clearly the case the matter is dealt with as appropriate for external counselling referral. The content of the supervision session is usually regarded as confidential. However, the supervisor will need to be able to report on an overview of the student's development and feed this into the weekly staff meeting.

Professional Development Group (Experiential Group)
The purpose of the professional development group is to share, examine and reflect together upon how the work affects the students on the programme as individuals. Each person brings to any pastoral encounter a personality (with strengths and growing edges), a personal history and the interpretation of that history, namely, one's story. All these are operative when genuinely encountering another person. The group provides a space for students to reflect on how they are affected through their encounters with patients and service users. The programme constitutes an institution with its own internal dynamics, and the group is the place where the playing out of internal dynamics can be observed, identified and contained.

The theoretical elements of the programme comprise the seminar content, as well as opportunities to learn from one another's approach to working in mental health ministry through the pastoral skills workshops. The quality of student participation in these elements depends very much on the individual's willingness to engage with the rather complex issue of reflective practice. We attempt to move students away from a dependent style of learning, and the fantasy that we can supply all the answers to everything they need to know to effect their ministry well.

We request students to read various articles in advance of the seminars and to produce written summaries regarding the ideas and themes presented in the reading, together with their reactions. We encourage students to take active part in the seminar discussion. The 'learning from experience' occurring via students' placements, as well as students' own life experience forms an important foundation for individual participation and group discussion.

Benefits for the Spiritual and Pastoral Care Team

The education programme is an ambitious undertaking for what is a relatively small and already rather over-stretched team operating as it does across four London boroughs. However, we consider the input to be worthwhile for two main reasons. First, we notice the benefits concerning increased staff team cohesion and collaboration. The three main tutors on the programme consist at present of the most senior chaplains in the team. However, there are opportunities for other team members to work on the programme, and to develop their skills concerning spiritual and pastoral education within the mental health context. On the back of the programme, we have introduced pastoral skills seminars for the main team, to which we invite our students and chaplaincy volunteers. These workshops have provided an invaluable space within the team for the sharing of different ways of working with religious and spiritual issues as they interface with mental health.

Second, the organization and management of students' placements has necessitated close collaboration with team leaders, who now welcome our students because of the benefits they bring on the whole to service user care, both in hospital and community contexts.

Dynamic structure

One aspect of particular importance concerns the dynamic interaction between student and staff groupings within the programme, which we discuss below with reference to supervision and the professional development group.

SUPERVISION

Traditionally, CPE saw the role of the supervisor as holding and containing every aspect of any individual student's experience of the course. We initially felt that it could be unhelpful for one person to have so much influence over the student's learning process. Therefore, we divided the traditional CPE supervisory function into two:

- the student's personal/professional development and the work

- the educational formation and overall course containment.

These functions are divided between the supervisors, the tutors, and the course director.

The strengths of this approach include the fact that students receive a variety of input and the experience of different personalities within the team. It separates out also the space for self-disclosure from the space for educational assessment, where students' personal and professional development can be viewed from within a broader framework of experience. It ensures that the supervisors are actually practising chaplains, as mentioned earlier, rather than CPE supervisors who may or may not have direct experience of the specific pastoral context within which the learning takes place.

However, we have discovered that this separation of functions places an increased importance on the cohesion between individuals within the staff team. We have observed two kinds of pressures on staff cohesion. First, the pressures of pastoral work in a healthcare setting, and particularly the mental health setting. These pressures can result in manipulation and splitting within the staff/student body reflecting the acute nature of the disturbances being worked with. Second, the opportunities for differences in emphasis and practice between staff, which we believe to be strengths in our programme, if unacknowledged, can lead to splitting within the student body. The students can pick-up on and act out these differences. This results in splitting (for example, good person and bad person), religious identifications and gender tensions around competition and authority. This leads to the erection of defensive behaviour and resistance to the task of learning.

THE PROFESSIONAL DEVELOPMENT GROUP

A common complaint about the group is that no one understands the nature of its function. This is partly based on it being one area of the course where there is no specified content/agenda. Therefore, its focus can only be on the individual participants of the course. Experience shows that it remains possible for students to avoid engaging with the relational tasks that the group seeks to foster. Whether this is the case or not, the group still fulfils its vital function.

We discovered this truth to our cost recently when we discarded the group as part of the structure for the final semester. The decision for this was partly in response to student criticism of the group and partly to reduce workload on staff. However, it resulted in a lack of containment evidenced by accusations of a lack of safety. It also resulted in negative projections focusing on one of the programme tutors who in her meetings with the student body remained the only point at which the whole of the course dynamic could be focused.

Conclusion

The early history of CPE indicates that there has always been a tension between mental health and other clinical contexts concerning pastoral education (see further, Sutherland 1994). It is easier in acute medical and prison contexts for the developmental process to be domesticated by conventional religious expectations – that is, the need of the church's ministry.

For Anton Boisen, the recognized father of the CPE movement, the central element of students' learning was not solely their educational needs but their observance of, and more importantly their encounter with others as *living human documents*. He believed that this required a suspension of the direct application of traditional theological models and understandings in order to allow for new insights to emerge that were particular to the immediate pastoral situation:

> The attention will be shifted from the past to the present; from books to the raw material of life. Experience will no longer be fitted to the system but system to experience... Studying the human personality

in health and in disease, in prosperity and in disaster, seeking patiently and systematically and reverently to discover the motive forces and the machinery which are involved and to formulate the laws which govern them, we may be able to lay the foundations of a new theology. (Boisen, in Asquith 1992, p.23).

The 'ultimate context' of our education programme can be seen in its objectives which include increased student competency in spiritual, religious and pastoral care, spiritual insight and awareness. Further, we hope to engender developing fluency in interpersonal facility and skill in healthcare and organizational contexts, as well as experience in team and collaborative working. Permeating the whole is the desire to encourage an experience of inclusive and non-discriminatory working relating to issues of ethnicity, faith, gender, sexual identity and orientation. Student feedback generally assures us that we have succeeded in these objectives, and that the students are pleased to have had the opportunity to develop more in terms of their personal and professional and spiritual lives, even though the journey at times might have been very challenging.

More fundamentally, we are aware that the time students spend with us is relatively short. We do hope, however, that their experience through the programme will sow seeds with them that will flourish in ways we may never get to hear about, but that will serve the wider community regarding appropriate responses to the religious and spiritual lives of people with mental health needs. Again, following Boisen, we trust that 'we may have been able to start something' leading to 'life-long devotion to patient, accurate, reverent exploration in all its range of that inner world with which religion is concerned' (Boisen, in Asquith, pp.30–31).

References

Boisen, A. (1992) 'The Challenge to Our Seminaries.' In G. Asquith (ed.) *Vision from a Little Known Country: A Boisen Reader*. Decatur, GA: Journal of Pastoral Care Publications.

Boisen, A. (1992) 'Theological Education via the clinic.' In G. Asquith (ed.) *Vision from a Little Known Country: A Boisen Reader*. Decatur, GA: Journal of Pastoral Care Publications.

Freire, P. (1972) *Pedagogy of the Oppressed*. London: Penguin.

Freire, P. (1974) *Education for Critical Consciousness*. London: Sheed and Ward.

Freire, P. (1985) *The Politics of Education: Culture, Power, and Liberation*. London: Macmillan.

Knowles, M. (1977) *Self-directed Learning*. New York: Association Press.

Knowles, M. (ed.) (1984) *Andragogy in Action*. San Francisco: Jossey-Bass.

Sutherland, M. (1994) *The Psychological Self as Educational Subject*. Unpublished MA Dissertation.

A Reflection on Recovery: Psalm 102:2–10, 28
Arthur Hawes

2   Hide not your face from me
    in the day of my distress.

3   Incline your ear to me;
    when I call, make haste to answer me.

4   For my days are consumed in smoke
    and my bones burn away as in a furnace.

5   My heart is smitten down and withered like grass,
    so that I forget to eat my bread.

6   From the sound of my groaning
    my bones cleave fast to my skin.

7   I am become like a vulture in the wilderness,
    like an owl that haunts the ruins.

8   I keep watch and am become like a sparrow
    solitary upon the housetop.

9   My enemies revile me all the day long,
    and those who rage at me have sworn together against me.

10 I have eaten ashes for bread
    and mingled my drink with weeping.

28 You change them like clothing, and they shall be changed;
    but you are the same, and your years will not fail.

Psalm 102, especially the opening verses, addresses the whole question of mental health. I want to reflect upon verses 2 to 10 and verse 28 printed above because here the writer faces mental illness head on.

At the beginning are the words 'in the day of distress…'. Immediately there is a recognition that mental illness causes suffering, pain, bewilderment and confusion. Distress captures all these experiences and more. The request, the prayer, the call, is for a rapid response and an answer to the problem and the pain. If broken bones can mend and at the point of breakage be stronger, why is it that broken spirits, tortured souls and shattered identities cannot be mended and healed within a month or two?

The Psalmist is aware of the severity of mental illness and identifies the following:

• 'My bones burn away' – as a spirit disintegrates, the experience and feeling is of one's very skeleton being under threat.

- 'I forget to eat' – eating is so often an indicator of the severity of the mental health problem. The pain and suffering are so all consuming that thoughts of food and balanced diets are not a priority.

The groaning described in verse 6 is an expression of the depth of anxiety and torment which is such that it cannot be expressed in words, but only groans.

The location for this anguish is described as living in a wilderness and among the ruins. In both places the familiar landmarks have disappeared. The only boundary in the wilderness is the horizon and the only identifiable object in the ruin has been shattered. Here is a metaphor for mental illness itself – life without boundaries and identifiable objects. The next verse reinforces this by powerfully describing the solitariness of the sufferer. Mental illness drives a person into their own inner world because of so many things – disturbed emotions, confused thoughts, loss of the familiar, and shattered identities are but a few.

Verses 9 and 10 move us from the inner world to the external world which is a place of fear and uncertainty. Here enemies are to be found, real or imagined. Here are ghosts which later become internalized and add to the confusion of the inner world. It is only when tears mix with drink, that we begin to capture something of the despair and futility of a mind under pressure, a person disorientated and a spirit disembodied.

The penultimate verse of the psalm reverses all of this. God may well be changeless but his creatures live with change. Change is a feature of mental states and what is offered through the grace of God and the spiritual dimension is hope where there is despair, joy where there are tears, glory where there is evil and destruction, and an inner peace and tranquility where there is confusion and distress.

CHAPTER 22

RESEARCHING SPIRITUALITY
AND MENTAL HEALTH: A
PERSPECTIVE FROM THE
RESEARCH

SECTION E
Research

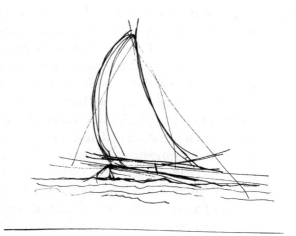

CHAPTER 22

RESEARCHING SPIRITUALITY AND MENTAL HEALTH – A PERSPECTIVE FROM THE RESEARCH

John Swinton

When the editors of this book asked me to write a chapter reflecting on the differences in the ways spirituality and mental health are researched in the US and the UK, I wasn't convinced that it was a good idea. This was partly for pragmatic reasons. Within the limitations of a short chapter it is not possible to do justice to the diversity of complex cultural nuances within the research literature. Certainly it might be possible to give a sense of what is happening, but an authentic comparative study would take up much more space than is available. But my reservations were deeper than simply the constraints of time and space. The research produced within the field of spirituality and mental health is so varied, that tying down particular cultural differences is not a straightforward task. I was not convinced that any one approach or methodology could be said to represent either the US or the UK. Both countries have produced research that is rich and very diverse in terms of the breadth of methodologies and approaches. This richness refuses to be tied down within tight conceptual categories or tidy methodological frameworks and cannot be confined neatly within cultural boundaries.

Nevertheless, as I began to look at some of the research that is emerging from the US and the UK, some interesting patterns, commonalities, themes, tensions and discontinuities did begin to emerge. I would not claim to have uncovered a single unified 'US model' or a readily identifiable 'UK model'.

Nevertheless, there are certain interesting cultural dynamics that impact on the way that the relationships between spirituality and health are investigated within these two countries and which do serve to separate their respective research agendas in ways that are potentially significant.

The cultural shape of research

What I offer in this chapter is not a systematic review of the literature, but rather a perspective that emerges from the literature that will allow us to begin to think about the impact of contrasting cultural assumptions on the ways in which we choose to do research. All of us seek to do research under the same banner: 'spirituality and mental health,' but the particularities of our cultural context deeply impacts on the way that we interpret the nature and the content of that task. In reflecting on some of the tensions and differences between the research agendas of the UK and the US, we will be able to examine aspects of these important cultural dynamics and develop perspectives that will guide us as we seek to understand the complex connections between culture and research.

A framework for analysis

In her paper 'Spirituality and Health: Towards a framework for exploring the relationship between spirituality and health', British researcher Joanne Coyle offers three approaches within which the research on spirituality and health can be examined and explored (Coyle 2002). She describes these approaches as:

- the structural-behavioural approach
- the value guidance approach
- the transcendent approach.

Here I will draw on two of these categories – the structural-behavioural approach and the value guidance approach – as rough categories that will enable us to highlight some important cultural differences between the two contexts we are focusing on. For the purposes of analysis I would like to suggest that the structural behaviourist model forms a significant aspect of the US approach to spirituality and healthcare in general and mental healthcare in particular, and that the value guidance approach is typical of the main body of research emerging from the UK.

The structural-behaviourist approach: A perspective from the US

The structural-behaviourist approach constitutes a significant stream of research activity in the US and focuses specifically on *religious* commitment and its implications for health and human well-being (Levin 2001). Here the emphasis is on the specific practices associated with organized communities of faith. Spirituality (for the most part understood in terms of formal religion) is assumed to aid health primarily by connecting people to religious communities where they learn certain beliefs and ways of viewing the world and use particular practices that provide structure to their lives and encourage forms of behaviour that are health enhancing and health promoting. These practices include such things as:

- church attendance
- religious affiliation
- social supports
- enhanced psychological states
- private religious involvement – (prayer, scripture reading, etc.)
- sense of place, belonging and identity within religious community. (Chatters 2000; Koenig 1998; Koenig, Larson and McCullough 2001).

The emphasis here is on the *function* of religious beliefs as shapers of behaviours and responses, rather than on the content of specific belief systems. The growing evidence base that has emerged from this approach indicates that religious behaviour can have a positive effect on physical and mental health. Such behaviour has been shown to be beneficial on a number of levels and in relation to a wide variety of conditions. Health benefits include:

- extended life expectancy
- lower blood pressure
- lower rates of death from coronary artery disease
- reduction in myocardial infarction
- increased success in heart transplants
- reduced serum cholesterol levels
- reduced levels of pain in cancer sufferers

- reduced mortality among those who attend church and worship services
- increased longevity among the elderly
- reduced mortality after cardiac surgery.

(Koenig *et al.* 2001)

Those working with this religiously focused model do at times speak about the more general term 'spirituality' (Koenig *et al.* 2001). However, it is clear that the majority of the research done within this approach emphasizes religion and for the most part the Christian religion.

A key aspect of this approach is the way in which it seeks to utilize the methods of science to show the relationship between religious practices and health. Standard scientific techniques such as randomized control trials, statistical analyses and modes of research that follow the principles of falsifiability, generalization and replicability (Swinton and Mowat 2006) mark this approach out as firmly within the paradigm of the so called hard sciences.

Beginning in the early 1990s (Miller and Thoresen 2003) researchers began to draw upon these methods to measure the relationships between religion and health in ways which were methodologically sophisticated and which sought to be credible not only to religious organizations, but also to the scientific community. Miller and Thoresen note that: 'Before the 1990s, the relationship between religion and health was largely a de facto area of research: researchers often buried religious variables in the methods and results sections of their studies without overtly highlighting them as legitimate areas of health research' (Miller and Thoresen 2003). After the 1990s there was a movement that sought to move this area of research from the peripheral to the mainstream of scientific enquiry. With the publication of several special issues on spirituality and health in professionally refereed scientific journals (American Psychologist 2003; Baumeister and Sedikides 2002; Thoresen and Harris 1999), the movement towards what we might describe as the 'religion and health movement', (Levin 2001) was well and truly underway. While there are a number of different perspectives on religion and health emerging from the US, it is this scientifically oriented approach with its mantra of 'religion is good for your health!' and its focus on structure and behaviour that has attracted most attention and the majority of the funding.

Religion, research and culture

This approach is not without its theological and scientific critics. (Schuman and Meador 2003), but it is not coincidental that the central focus of the structural-behaviourist approach as it has worked out within the US is primarily on religion. Demographic studies indicate strongly that in comparison with the UK, the US is a very religious country. In an ICM survey (2004) conducted for the BBC, researchers discovered that 67 per cent of the US citizens who were polled claimed that they prayed regularly. This was compared with UK citizens of whom 28 per cent claimed to pray regularly. This same survey found that 54 per cent of those polled in the US regularly attend organized religious services, compared with 21 per cent in the UK (ICM, 2004). Furthermore, *Time* magazine (Wallis 1996) found that 82 per cent of Americans believed that prayer heals. To date no such survey appears to have been carried out in the UK.

The overwhelming majority of Americans claim to be religious with 80 per cent identifying themselves as Christians. The US hosts 300,000 worshipping congregations spread out between more than 4000 denominations. Viewed from this perspective the reasons why the research focuses on religion and not primarily on the less tangible concept of 'spirituality' are not difficult to understand. It is of course very difficult to research the actual content of religious beliefs and how they may or may not impact upon health. However, researching religious *behaviour* is methodologically and culturally more of a possibility. Consequently the structural-behaviourist model fits well within the more religious context of the US and with the preferred methods and goals of science.

Religion is good for your mental health

Within this developing evidence base there is a growing body of research that suggests that religion is beneficial for mental health. (Koenig 1998, 2005) A number of systematic reviews of the research literature have consistently reported that involvement with religious communities can be beneficial for mental health (Bergin 1983; Gartner, Larson and Allen 1991; Koenig, Larson and Weaver 1998; Larson, Pattison, Blazer *et al.* 1986). We are discovering that a healthy religion makes us happier (Witter, Stock and Haring 1985), protects us from depression (McCullough and Larson 1999), makes us more secure, less anxious (Shreve-Neiger and Edelstein 2004), and provides us with a stronger sense of self (Pollner 1989). Also, if our religion is manifested within a religious community, this in turn has significant health benefits (Brown and Prudo 1981; Brown, Ndubuisi and Gary 1990;

Strawbridge, Cohen, Shema *et al*.1997). It is becoming clear that, if properly understood and effectively utilized, a person's religion can be a beneficial dimension of the caring process.

Of course, there is also evidence to suggest that the religion–health connection is not always healthy or verifiable. For example, a study by Speck and King (1999) indicated that strong spiritual belief was predictive of poor clinical outcome. Again, Levin and Vanderpool (1987) conclude that there is insufficient evidence to confirm that religion and health are positively and significantly related. Nevertheless, the majority of the religion and health studies appear to indicate varying degrees of positive correlation between religion and positive mental and physical health.

Why is religion good for your health?

The explanation for the connection between religion and health in the structural-behaviourist model of research is primarily cognitive and behavioural. Levin highlights five possible mechanisms that might be at work:

1. *Regulation of individual lifestyles and health behaviours.* Most religious systems have prohibitions on certain ways of behaving and living (e.g. the prohibition on alcohol, smoking, etc), all of which have health benefits for participant.

2. *Provision of social resources* (e.g. social ties, formal and informal support). There is a recognized connection between mental health and well-being and effective social support structures. Social support can tie people into supportive relational networks which are both protective against mental illness (Brown and Prudo 1981) and healing of it when it develops (Swinton 2000).

3. *Promotion of positive self-perceptions.* Religion can promote self-esteem by incorporating people into secure relational networks that are affirming and accepting (Swinton 2000). It can also engender feelings of personal mastery in ways that can be supportive and health promoting (Pelzer and Koenig 2005).

4. *Provision of specific coping resources* (i.e. particular cognitive or behavioural responses to stress). Adherence to a particular faith tradition realigns a person's thinking and can enable then to cope constructively with trauma and illness. The signs, symbols, rituals and narratives of faith communities provide the resources for individuals to re-form their life-worlds in significant ways (Pargament 1997).

5. *Generation of other positive emotions* (e.g. love, forgiveness). The growing body of literature for example within the area of forgiveness research (Worthington 1998) indicates that religion can generate particularly positive emotions which have the potential to be health enhancing.

6. *Additional hypothesized mechanisms, such as the existence of a healing bioenergy.* The growing literature within the area of prayer studies is indicative of the possibility that there may be supra-empirical dimensions to religion and spirituality that are currently not understood but which may have healing capacities (Dossey 1993).

From this necessarily brief and selective overview of the current research that falls within the structuralist-behavioural approach, it is clear that traditional types of religious belief and practice continue to have considerable beneficial therapeutic potential. This approach fits well within the US social and spiritual context and continues to be one of the major strands of research that has emerged from within that context.

The value guidance approach

Turning to the research being carried out within the UK, while some are researching within the model of the structural behaviourists (Francis *et al.* 2004; Loewenthal, Macleod, Goldblatt *et al.* 2000; Maltby, Lewis and Day 1999), the majority of the work falls within Coyle's second category: the value guidance approach. The value guidance approach assumes that spirituality is not necessarily worked out within a system of religion. Rather it assumes that spirituality is worked out primarily through an individual striving to attain a higher value, meaning or goal for their lives. (Dyson, Cobb and Foreman 1997). Oldnall points out that within approaches to spirituality which adopt this type of position:

> [t]he concept of god does not constitute a transcendent being or a set of religious beliefs. Instead, the person has consciously or unconsciously chosen a set of values which become the supreme focus of life, and/or around which life is organized... From this perspective it may be argued that the perceived values embraced by the individual have the ability to motivate the individual's life style towards fulfilment of their individual needs, goals and aspirations. Leading to the ultimate achievement of self-actualization. (Oldnall 1996)

This approach assumes that spirituality relates equally and arguably primarily to values, principles and ideals that do not necessarily relate to belief in the transcendent. From a value guidance perspective, 'the content of beliefs is irrelevant so long as they give the individual values to guide life' (Coyle 2001). Unlike the more religiously oriented structural behaviourist approach, there is no necessity for the Divine or for particular communities that claim to have the Divine at the centre of their identity and existence.

This model presents a perspective within which *all* people are assumed to be spiritual and to have a spirituality with *some* choosing to express this through the structures of formal religion. This approach has in many ways become representative of the way in which researchers within the UK have approached spirituality, particularly within the field of nursing where the majority of the research on spirituality and health has been done. This view of spirituality fits well with the rapidly secularizing social context in the UK and relates in interesting ways to the ongoing reconstruction of spirituality that seems to be occurring in the light of this.

Reconstructing the spirit

Within the UK the post-war period has seen a sharp decline in adherence to institutional religion. This decline has carried on into the new millennium. However, although people within the UK may be becoming less *religious*, it would be a mistake to assume from that that they were necessarily becoming less *spiritual* (Hay and Hunt 2000; Heelas and Woodhead 2005). It seems that relatively few people have opted out of some sort of belief. Experiences of the sacred and or the spiritual remain widespread even though religious practice appears to be declining. (Davie 2002). While many people within contemporary UK culture wish to *believe* in the spiritual dimensions of life, they are less inclined to want to *belong* to religious organizations or participate in religious communities. This migration of spirituality from the religious to the secular has led to an opening up, or perhaps better a reconstruction of traditional understandings of spirituality to include dimensions which may be functionally similar to the traditional religious quest, but which are epistemologically variegated, qualitatively different and which no longer locate themselves within any form of religious practice, tradition or system. Spirituality is viewed as a general human need that can be met without any necessary reference to the transcendent and with no necessity for involvement in formal religious structures. Rather than being perceived as a divine gift or a consequence of sustained interaction with God or a religious community, spirituality has come to be understood as a *personal* quest for *personal* value and fulfilment which is carried out by *individuals*, sometimes with the help of others but often alone, or at least without any formal connection to a supportive community.

This is not to say that religion is not significant for a substantial number of people. Religion remains a vital primary source of spiritual expression for many people within the UK. Indeed, certain forms of religion, particularly black and evangelical churches, have not only survived the decline but are showing significant growth. The point to bear in mind here is that, within a British context, certain forms of institutionalized religion seem to have lost their meaning, significance and attraction to a significant number of people who are now working out their spiritual impulses in different ways. The values guidance model can thus be seen to fit well with the spiritual climate of British culture.

From spiritual communities to spiritual individuals

One result of this process of this changing understanding of spirituality has been a significant shift in the *location* of spirituality. Religious spirituality is something that a person learns and discovers through interaction with specific others over a sustained period of time, normally within some form of faith community. Religious spirituality tends to have an external referent, i.e. it is something that is perceived as given to individuals and communities from outside of themselves (divine revelation), rather than something they engender from within themselves. Traditional religions are normally associated with some kind of formal community involvement, a set of fixed beliefs, narratives, rituals and behaviours that, as we have seen, have implications for health and well-being.

The wider understanding of spirituality that is represented in the value-guidance approach differs significantly in that it is dependant primarily on individual choices focused on unique individuals. In other words, it tends to focus on the immanent rather than the transcendent dimensions of human spirituality. Spirituality is considered a personal possession, a commodity which people *individually* seek to develop in order that they can find *personal* meaning, hope, purpose, happiness, comfort and so forth. Approaches to research and the practice of spiritual care that base themselves on this approach similarly embark on developing ways in which individuals can develop their personal spirituality without any necessary reference to or connection with any form of community. The transcendent and religious dimension is certainly present within certain perceptions and definitions of spirituality (Cook 2004; Tanyi 2001), but it remains possible to achieve that sense of transcendence without reference to a transcendent Other.

My intention in delineating the wider approach to spirituality in this way is not to deride or downgrade it. My point is that the specific nature of the 'new spirituality' has significance in terms of interpreting and applying the research data. Many of the health benefits noted in the structural-behavioural studies are not available to those who perceive spirituality in individualistic, personal terms. There may well be health benefits involved with the wider understanding of spirituality, but as yet there is a minimal evidence base to support such claims. We therefore need to be very careful when making claims about what the literature says about the health benefits of forms of spirituality which in fact relate to religion and religious communities, and then uncritically applying these claims to a UK context where most people have little or not religious involvement.

The UK research approach

This wider perspective on spirituality that has emerged within the UK healthcare literature helps us to understand why the general research approach to spirituality within the UK tends to be different from that which is presented by structural-behaviourists in the US. It is interesting to note that much of the UK research on spirituality and health seems to be written *in reaction* to the heightened claims of science. While the US approach pushes for the importance of science for the development of our understanding of the role of a spirituality within healthcare, the UK approach tends, to varying degrees, to stand *against* science at least in its more reductionist forms. This emphasis combined with the broader understanding of spirituality leads to significant differences in research approaches.

The UK focus tends not to be on whether religion is good for your health as defined by scientific assessment of health and well-being. Rather the UK literature tends to focus on such things as:

- what does it mean to offer spiritual care? (Thomson 2002)
- the personal meaning of spirituality for the client (Swinton 2001)
- the significance of spiritual assessment for effective spiritual intervention (Culliford 2002)
- respect for the individual's beliefs (McSherry and Ross 2002)
- conceptual issues around the definition of the spiritual (McSherry and Ross 2002)
- cultural issues surrounding spiritual care (Narayanasamy 1999)
- ways in which practitioners can engage with religious beliefs (Dein 2004).

The focus within the UK research literature is thus seen to be more qualitatively oriented and person-centred, aimed at recognizing the uniqueness of individuals and enhancing good practice that will enable the individual to achieve their spiritual goals and journey and facilitate better care for the individual spiritual needs of people in the midst of their distress. The structural behaviourist approach focuses more widely on broad categories and diagnoses (addiction, depression, suicide, religious practices, religious communities etc) with less attention being paid to the lived experience of the issues of specific caring practices. In this sense the research agenda seems, not surprisingly, to match the cultural climate.

There is therefore an interesting difference in approach and style with the UK-based studies tending to focus on research that is primarily aimed at practice which, at times reacts strongly against the methods and assumptions of science, and the US where the emphasis is on the credibility and importance of science for helping us to understand the health benefits of religion. This is of course a broad stroke analysis and there are exceptions on both sides of the Atlantic. However, broad as the analysis is it nonetheless brings certain interesting cultural dynamics to our attention.

Spirituality and mental health

When one turns to the UK literature that looks specifically at *spirituality* and mental health, one is immediately struck by the fact that there isn't much of it! In comparison with the amount of research done on spirituality within other areas of healthcare, the volume of empirical research that focuses specifically on spirituality and mental healthcare is very small. There are a number of useful reflective pieces that draw together thinking, ideas, concepts and approaches drawn from elsewhere (Culliford 2002; Thomson 2002). However, when it comes to actual original research that looks specifically at spirituality and mental health, the field is sparse. The exception to this is the emerging body of user-led research that will be explored in detail in the next chapter. There we do find original research and new perspectives that are unavailable elsewhere. However with regard to the type of research into the relationship between spirituality and mental health similar to the data produced by the cognitive behaviourists, the field is significantly under-developed. It is therefore rather unclear as to whether spirituality (as opposed to religion) is actually good for one's mental health. The evidence is indicative; it may well be; but it is far from proscriptive. There remains a real need for further research and reflection within this area within a UK context.

Conclusion

In this chapter I have tried to capture something of the significance of the cultural dynamic that underlies the research approaches within the UK and the US. In drawing out tensions and comparisons between the US and UK experiences, it has not been my intention to suggest that one is better than the other. Spirituality and religion are complex and difficult subjects to research. The more tools we have to help us to achieve that task the more effectively we will be able to understand and deal creatively with these vital dimensions of people's experiences. Nevertheless, we do need to recognize the significance of cultural differences for the ways in which we collect, understand and implement the research data. What is appropriate evidence within US culture may not be appropriate within the context of the UK and vice versa. We need to retain a realistic humility about the healing potential of 'spirituality' until the research has been done. Taken together, if we recognize them and learn to use them thoughtfully and creatively, the two approaches highlighted in this chapter offer fascinating challenges and possibilities for the future. The only real question is whether or not we are prepared to take up that challenge?

Bibliography

American Psychologist: Journal of the American Psychologists Association. [Special Issue: Health and Religious Beliefs] (2003) Vol. 58. No. 1.

Astin, J.E., Harkness, E. and Ernst, E. (2000) 'The efficacy of "distant healing": a systematic review of randomized trials.' *Annals of Internal Medicine 132*, 903–910.

Baumeister, R.F. and Sedikides, C. (eds) (2002) *Psychological Inquiry: An International Journal of Peer Commentary and Review. Special Issue: Religion and Psychology 13*, 3.

Bergin, A.E. (1983) 'Religiosity and mental health: a critical reevaluation and meta-analysis.' *Professional Psychology: Research and Practice 14*, 170–84.

Brown, D.R., Ndubuisi, S.C. and Gary, L.E. (1990) 'Religiosity and psychological distress among blacks.' *Journal of Religion and Health 29*, 1, Spring, 55–68.

Brown, G.W. and Prudo, R. (1981) 'Psychiatric disorder in a rural and an urban population:1 Aetiology of Depression.' *Psychological Medicine 11*, 581–99.

Chatters, L.M. (2000). 'Religion and health: public health research and practice.' *Annual Review of Public Health 21*, 335–67.

Cook, C.H. (2004) 'Addiction and spirituality.' *Addiction 99*, 539–51.

Cotterell, P. (1990) *Mission and Meaninglessness.* London: SPCK.

Coyle, J. (2001) 'Spirituality and health: towards a framework for exploring the relationship between spirituality and health.' *Journal of Advanced Nursing 37*, 6, 589–97.

Culliford, L. (2002) 'Spiritual care and psychiatric treatment: an introduction.' *Advances in Psychiatric Treatment 8*, 249–61.

Davie, G. (2002) *Europe: The Exceptional Case.* London: DLT.

Dein, S. (2004) 'Working with patients with religious beliefs.' *Advances in Psychiatric Treatment 10*, 287–95.

Dossey, L. (1993) *Healing Words.* San Francisco: Harper Collins/Harper San Francisco.

Dyson, J., Cobb, M. and Foreman, D. (1997) 'The meaning of spirituality: a literature review.' *Journal of Advanced Nursing 26*, 1183–8.

Ellison, C.G. and Levin, J.S. (1998). 'The religion-health connection: evidence, theory and future directions.' *Health Education and Behavior 25*, 700–720.

Francis, L.J.M., Robbins, C.A., Lewis, C.F., Quigley C.F. and Wheeler, C. (2004) 'Religiosity and general health among undergraduate students: a response to O'Connor, Cobb and O'Connor.' *Personality and Individual Differences 37*, 485–94.

Gartner, J., Larson, D.B. and Allen, G. (1991) Religious commitment and mental health: a review of the empirical literature. *Journal of Psychology and Theology 19*, 1, 6–25.

Greasley, P., Chiu, F.L. and Gartland, M. (2001) 'The concept of spiritual care in mental health nursing.' *Journal of Advanced Nursing 33*, 5, 629–37.

Hay, D. and Hunt, K. (2001) 'Understanding the spirituality of people who don't go to church: A report on the findings of the adults' spirituality project at the University of Nottingham.' Available at www.facingthechallenge.org/nottingham.php (accessed 19 October 2007).

Hay, D. and Nye, R. (2006) *The Spirit of the Child.* London: Jessica Kingsley Publishers.

Heelas, P. and Woodhead, L. (2005) *The Spiritual Revolution: Why Religion is Giving Way to Spirituality.* London: Blackwell.

Highfield, M.F. (1992) 'Spiritual health of oncology patients: nurse and patient perspectives.' *Cancer Nursing 15*, 1–8.

ICM Research Limited (2004) *What the World Thinks of God.* Available at http://news.bbc.co.uk/1/hi/programmes/wtwtgod/pdf/wtwtogod.pdf (accessed 20 April 2006).

King, M., Speck, P. and Thomas, A. (1999) The effect of spiritual beliefs on outcome from illness. *Social Science and Medicine 48*, 9, 1291–99.

Koenig, H.G. (2005) *Faith and Mental Health: Religious Resources for Healing.* West Conshohocken, PA: Templeton Foundation Press.

Koenig, H.G. (ed.) (1998) *Handbook of Religion and Mental Health.* San Diego: Academic Press.

Koenig, H.G. and Larson, D.B. (2001) 'Religion and mental health: evidence for an association.' *International Review of Psychiatry 13*, 67–78.

Koenig, H.G., Larson, D.B. and McCullough, M.E. (2001) *Handbook of Religion and Health.* New York: Oxford University Press.

Koenig, H.G., Larson D.B. and Weaver, A.J. (1998) 'Research on religion and serious mental illness.' In R.D. Fallott (ed.) *Spirituality and Religion in Recovery from Mental Illness.* San Francisco: Jossey-Bass.

Larson, D.B., Pattison, E.M., Blazer, D.G., Omran, A.R. and Kaplan, B.H. (1986) 'Systematic analysis of research on religious variables in four major psychiatric journals, 1978–1982.' *American Journal of Psychiatry 149*, 329–34.

Levin, J. (2001) *God, Faith, and Health: Exploring the Spirituality-Healing Connection.* New York: John Wiley.

Levin, J.S. (1996) 'How prayer heals: a theoretical model.' *Alternative Therapies Health and Medicine 2*, 1, 66–73.

Levin, J.S. and Vanderpool, H.Y. (1989) 'Is religion therapeutically significant for hypertension?' *Social Science and Medicine 29*, 69–78.

Loewenthal, K.M., Macleod, A., Goldblatt, V., Lubitsh, G. and Valentine, J.D. (2000) 'Comfort and joy? Religion, cognition, and mood in Protestants and Jews under stress.' *Cognition and Emotion*, 14, 3, 335–374.

Maltby, J., Lewis, C.A. and Day, L. (1999) 'Religious orientation and psychological well-being: the role of the frequency of personal prayer.' *British Journal of Health Psychology 4*, 4, 363–78.

McCullough, M.E. and Larson, D.B. (1999) 'Religion and depression: a review of the literature.' *Twin Res 2*, 2,126–36.

McSherry, W. and Ross, L. (2002) 'Dilemmas of spiritual assessment: considerations for nursing practice.' *Journal of Advanced Nursing 38*, 5, 479–88.

Miller, W.R. and Thoresen, C.E. (2003) 'Spirituality, religion and health: an emerging research field.' *American Psychologist 5*, 1, 24–35.

Narayanasamy, A. (1999) 'Transcultural mental health nursing 1: benefits and limitations.' *British Journal of Nursing 8*, 10, 664–68.

Oldnall, A. (1996) 'A critical analysis of nursing: meeting the spiritual needs of patients.' *Journal of Advanced Nursing 23*, 138–44.

Pargament, K.I. (1997) *The Psychology of Religion and Coping: Theory, Research, Practice.* New York: Guilford Publications.

Peltzer, K. and Koenig, H.G. (2005) 'Religion, psychology and health.' *Journal of Psychology in Africa 15*, 1, 53–64.

Pollner, M. (1989) 'Divine relations, social relations, and well-being.' *Journal of Health and Social Behaviour 30*, 92–104.

Schuman, J.J. (2003) *Heal Thyself: Spirituality, Medicine, and the Distortion of Christianity.* Oxford University Press.

Schuman, J. and Meador, K. (2004) *Heal Thyself: Spirituality, Medicine and the Distortion of Christianity.* New York: Oxford University Press.

Shreve-Neiger, A.K. and Edelstein, B.A. (2004) 'Religion and anxiety: a critical review of the literature.' *Clinical Psychology Review 4*, 379–97.

Strawbridge, W.J., Cohen, R.D., Shema, S.J. and Kaplan, G.A. (1997) 'Frequent attendance at religious services and mortality over 28 years.' *American Journal of Public Health 87*, 957–61.

Swinton, J. (2006) *Practical Theology and Qualitative Research.* London: SCM Press.

Swinton, J. (2001) *Resurrecting the Person: Friendship and the Care of People with Mental Health Problems.* Nashville: Abingdon.

Swinton, J, and Mowat, H. (2006) *Practical Theology and Qualitative Research.* London: SCM Press.

Tanyi, R.A. (2002) 'Towards clarification of the meaning of spirituality.' *Journal of Advanced Nursing 39*, 5, 500–509.

Thomson, I. (2002) 'Mental health and spiritual care.' *Nursing Standard 17*, 9, 33–8.

Thoresen, C.E. and Harris, A.H.S. (eds) (1999) 'Spirituality and health.' *Journal of Health Psychology 4*, 291–300.

Wallis, C. (1996) 'Faith and healing.' *Time Magazine*, Monday 24 June. Available at www.time.com/time/magazine/article/0,9171,984737,00.html (accessed 20 September 2007).

Witter, R.A., Stock, W.A. and Haring, M.J. (1985) 'Religion and subjective well-being in adulthood: a quantitative synthesis.' *Review of Religious Research 26*, 332–42.

Worthington, E.L. Jr. (ed.) (1998) Dimensions of forgiveness: psychological research and theological perspectives (pp.321–339). Philadelphia: Templeton Foundation Press.

Reflection: A Small Piece from a Spiritual Journey

Basia Spalek

As a researcher I am committed to working actively with communities and organizations, particularly those occupying marginalized positions within wider society, so as to give space to previously unheard or hidden voices and experiences. Since 1999 I have been working with Muslim individuals and organizations on a wide range of issues in relation to the criminal justice sector. This work has played an instrumental role in a personal (spiritual), as well as professional, journey that I am continuing to make.

Listening to accounts from individuals whose identities include religious and spiritual dimensions has acted as a powerful impetus to my critiquing the dominance of a positivist, scientific tradition, that historically gained ground in modern Western society under Enlightenment philosophy, which has valued knowledge characterized by 'rationality' and 'objectivity' over other knowledges. A false dichotomy has been created between the secular and the sacred, with the former being valorized and given public space, the latter viewed as the illegitimate 'Other', rarely given much attention by researchers and policy makers.

This so-called regime of rationality creates a situation where researchers, to be viewed as legitimate, have to conceal their identities, particularly those spiritual and/or religious aspects of themselves. Although self-reflexivity is gaining increasing prominence within social scientific research methodology, particularly within methods arising from feminist work, this has to be carefully stage-managed because to show a deeper emotional, spiritual and therefore human side risks the researcher's work being devalued due to its perceived lack of 'objectivity'. I wish to make clear here that as a non-Muslim, my work with Muslim communities has played an important role in my undertaking a spiritual journey, which has included and involved questioning aspects of myself which can be linked to perpetuating dominant knowledge constructions and power relations that can serve to oppress people.

It has been argued that good research requires active involvement with organizations and individuals in order to understand and portray their worldviews and lifestyles. The question that I wish to pose here is, what do we mean by 'active involvement' and is there a safe space in contemporary Western society within which to claim that active involvement can include the researcher undertaking a spiritual journey that leads to more reflective, and in my opinion more interesting, research?

CHAPTER 23

RESEARCHING THE SOUL: THE SOMERSET SPIRITUALITY PROJECT

John Foskett and Anne Roberts

Introduction or setting the scene

In this chapter the authors record their experience of the founding and development of spiritual and religious care for people in the context of the mental health services and religious and spiritual groups in Somerset. Anne Roberts is a service user/survivor and a member of an Anglican Church and John Foskett is Adviser on spirituality and religion to the Somerset Partnership Social Care and NHS Trust, a retired Anglican priest and mental healthcare chaplain. The Adviser was first called upon to help with a consultation process following the closure of the two large psychiatric hospitals in the county and with them the loss of the hospital chapels and the chaplaincy service in the mid-1990s.

The NHS Trust invited service users and carers, professionals and religious leaders to meet and consider how best to respond to the spiritual and religious needs of both users and staff. In common with other policies the Trust was keen to work in partnership with the appropriate groups in the county and contacted the Churches Together in Somerset to help facilitate this. The consultation took 18 months and involved over 200 people. We quickly recognized what a mixed religious history Somerset has. Villages still remember which side they were on in the civil war and countless tea rooms and pubs lay claim to the patronage of Judge Jeffries and his bloody assizes. Churches including the Cathedral in Wells were used as religious prisons and the last Bishop of the diocese when seeking cooperation with other denominations was firmly reminded that ecumenism required Anglican repentance first.

In the end the consultation resulted in the appointment of four Chaplain Co-ordinators to the four localities in the county. These individuals were appointed to develop a service on the lines reached in the consultation. They were not expected to fulfil the traditional function of hospital chaplains, they were paid for only one session a week, but to provide a focal point for service users/survivors and carers, staff and religious/spiritual leaders and groups of all faiths and none. They were to encourage everyone to play their part in the provision of spiritual and religious care in the context of mental health and treatment.

The four appointed by the Trust and commissioned by the Churches Together included two clergy, one Anglican and one United Reformed, and two lay women, one Catholic and one Anglican. The aim was to have chaplain co-ordinators who already knew their localities and the likely spiritual resources available to the project. The four appointed established themselves and their regular presence in the acute and secure services of the Trust where it was recognized that service users had the least contact with local religious and spiritual groups. They also made contact with the local Churches Together and other voluntary groups interested in spirituality in order to build up community resources which everyone could explore and develop. Each chaplain co-ordinator was supported by the Adviser and by a group representative of the Churches Together and the Mental Health Trust in their locality (Foskett 1999). As the service developed the need for more chaplaincy time became apparent and was extended to two sessions a week, including training opportunities within the Trust and through the national chaplaincy organizations. After four years it seemed opportune to assess the value of the services to users/survivors, carers, staff and religious and spiritual groups and to identify how best to develop it in the future. So a research programme was planned.

Spirituality and religion among mental health professionals and religious leaders

The first stage in the research was to investigate how mental health professionals regarded spirituality and religion and the impact that the chaplaincy had had upon them. Questionnaires similar to those used in a major study of psychiatrists in London (Neeleman and King 1993), were sent to all the staff in one of the Trust's localities and two-thirds replied. These included representatives from all the professions. A similar questionnaire was given to representatives of the Churches Together and again a third replied. The full results of these two studies are recorded in the journal *Mental Health, Religion and Culture* (Foskett, Marriott and Wilson-Rudd 2004a).

There were significant parallels between both groups. The majority recognized the importance of religion and spirituality to people's mental well-being, however their lack of training and expertise in each other's disciplines made them cautious of engaging in this area of care. Both groups were uncertain about how and why religion and spirituality helps some people and harms others. At the same time there was evidence of their reluctance to use each other's expertise. Referrals to the Trust's chaplains were rare and their role questioned. However both professions were more confident when service users/survivors and carers were clear about the spiritual care they needed and that which they could contribute to from their own resources. Under these circumstances both professions did refer to one another. The mental health professionals were moderately more interested in further training than were the clergy.

Service users'/survivors' and carers' research

We decided to approach research among service users/survivors and carers in a different way. The Mental Health Foundation's programme Strategies for Living provided a model for user-led and applied research. Their first project *Knowing our own minds* (Mental Health Foundation 1997) indicated how important religion and spirituality were to more than half of those in a national survey. For the majority religion had been a positive resource and for a minority it was clear what had been unhelpful. The Adviser, encouraged by this resource and the obvious confidence and dignity it had afforded the service users/survivors who had done the research, invited a group of service users in Somerset to do a more detailed user-led study of spirituality and mental health in the county. At first the group was very suspicious both of the subject and of the research, echoing the taboo revealed among staff and religious leaders. Would they be contributing to yet another means of defining and stigmatizing themselves?

> The very first meeting seemed to be a room full of dog collars, plus thankfully Anne! I remember wondering how any sort of user-led research was going to emerge from this…we moved a long way from there.

> I didn't understand the process or the mechanisms. I was suspicious of this 'band of brothers' wanting to spread the good word by attaching something to users. I wondered what they are *really* after? What's it *really* about? (Mental Health Foundation 2002, p.60)

However Vicky Nicholls and Alison Faulkner, service user researchers from the Strategies for Living Project, met these fears by explaining how much user-led research was contributing to people's understanding of mental health (Townsend and Braithwaite 2002). The group took control of the idea and began to explore the kind of research it wanted to do. We interviewed one another, learnt how much we had to share and how supportive it was to do this. The Trust and the Mental Health Foundation provided funds, with which we could pay both interviewers and interviewees and the Somerset Spirituality Project was born. First we learnt about qualitative research techniques and then practised on our friends. This process refined the questions and areas for our research and how we could help interviewees express themselves as they wanted rather than as we expected.

In 2000 we began interviewing some 30 service users/survivors and carers, who had responded to our invitation through the mental health service, voluntary groups, churches and the local media. Twenty-five interviews were eventually used in the research covering a mix of genders, ages, faith traditions and diagnoses for major mental illnesses. The six of us who had trained shared these interviews between us and supported one another at regular meetings. The user author to this chapter put it like this:

> I can remember thinking at the very beginning that we would do well if we could relate to one another, let alone work together. We are all so different and come from very different backgrounds and experience. How wrong you can be?! As a group we get on remarkably well. I have found the team very kind and very supportive (and 'forgiving' when I have 'slipped up'). We have developed trust and closeness within the group and perhaps most surprising of all, to balance out the very nature of the work, we have had great FUN just being in one another's company. (Mental Health Foundation 2002, p.60)

All those interviewed could read the typescript of their interview and amend it wherever they wanted. Then we worked on the transcripts with at least two of us reading each. We identified themes and conclusions to be drawn from them. With these we invited all the interviewees to a meeting to discuss our findings and to see how far they met with their wishes and hopes. Finally we got down to writing a report of the research in which all of us took a part and read each other's contributions. Wherever we could we used the words of the interviewees as evidence for any conclusions or recommendations which the report included. These were divided into five chapters.

JOURNEYS

How do service users/survivors experience and manage their mental health problems and their religious and spiritual gifts and needs? The interviews had born witness to a theme of journeys and pilgrimages in the experience of service users. So this seemed a good way of expressing the overall conclusions of the research.

> We're on a journey, each one of is on a journey, we either regress or we develop (Mental Health Foundation 2002, p.10)

MENTAL HEALTH SERVICES AND CHURCHES

The next two chapters dealt with two of the main areas in the research. First, how have mental health services helped or hindered the spiritual and religious life of users/survivors? And second, in what ways have churches been helpful and unhelpful to service users and survivors? In the former it was clear that mental health professionals' uncertainty about religion and spirituality affects service users'/survivors' ability to express how important their spirituality is to their well-being.

> A human being can have an organic crisis with all sorts of disorders and disruptions to their life which is actually a very valuable experience and not something to be knocked out of them by medication. (Mental Health Foundation 2002, p.24)

However when they were open to the spiritual and took users/survivors' faith seriously, then everyone benefited from this more holistic approach.

> I think it was combination of my GP, the medicine and my spiritual life. In some incredible way they all came together and I think it was the spiritual element that was the glue that held it all together. (Mental Health Foundation 2002, p.24)

The Churches came in for affirmation and criticism on similar lines. There was the same desire for acceptance and understanding, and appreciation for spaces and places which are holy and sacred and in which users and survivors could just be. The new community units have very few of these and the old hospital chapels were missed.

> I felt very alone and isolated in a strange environment. I wanted some kind of stability within that and that was why my faith and religion were coming in at that time... I wanted to identify with it as soon as possible... Being very vulnerable and feeling you've got that (religious) support...I hope I can get that over to people that are looking after me so that they can understand that. (Mental Health Foundation 2002, p.20)

Interviewees spoke of the support they had from their local churches and Christian friends but also of their problems with the doctrines and teachings of the church when these conflicted with their own beliefs and doubts.

> (Clergy) lean you on the side of their beliefs rather than look at yours... You always got to be preached to rather than you are a person and you've got a right to have your own beliefs. (Mental Health Foundation 2002, p.36)

The service users were aware of the problems that both religious and mental health professionals had when addressing spirituality in this context. They suggested that staff and clergy needed to explore their own spiritualities as a basis for their work.

> I think they need to believe in their own profession and they need to believe in themselves as therapists...perhaps it is scary to admit that there may be vast areas and infinite degrees of beingness beyond what they feel comfortable with. (Mental Health Foundation 2002, p.25).

Thus it was reassuring to find that the chaplaincy service was recognized as a very positive resource.

> He seemed to there right from the beginning... Not knowing him but recognizing him by his dog collar. I think the work they do on the site is so important and they are open to everybody. (Mental Health Foundation 2002, p.22)

In contrast one believer wanted more than just sympathy and comfort. 'The thing I dread is that some well-meaning chaplain would come to see me and never impart any Christian content' (Mental Health Foundation 2002, p.23). One of the research team summed up the importance of the chaplains in this way:

> There's a major gap and no-one with specific responsibility to bridge that gap...how much can you achieve in one morning or afternoon session (like the sessional chaplains)... If one person can make that much difference (as people have reported in the research) in a few hours, how much more could be done with a lot more time? (Mental Health Foundation 2002, pp.60–61)

ACCEPTANCE

The next chapter took up the theme of 'acceptance' which recurred often in the interviews and was fundamental to the spiritual well-being of both users/survivors, carers and staff. There were stories of the difference that acceptance made especially when people were at their lowest, or behaving most erratically and anxiously. There was also the recognition of how debilitating to the soul stigma is and how liberating acceptance can be.

> I would make very good friends with someone and they would find out either from me or somebody else about my mental illness, and in an instant nobody wanted to know: It's laughable really. (Mental Health Foundation 2002, p.45)

> The community nurse was terrific. Although he was not a Christian, he asked me very, very pertinent questions about how I reconciled my faith with what was happening to me and what God meant to me. (Mental Health Foundation 2002, p.23)

SPIRITUALITY AND PSYCHOSIS

The final chapter dealt with the question, what is the relationship between 'psychotic' and mystical experience? We were tentative in addressing this very sensitive area but some of the interviewees brought the subject up themselves.

> The experience was of both hell and heaven... I felt as if I was being physically crucified and it was not just the sort of experience of crucifixion, it was all deaths that man has ever known and all that I could ever imagine.

> I think we are all linked at an unconscious level and that's where I was when I was psychotic... There were various insights I carried forward. I hallucinated the book I hope I'll get published. (Mental Health Foundation 2002, p.50)

We were fortunate in finding one service user/survivor, who had the research expertise to analyse half of the interviews with a grounded theory approach (MacMin and Foskett 2004). She was able to identify the times, places and contexts in which service users and survivors were most open to and most in need of their spiritual and/or religious resources, and conversely how much they suffered if these were not available to them. A mental health crisis and/or admittance to a mental health service are often the most critical times, when people's faith is most in need of attention. This is then repeated at many stages in the experience of severe and continuing mental distress.

> When I went into the unit it was the most desolate period in my life. I would have been pleased to see almost anybody, especially somebody that had some Christian input, some contact with the real world (Mental Health Foundation 2002, p.20)

From research to practice

Following the publication of the user-led research report in 2002, Somerset Partnership NHS Trust called a conference to review all three research studies with representative constituencies of service users, carers, mental health and religious professionals. That conference explored the conclusions and recommendations from all the reports and set itself a programme involving all these constituencies in the development of spiritual and religious care. Four years later it is amazing to see what has grown from the seeds sown by the research. The user quoted above has published her hallucinated book together with contributions from her family and from some of the staff who cared for her (Harvey 2003). Of course the ripening has been mixed with many windfalls and damaged fruit lost along the way. Initially the enthusiasts hoped for dramatic changes. We expected service users/survivors and carers to have much more confidence in expressing their needs and showing the potency of their spiritual and religious resources. A leaflet with texts from the user-led report was distributed widely throughout the Trust and local churches, and this had some effect in raising people's consciousness about spirituality. We anticipated that mental staff and units would now be ready to accept service users' spiritual requests and make more use of the chaplains. In practice it has proved uphill work. Even to introduce some rudimentary form of spiritual and religious self-assessment, and the provision of a few sacred spaces to replace the chapels has taken much time and effort to achieve (Foskett, Matthews, MacMin *et al.* 2004b).

More disturbing has been the current pressure to downsize and curtail creative services. In many units there are not the resources to offer anything like a holistic service or for staff and users to spend sufficient time with one another to foster and develop people's spiritual resources. The chaplaincy time could easily be doubled and still not meet the demands made upon it. Units which have the least resources and manage the most traumatic experiences are not as attractive to holistically orientated staff as are outreach and crisis units. After the early funding for the research we have had an enormous struggle to recompense service users/survivors and carers for their massive contribution to this work. Professionals are paid both their salary and their expenses, but it has proved much harder to secure either for service users and carers. The inequity in this must affect the spiritual efficacy of all we do. All faith traditions recognize that spirituality separated from ethics and justice degenerates into pietistic rituals and rhetoric.

On the more positive side, more chaplaincy time has been found, referrals are much more common and more units now have the services of local clergy and laity as Honorary Chaplains. A quarterly open spirituality forum, some inspiring user produced publications (Speak Up Somerset, or SUS), two resource centres specializing in holistic care, a number of conferences and a retreat have helped develop understanding and expertise among service users/survivors, carers, staff and religious leaders. The last conference in 2005 (Somerset Partnership) entitled 'Embracing Diversity' went furthest in bringing together New Age, Shamanistic and the Pagan beliefs, so valued in Somerset, with different Christian traditions. We shared an illuminating hour of silence together, which embraced our diversities so much more effectively than words seem to do. As a result of these developments the service user author has been directly involved with the NIMHE national spirituality project and Somerset is one of its sites of good practice.

All of this provided grounds for the Chief Executive of the NHS Trust to produce a policy statement for all staff, service users/survivors and carers. This underlines the importance of spirituality and religion to some users/survivors, carers and staff and the need for adequate provision for these in care plans and in the Trust's facilities. To reinforce this policy the Trust plans to role out a new training programme for all staff involving service users/survivors and carers and religious and spiritual leaders, together with a more in-depth training for those who want professional education in this area of care.

In all these developments the research has proved a most valuable resource to help persuade those who remain sceptical about spirituality and religion in mental health, to identify ways in which services can be improved and as a constant reminder of how easily people's faith can be undermined and their spiritual care neglected. The chaplaincy regularly looks back to the evidence of what was wanted and how best to deliver it within the current constraints of time and funding. To this end one of the Chaplain Co-ordinators contributed to the Mentality/Church of England's (2005) mental health resource pack for local churches and congregations and her colleague has developed a popular induction course for all staff and a course about mental health and the major faiths.

Conclusion

The story of this research and its developments, has been remarkable in a number of ways. To explore this sensitive subject from the four perspectives of service users/survivors, carers, mental health professionals and religious and spiritual leaders at the same time and in the same context is unique. This gave us confidence in working together and in learning how to cooperate when applying the results of the research. At the same time the work has caught a universal wave of interest in the spiritual. Spirituality and religion matter for good and ill in our society. The desire to learn and understand more is the most satisfying of the many consequences of this research and a real encouragement to people from all constituencies to go on learning together. The work is 'taken as seriously' as those who inspired it wanted and hoped.

> I am tired of being talked about,
> Treated as a statistic,
> Pushed to the margins of human conversation.
> I want someone who will have time for me,
> Someone who will listen to me,
> Someone who has not already judged
> Who I am or what I have to offer.
> I am waiting to be taken seriously.

(Mental Health Foundation 2002, p.1)

References

Foskett, J. (1999) 'Soul searching within the service.' *Mental Health, Religion and Culture 2*, 1, 11–18.

Foskett, J., Marriott, J. and Wilson-Rudd, F. (2004a) 'Mental health, religion and spirituality: attitudes, experiences and expertise among mental health professionals and religious leaders in Somerset.' *Mental Health, Religion and Culture 7*, 1, 5–22.

Foskett, J., Roberts, A., Matthews, R., MacMin, L., Cracknell, P. and Nicholls, V. (2004b) 'From research to practice: the first tentative steps.' *Mental Health, Religion and Culture 7*, 1, 41–58.

Harvey, S. (2003) *Sheila's Book: A Shared Journey through Madness.* Taunton: Somerset Virtual College Publications.

MacMin, L. and Foskett, J. (2004) '"Don't be afraid to tell." The spiritual and religious experience of mental health service users in Somerset.' *Mental Health, Religion and Culture 7*, 1, 23–40.

Mental Health Foundation (1997) *Knowing our own Minds.* London: Mental Health Foundation.

Mental Health Foundation (2002) *Taken Seriously: The Somerset Spirituality Project.* London: Mental Health Foundation.

Mentality/Church of England (2005) *Promoting Mental Health: A Training Resource for Spiritual and Pastoral Care.* Available at www.mentality.org.uk (accessed 20 September 2007).

Neeleman, J. and King, M. (1993) 'Psychiatrists' religious attitudes in relation to clinical practice.' *Acta Psychiatrica Scandinavica 88*, 420–24.

Somerset Partnership (2005) *Embracing Diversity, Meeting Spiritual Needs in Mental Health: A Conference Report.* Bridgwater: Somerset Partnership Social Care and NHS Trust.

Townsend, M. and Braithwaite, T. (2002) 'Mental health research – the value of user involvement.' *Journal of Mental Health 11*, 117–19.

SUS (Speak Up Somerset) has published a number of books including: *Positive Steps Diary, A Journal of Hope, The Art of Recovery: Poetry Anthology.* SUS, PO Box 3484, Yeovil BA21 5ZH.

Just Be

My mind was troubled
I couldn't sleep,
'Worry not'
I kept repeating.
It was not good enough
My worries would not disappear.
I tossed and turned
And turned and tossed
Asking myself questions
Over and over again,
That I had no answers to.
Which was the right way to go?
I seemed to have lost direction.
Why was making a decision so painful?
I wanted to spare the pain
Of myself and others.
Was I really capable of doing that?
My mind tumbled over this.
I spoke to God
My Father in Heaven,
I felt His gentle touch
Reassuring me
Holding me close,
'Just be', He whispered,
'Just be yourself.'

Sue Holt

CHAPTER 24

CONCLUDING THOUGHTS

Mary Ellen Coyte, Peter Gilbert and Vicky Nicholls

The boat

It would be impossible, and perhaps unhelpful, to summarize the material in the book, contributed by such a wide variety of people in many styles of discourse and written for a diverse audience. The experience and background of each reader will bring its own wisdom to bear.

We hope that what the contributions do is reflect the diversity and open-endedness of spirituality; attributes of not knowing and the unpredictable nature of synergies and connections. The image of the sailing boat which has travelled these pages carries with it a sense of journey, discovery, knowing and unknowing. These can be frightening but an emphasis on the opposite, trying to nail mental ill health in one box or another, can be the death of spiritual values and, unfortunately, the breaking of the spirit of many people with mental health difficulties and those who work with them.

In mental health we are dealing with some of the most acutely painful, enduring and mystifying experiences. No wonder people want answers. Trying to tame the mystery with science or religion does not necessarily end the suffering, but that does not stop us seeking solutions and understanding. Those very same qualities represented by the boat which can underpin fear and insecurity might also be the key to excitement, wonder, stimulation and creativity – attributes which give us hope, which keep us going and which might prompt research and a wish to make sense of that world which is spirituality and mental health.

The mandala

Because of the complex nature of spirituality and mental health any writing on the subject is unlikely to be a step-by-step manual. It is further complicated because of that element which is about relationship to an 'other' of some sort, for example: to another human, to oneself, a Deity, or a dis-ease. There are many variables at play.

However these are the very reasons that we might need calm and peace and the mandalas, which open and close this volume, are intended to give a sense of containment and arrival. Mandalas traditionally represent the universe or cosmos, sometimes containing an attribute to a deity and, in Jungian terms, represent the effort to unify the self. They hold all this in their stable geometric forms.

Among these pages there are many pointers and suggestions which we hope will demystify, endorse or improve existing practice, or provide new ideas and support for individuals and organizations who wish to reach out and find their own centred ways to fulfil their role.

The poems and the stories

Art, poetry and story are rich symbolic languages. They are ways of both containing and revealing mystery and that is why it was necessary for this book to give space to poems, people's stories, artwork and to refer to the languages of physical expression. These contributions are also a statement about the need for respect and understanding of the symbolic. These representations of existence are as valuable as any diagrams which support more formal academic input.

The richness of these symbolic languages transmits information about experience and the spiritual which transcend formal explanations. The complexity of spirituality makes these languages necessary.

Those with mental health needs can often feel the inexplicable within themselves and know it defies explanation in ordinary words. They can also use language which is misunderstood and so adds to their diagnosis of dis-order. When the language is properly heard, or even if there is a hesitant attempt to understand it, it carries the potential for deep understanding and healing. Those who want to help those in mental distress might also need to have gifts and experience which cannot be put into words of everyday language.

Jewels for the journey

It may feel impossible to work with such lack of clarity and, in our so called rational society, with risk assessment high on the agenda, who can blame practitioners and carers for wanting clear-cut guidelines for themselves. When so much paperwork is based on getting boxes ticked why can't there be a simple tick list of options and procedures? Service users, too, often yearn for a simple solution. But where spiritual values are part and parcel of an individual's or organization's way of life, where these seemingly nebulous qualities are valued and endorsed, people often find that, paradoxically, they are then more likely to tick all the right boxes, but in a natural way, as part of the ongoing journey.

People may want to be shown the way but, often, when they are allowed to find their own way in a supportive environment they nurture their own spiritual skills and values.

This book has allowed individual expression, personal jewels, within a framework of meaning. It gives ideas, points of resonance, a mixture of styles and language. We hope that some of these gems will be useful companions adding brilliance and illumination to your own journey.

When all is Said and Done

When all is said and done,
Love.
Love above us, love below
Love to enfold us in Her arms
Love to give us a voice.
When the carrion crows have fed their fill
Of human flesh
And there seem to be nothing but bones -
Love will find a way through;
Will send up a new shoot of hope;
Will insist that everything passes
But that life never ends.

Vicky Nicholls, October 2007

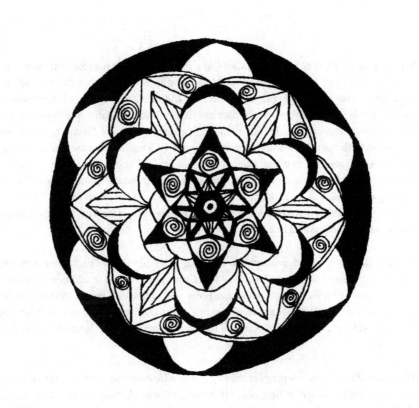

CONTRIBUTORS

Sarajane Aris is Head of Emergency Care Clinical Psychology Services for Derbyshire MH Services NHS Trust. She has worked for Mental Health Services within the NHS for 27 years. She is also a transpersonal psychotherapist and held the first official transpersonal clinical psychology post created within the AWP Trust in Bath. She founded the Transpersonal Network for clinical, counselling psychologists and therapists, under the auspices of both the transpersonal section within the BPS and the division of clinical psychology. She is involved in organizational development, and also governance work for the Health Commission. She seeks to 'bridge', bringing a transpersonal/spiritual note and sense of being to this work and a moment-to-moment awareness in her life in general. Her work and life is informed by a spiritual journey located within transpersonal psychology, Tibetan Buddhism and the mystical traditions.

Frances Basset is an independent transpersonal psychotherapist. She trained with the Psychosynthesis and Education Trust. She sees clients privately and in addition works as a volunteer counsellor for Brighton and Hove Federation of Disabled People. She also works as a Senior Lecturer at the Institute of Nursing and Midwifery, University of Brighton. Frances worked as a nurse for 15 years and has always been interested in spirituality within healthcare.

Thurstine Basset is an independent training and development consultant and runs his own company, which is based in Brighton. He works for national voluntary agencies, such as Mind, Together and the Mental Health Foundation. At the Richmond Fellowship, he is the joint course leader for their Diploma in Community Mental Health, which is accredited by Middlesex University. He has published widely in the field of mental health training and education. He has written a number of learning packages and materials, many of which are published by Pavilion Publishing, with whom he works in an advisory role. He likes to walk for exercise, relaxation and spiritual well-being.

Sarah Carr works as a research analyst for the Social Care Institute for Excellence in London, specializing in service user/survivor participation in research and service development. She has had lifelong experiences of mental distress, with several diagnoses and treatments along the way. Sarah studied Theology to Master's level. She is a trustee of PACE, a

London-wide organization which responds to the emotional, mental and physical health needs of lesbians and gay men in the Greater London Area. Sarah has written on both mental health and service user participation. Her publications include:

'The sickness label infected everything we said: lesbian and gay perspectives on mental distress.' In: Tew, J. (ed) *Social Perspectives in Mental Health: Developing Social Models to Understand and Work with Mental Distress.* London: Jessica Kingsley Publishers.

SCIE Position Paper 3: *Has Service User Participation Made a Difference to Social Care Services?* London: SCIE/Policy Press.

'Participation, power, conflict and change: theorizing dynamics of service user participation in the social care system of England and Wales.' In: *Critical Social Policy 27*, 2, May 2007 (forthcoming).

Paul Chapple is Honorary Chaplain at St George's Park, a new hospital for the treatment of mental disability and part of the Northumberland, Tyne, and Wear NHS Trust. He headed up hospital pharmacy in Northumberland for many years but felt able to express his dissatisfaction with the strictly 'medical model' through the Leeds MA in Healthcare Chaplaincy. He retains his professional interest, however, by taking the pharmaceutical lead in drug misuse work throughout Northumberland.

Mary Ellen Coyte has experience of long-term mental distress and came to realize that finding her solution to this was a spiritual exploration. She has worked in health and mental health for nine years, specializing as a trainer and researcher in user involvement, service development and spirituality. Having trained with the Department of Spiritual and Pastoral Care at London's Maudsley Hospital she now volunteers as a lay mental health chaplain in another London hospital. She is also a community dance leader whose approach draws on the use of movement, creativity and relationship in fostering and maintaining good mental health. She is editor of *A Pocket Book of Spiritual Strategies* (Speak Up Somerset; forthcoming), a collection gathered from service users and survivors.

Veronica Dewan is a 50-year-old woman of Indian, Punjabi and Irish heritage who draws on her personal experiences of transracial adoption, catholicism, the care system and mental health services in writing fiction and non-fiction prose.

Wendy Edwards has used mental health services for the past 12 years. She has previously been employed in a variety of jobs including working in a rubber band factory; a guide and tourist facility worker at York Minster; a volunteer co-ordinator and community development worker for a charity in Hackney; a carer, and a Housemistress at two boarding schools. She is also a former member of an Anglican Religious Community. Wendy is now involved locally in Oxford as a mental health consultant and trainer and has a particular interest in spirituality and mental health. In 2005 Wendy formed IMPACT a service user-led mental health campaign group for Oxfordshire.

Suman Fernando has lectured and written widely on issues of race and culture in mental health. His books include *Mental Health, Race and Culture* (2nd edition, 2002) and *Cultural Diversity, Mental Health and Psychiatry: The Struggle against Racism* (2003). He is involved in voluntary organisations serving black and minority ethnic (BME) communities in London and is Vice-Patron of a non-governmental organisation (NGO) providing social and mental health care in Sri Lanka. He is also consultant to a multi-centre program for capacity building for mental health care in low income countries affected by conflict and natural disasters. He is currently Honorary Senior Lecturer at the European Centre Migration and Social Care (MASC) at University of Kent and Honorary Professor in the Department of Applied Social Studies, London Metropolitan University. His personal website: http://www.sumanfernando.com

The Revd Canon **John Foskett** is an Anglican priest, pastoral counsellor and consultant. Currently he is an Adviser on Religion and Spirituality to the Somerset Partnership Social Care and NHS Trust. He has helped the Trust develop its service over the last 12 years and together with Anne Roberts and others has done research into spirituality, religion and mental health in Somerset among service users and carers, religious and mental health professionals. He is President of both the Association for Pastoral and Spiritual Care and Counselling and of the British and Irish Association for Practical Theology. He is a Fellow of the British Association for Counselling and was for 18 years chaplain at the South London and Maudsley NHS Trust. He worked for and taught at the Richmond Fellowship College. He is the author of two books and many articles and chapters on mental health and pastoral care.

Bill (K.W.M.) Fulford is Professor of Philosophy and Mental Health in the Medical School and the Department of Philosophy, University of Warwick, where he runs a Masters, PhD and research programme in Philosophy, Ethics and Mental Health Practice. He is also an Honorary Consultant Psychiatrist in the Department of Psychiatry, University of Oxford, and Visiting Professor in Psychology, the Institute of Psychiatry and King's College, London University. He is the founder and Co-Editor of the first international journal for philosophy and mental health, *PPP – Philosophy, Psychiatry, and Psychology*, and of a new book series from Oxford University Press on International Perspectives in Philosophy and Psychiatry. A recent book in the series is his *Oxford Textbook of Philosophy and Psychiatry* co-authored with Professors Tim Thornton and George Graham. He is currently seconded part-time to the Department of Health in London as Special Adviser for Values-Based Practice. With Professors Kamlesh Patel and Chris Heginbotham, he has recently established an international Institute for Philosophy, Diversity and Mental Health at the University of Central Lancashire in England.

Peter Gilbert is Professor of Social Work and Spirituality at Staffordshire University and NIMHE Project lead on Spirituality and Mental Health. He is an associate consultant with the National Development Team. A practising social worker for 13 years, Peter managed services for a range of user groups; was Director of Operations for Staffordshire Social Services; and Director for Worcestershire County Council. He graduated in Modern History from Balliol College, Oxford, and has a Masters degree in Social Work and an MBA from Sussex University.

In the past few years Peter has specialized in work in mental health, with people with learning disabilities, and in the field of ethical leadership. He was NIMHE/SCIE Fellow (with Professor Nick Gould) from 2003–2006, and is a member of various national boards. Each year he runs a number of retreats at the Benedictine Abbey of Worth. Peter is the author of a number of books, most recently: *The Value of Everything* (2003) and *Leadership: Being Effective and Remaining Human* (2005).

Tom Gordon has been chaplain at the Marie Curie Hospice, Edinburgh, for 12 years having previously worked as a Church of Scotland parish minister for 20 years. He has advised Marie Curie Cancer Care on spiritual issues, and writes and lectures on spiritual and religious care, all aspects of chaplaincy, and loss, grief and bereavement, including involvement with ministers in training and in-service training. He also serves on the editorial board of the *Journal of the Scottish Association of Chaplains in Health Care*. His book, *A Need for Living*, published in 2001, offers insights into the understanding and delivery of spiritual care through reflections on images and ideas utilized in his chaplaincy. His second book, *New Journeys Now Begin*, on aspects of grief and loss, was published in June 2006. Both books are published by 'Wild Goose Publications' – www.ionabooks.com – and contain examples of Tom's poetry. He is married with three grown-up children, and lives in East Lothian.

Ali Jan Haider is Deputy Director of Equality and Diversity within Primary Care, NHS, at Bradford. He has a background in social work practice, and extensive experience as a management and organizational development consultant specializing in change and diversity. Ali Jan also acts as a consultant to the local mental health care trust on diversity and equality, and he oversees the work of the 'delivering race equality in mental health' which Bradford has been chosen to spearhead.

Julia Head is Bishop John Robinson Fellow in Pastoral Theology and Mental Health, and Specialist Chaplain, South London and Maudsley NHS Trust. She is currently studying for a post-graduate diploma in counselling.

Azim Kidwai is a Director of Q Consulting, a leading management consultancy providing policy support to numerous government departments, including the Department of Health and Home Office. He is an associate fellow at the University of Ain Shams, Cairo, Egypt, where he is currently lecturing on Mental Health and Spirituality. An experienced project manager he has held a range of posts across the public sector, from the National Health Service to the Government Communications Head Quarters.

In recent times Azim has began to specialize in working with organizations to establish Cultural Capability and Spiritual Sensitivity. He is currently a Trustee at IslamBradford, a social welfare organization improving access to Islam for Muslims and non-Muslims. He is also the principle consultant for Health and Offender Partnerships at the Department of Health and is leading on their equality programme 2006–2007. At the time of writing the chapter for the book Azim was Modernization and Diversity Project Manager for Bradford District NHS Care Trust.

Cameron Langlands has been Head of Chaplaincy Services for NHS Greater Glasgow and Clyde Mental Health Partnerships for seven years having previously worked as a Church of Scotland parish minister. Cameron is a member of the editorial board of the *Scottish Journal of Healthcare Chaplaincy* and serves on a number of working parties including NHS Education for Scotland Standards for Healthcare Chaplaincy. Currently studying for his PhD, Cameron's areas of interest are mental health, sexuality and gender issues and he presents sessions and has published on the subjects of HIV, spirituality and sexuality.

Christopher MacKenna is Director of St Marylebone Healing and Counselling Centre. He is an Anglican clergyman and a Senior Member of the Jungian Analytic Section of the British Association of Psychotherapists. He has been involved in pastoral care, counselling and psychotherapy for over 35 years, and has published a number of papers on the relationship between psychotherapy and religion.

Mariyam Maule was a poet, historian, human rights activist and mental health service user who died tragically in 2005. Mariyam was of Egyptian origin, transracially adopted and brought up in Scotland. She lived the last 13 years of her life in London, graduating in African History from The School of African and Oriental Studies in 1994. It was at this time that Mariyam first came into contact with mental health services, and in the years that followed described her experiences in powerful poems about the nature of despair, injustice in the world and neglect and abuse within the psychiatric system but also about love and hope, acknowledging both the deep love she had for her adopted family and her despair at being separated at birth from her Egyptian cultural roots. In 1998, Mariyam co-founded SIMBA (a Black MH service user group) and her inspiration, energy, passion, humour, intellect and loyalty was central to the group's development over the next seven years. In 2006, several of Mariyam's poems were published post-humously in *In Search for Belonging, Reflections by Transracially Adopted People* (Ed Perlita Harris). In this book, publication of her actual words (spoken at a Mental Health conference on spirituality in 2003) will enable her valuable insights to continue to be shared so others may learn.

Nigel Mills trained as a Clinical Psychologist at the Institute of Psychiatry in London. He has worked in the NHS, for the past 22 years in Manchester, Cambridge, Surrey and South Wales. Alongside his psychological training Nigel has also undertaken many years of training in QiGong/Chigung. His main influences in this respect have been Bruce Kumar Frantzis and Zhxing Wang. Nigel has also trained as a Cranio-Sacral Therapist. He currently works part time for Hereford Primary Care Trust as a Clinical Psychologist and is also part time self-employed utilizing a combination of Cranio-Sacral Therapy, Psychological Therapy and QiGong. He has written many articles on the combination of psychological and body-based approaches to therapy.
Website: www.nigelmillstherapies.co.uk

David Mitchell has recently returned to parish ministry in the Church of Scotland following 15 years' service at the Marie Curie Hospice as chaplain and lecturer in palliative care. He has a particular interest in developing spiritual care and the role of the chaplain within healthcare and has served on working parties preparing the Clinical Standards for Specialist

Palliative Care, Standards for Hospice and Palliative Care Chaplaincy, Spiritual and Religious Care Competencies for Palliative Care, and NHS Scotland standards for healthcare chaplaincy. David co-edits the *Scottish Journal of Healthcare Chaplaincy*, has contributed chapters to a number of palliative care textbooks, and regularly presents teaching and conference sessions for a variety of healthcare professionals.

Vicky Nicholls is the joint coordinator of the Social Perspectives Network for Mental Health (SPN) and a freelance trainer and researcher in health and social care, specialising in spirituality and mental health. She also currently coordinates a Parental Mental Health and Child Welfare Network on behalf of SPN. She was previously a Project Coordinator at the Mental Health Foundation where she managed a national Spirituality and Mental Health Project in partnership with NIMHE and Strategies for Living Phase II, a UK-wide series of user-led research projects. Her life has been made unmeasurably richer by being the mother of a thriving three year old son.

Barbara Pointon was a principal lecturer in music at Homerton College, Cambridge, until she retired early to care for her husband, Malcolm, diagnosed with Alzheimer's disease in 1991 at the age of 51. They were the subjects of the award-winning TV documentary *Malcolm and Barbara…A Love Story*, and a sequel is currently being filmed. She campaigns nationally and internationally for a better deal for people with dementia and their carers. The Alzheimer's Society presented her with a 25th Anniversary Award in 2004 and she was awarded an MBE in the Queen's 80th Birthday Honours.

   Malcolm died peacefully at home earlier this year, cared for by Barbara till the end.

Andrew Powell graduated from the University of Cambridge with distinction in medicine and specializing in psychiatry and psychotherapy at the Maudsley Hospital, London. He was Consultant and Senior Lecturer at St George's Hospital, London for 11 years before moving to Oxford, where he continued to work in the National Health Service until 2000. Andrew is a member of the Royal College of Physicians and a fellow of the Royal College of Psychiatrists. He has served on the Council of the Scientific and Medical Network, and is an Associate of the College of Healing and Founding Chair of the Spirituality and Psychiatry Special Interest Group of the Royal College of Psychiatrists, UK. His publications on spirituality and mental health can be accessed on www.rcpsych.ac.uk/college/sig/spirit/publications/index.htm

Anne Roberts is currently a member of the Resident Community at the Ammerdown Centre, a Conference and Retreat centre in Somerset. She has been a teacher and is also active in her local church. She has been supported by outpatient care in the mental health services at different times in her adult life. In 2000 she became part of a small group comprising largely service users, which was responsible for planning and carrying out some research into people's experience of spirituality and mental health. The findings were published by the Mental Health Foundation in 2002, 'Taken Seriously. The Somerset Spirituality Project'. After writing one of the chapters for the report Anne wrote short articles for two other publications. She has been part of conference planning in Somerset, has spoken at various conferences and been a member of the steering group of the National Spirituality and Mental

Health Project. Anne's work is grounded in an interest in her own spiritual journey and its relation to her own mental health.

Mark Sutherland is Presiding Chaplain, South London and Maudsley NHS Trust, Psychotherapist and Supervisor.

John Swinton holds the chair in Practical Theology and Pastoral Care at the University of Aberdeen, Scotland, UK. He is also an honorary Professor at Aberdeen's Centre for Advanced Studies in Nursing. Professor Swinton worked as a registered nurse specializing in psychiatry and learning disabilities. He also worked for a number of years as a community mental health chaplain. His areas of research include the relationship between spirituality and health and the theology and spirituality of disability. His publications include *Spirituality in Mental Health Care: Rediscovering a Forgotten Dimension* (2001) London: Jessica Kingsley Publishers, and *Resurrecting the Person: Friendship and the Care of People With Severe Mental Health Problems.* (2000) Nashville: Abingdon Press.

In 2004 Professor Swinton founded the *Centre for Spirituality, Health and Disability* at the University of Aberdeen (www.abdn.ac.uk/cshad). The centre has a dual focus on: (a) the relationship between spirituality and contemporary healthcare practices, and (b) the theology and spirituality of disability. It is a multi-disciplinary project which aims to enable researchers, practitioner and educators to work together to develop innovative and creative research projects and teaching initiatives.

Neil Thompson is an independent consultant and author who has published widely on matters relating to social and occupational well-being. He also holds a part-time professorship in social work and well-being at Liverpool Hope University. His recent books include *People Problems* (Palgrave Macmillan, 2006), *Promoting Workplace Learning* (The Policy Press, 2006) and *Power and Empowerment* (Russell House, 2007). He has been a speaker at conferences and seminars in the UK, Ireland, Spain, the Netherlands, Norway, Greece, Hong Kong, Australia, Canada and the US. His website is www.neilthompson.info

Brian Thorne is an international figure in the world of person-centred therapy and has published extensively. He is Emeritus Professor of Counselling at the University of East Anglia, Professor of Education with the College of Teachers, Co-founder of the Norwich Centre and a lay canon of Norwich Cathedral.

Premila Trivedi is an Asian woman, born and brought up in London within a very traditional Hindu family with all the benefits and challenges that that brings. She has used MH services for many years and over the last decade has moved from being a passive, compliant patient to being a more 'troublesome' active survivor/user campaigning for improvement in MH services. With other black service users, Premila helped set up SIMBA (a black user group that uses its creativity to campaign for improvements in MH services for people from black communities) and, within the SIMBA family, has been enabled to explore some of cultural and spiritual issues she struggles with. Premila is currently employed part-time as an Education and Training Adviser for service user involvement at the South London and

Maudsley NHS Foundation Trust and also works freelance using her experience of life and mental health services to inform others, e.g. through writing chapters and articles and delivering training to MH professionals, particularly around MH, race and culture. Premila still struggles at times but with the crucial friendship and support of other survivors (and some aware MH professionals) endeavours to continue her journey – to wherever it may lead!

Andrew Wilson has been Chaplain for Mental health services in Croydon since 1989, within the South London and Maudsley NHS Foundation Trust. Before this he was a parish priest in South London for 18 years. Since his appointment at the time of the Community Care Bill, he has worked closely within the community as well as in the hospital setting.

Kim Woodbridge is Operational Manager for a joint Adult Mental Health Service at Milton Keynes PCT. Although originally training as a learning disabilities nurse and then mental health nurse, Kim has worked in many roles including, researcher, senior lecturer, a psychological therapist and psychotherapist. While working at the Sainsbury Centre for Mental Health, she led developments in the application of values-based practice to training, practice and organizational development.

She is currently completing her doctorate in values-based practice, which has included the development and evaluation of service user leadership training, a study of how a Crisis Home Treatment Team works with values and the development of a values-based practice curriculum for clinical practice and organizational development. She has had several publications in relation to values-based practice including the *Whose Values?* workbook, with Bill (K.W.M.) Fulford.

SUBJECT INDEX

AUTHOR INDEX